CONTENTS

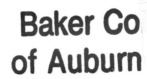

Baker Co
of Auburn

Surgery

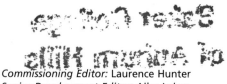

Commissioning Editor: Laurence Hunter
Senior Development Editor: Ailsa Laing
Project Manager: Elouise Ball
Designer: Kirsteen Wright
Illustrations Manager: Gillian Richards

Surgery

Andrew T. Raftery BSc MD FRCS(Eng) FRCS(Ed)

Formerly Consultant Surgeon, Sheffield Kidney Institute, Sheffield
Teaching Hospitals NHS Foundation Trust, Northern General
Hospital, Sheffield; Member (formerly Chairman), Court of
Examiners, Royal College of Surgeons of England; Formerly Member
of Panel of Examiners, Intercollegiate Specialty Board in General
Surgery; Formerly Member of Council, Royal College of Surgeons of
England; Formerly Honorary Clinical Senior Lecturer in Surgery,
University of Sheffield, UK

Michael S. Delbridge MBChB (Hons) MD MRCS(Eng)

Specialist Registrar in Surgery, Yorkshire and Humberside Deanery,
UK

Marcus J. D. Wagstaff BSc PhD FRCS(Plast)

Specialist Registrar in Plastic and Reconstructive Surgery, East
Midlands Deanery, UK

FOURTH EDITION

CHURCHILL
LIVINGSTONE

ELSEVIER

EDINBURGH   LONDON   NEW YORK   OXFORD
PHILADELPHIA   ST LOUIS   SYDNEY   TORONTO   2011

CHURCHILL
LIVINGSTONE
ELSEVIER

First edition 1996
Second edition 2001
Third edition 2006
Fourth edition 2011

ISBN: 978-0-7020-3993-5
International Edition ISBN: 978-0-7020-3994-2

British Library Cataloguing in Publication Data
A catalogue record for this book is available from the British Library

Library of Congress Cataloging in Publication Data
A catalog record for this book is available from the Library of Congress

Notice
Knowledge and best practice in this field are constantly changing. As new research and experience broaden our understanding, changes in research methods, professional practices, or medical treatment may become necessary.

Practitioners and researchers must always rely on their own experience and knowledge in evaluating and using any information, methods, compounds, or experiments described herein. In using such information or methods they should be mindful of their own safety and the safety of others, including parties for whom they have a professional responsibility.

With respect to any drug or pharmaceutical products identified, readers are advised to check the most current information provided (i) on procedures featured or (ii) by the manufacturer of each product to be administered, to verify the recommended dose or formula, the method and duration of administration, and contraindications. It is the responsibility of practitioners, relying on their own experience and knowledge of their patients, to make diagnoses, to determine dosages and the best treatment for each individual patient, and to take all appropriate safety precautions.

To the fullest extent of the law, neither the Publisher nor the authors, contributors, or editors, assume any liability for any injury and/or damage to persons or property as a matter of products liability, negligence or otherwise, or from any use or operation of any methods, products, instructions, or ideas contained in the material herein.

PREFACE

The authors (ATR and MSD) are grateful to the publishers, Churchill Livingstone, for the invitation to produce a fourth edition of the *Pocketbook of Surgery*. It was felt that a further younger co-author would be helpful in bringing the book up-to-date. I am pleased that Marcus Wagstaff, Specialist Registrar in Plastic and Reconstructive Surgery, has agreed to fill the role as co-author. Together we are reassured that in these days of self-directed, student-centred, problem-based learning, led by medical educationalists, there is still a place for a small book offering a didactic approach to the acquisition of surgical knowledge.

It is now nearly 15 years since the first edition, 10 years since the second and 5 years since the third. Much has changed in that time and most of the chapters have been updated. When this book was written initially, it was aimed at medical students, but more recently it has been used by foundation year doctors and those in the early years of specialist training and also as a revision book for the MRCS. With this in mind, we have added sections on such topics as clinical governance, audit and the medico-legal aspects of surgery, together with a section on basic practical procedures. An outline of the important steps in a number of common operations has been added in the relevant chapters. The chapter in previous editions on conditions of the skin has been amalgamated in this edition with the chapter on plastic surgery, and basic ENT has been added to the chapter on Head, neck and otorhinolaryngology. A new chapter on gynaecology has also been added to outline conditions which the surgeon may encounter in the diagnosis of abdominal masses or the acute abdomen.

The aim of this small volume, however, remains the same. Namely, to provide a concise and didactic account of the essential features of the more common surgical disorders at both a size and a price to suit the pocket. The book covers fundamental principles, as well as providing basic information on aetiology, diagnosis and management, including preoperative and postoperative care. The text covers the field of general surgery but aims also to cover the basic needs of the undergraduate and those in the early years of postgraduate training in surgery as far as the surgical specialities are concerned. It will give the student some idea of history-taking, what physical signs to elicit, the differential diagnosis, what investigations to order and how to treat the patient.

Read in conjunction with *Churchill's Pocketbook of Differential Diagnosis*, it will provide almost everything the undergraduate needs to know and will also have sufficient information for postgraduates studying for the MRCS.

We must apologize to the medical educationalists that there is no mention of procedural knowledge, procedural improvisation knowledge, propositional adaptational knowledge or metacognitive knowledge anywhere in this book. However, the basis of this book is to supply didactic information and we make no apology for this. We hope it will continue to help you on the wards and in the clinics – and in examinations.

Sheffield, 2011

A T R
M S D
M J D W

ACKNOWLEDGMENTS

We wish to gratefully acknowledge the help, advice and criticisms of the following people who kindly read sections of the book: Mr T J Locke, Consultant Cardiac Surgeon, Northern General Hospital, Sheffield; Mr B J Harrison, Consultant Endocrine Surgeon, Royal Hallamshire Hospital, Sheffield; Mr R Lonsdale, Consultant Vascular Surgeon, Northern General Hospital, Sheffield; Mr John Anderson, Consultant Urological Surgeon, Royal Hallamshire Hospital, Sheffield; Mr James Hahnel, Specialist Registrar in Orthopaedics, Yorkshire and Humberside Deanery; Mr R D E Battersby, Consultant Neurological Surgeon, Royal Hallamshire Hospital, Sheffield; Miss J Walker, Consultant Paediatric Surgeon, Sheffield Children's Hospital, Sheffield; Mr A J Parker, Consultant ENT Surgeon, Royal Hallamshire Hospital, Sheffield; Dr Susan Snape, Specialist Registrar in Microbiology and Infectious Diseases, Nottingham University Hospitals NHS Trust; Mr B M Shrestha, Consultant General and Transplant Surgeon, Northern General Hospital, Sheffield.

Any errors that may have crept in, however, remain our responsibility and not theirs. We would also like to thank Dr Matthew Bull, Consultant Radiologist, Northern General Hospital, Sheffield; Dr Sam Euinton, Consultant Radiologist, Chesterfield and North Derbyshire Hospital, Chesterfield; Dr Peter Brown Consultant Radiologist, Northern General Hospital, Sheffield, and Dr Alan Sprigg, Consultant Radiologist, Sheffield Children's Hospital, Sheffield, for providing X-rays for the various editions of the book. We would also like to thank our former teachers, colleagues and students who have all contributed in some way to this book. We would particularly like to thank our wives for their patience and encouragement throughout the production of this book. Finally, we would like to thank Mrs Denise Smith for the hard work and long hours that she has put into typing and re-typing the manuscript.

Sheffield, 2011

A T R
M S D
M J D W

CONTENTS

ABBREVIATIONS

ABG	arterial blood gases		**CEA**	carcinoembryonic antigen
ACE	angiotensin-converting enzyme		**CML**	chronic myeloid leukaemia
ACTH	adrenocorticotrophic hormone		**CMV**	cytomegalovirus
ADH	antidiuretic hormone		**CNS**	central nervous system
A&E	Accident and Emergency		**COPD**	chronic obstructive pulmonary disease
AF	atrial fibrillation		**Cr**	creatinine
AFP	α-fetoprotein		**CRF**	chronic renal failure
AIDS	acquired immunodeficiency syndrome		**CRP**	C-reactive protein
ALG	antilymphocyte globulin		**C&S**	culture and sensitivity
ALT	alanine transaminase		**CSF**	cerebrospinal fluid
ANF	antinuclear factor		**CT**	computerized tomography
APTT	activated partial thromboplastin time		**CVA**	cerebrovascular accident
ARDS	adult respiratory distress syndrome		**CVP**	central venous pressure
ARF	acute renal failure		**CVVH**	continuous veno-venous haemofiltration
ATLS	advanced trauma life support		**CXR**	chest X-ray
ASD	atrial septal defect		**DDH**	developmental dysplasia of the hip
AST	aspartate transaminase		**DIC**	disseminated intravascular coagulation
ATG	antithymocyte globulin		**DIVA**	digital intravenous angiogram
ATN	acute tubular necrosis		**DM**	diabetes mellitus
AV	arteriovenous		**DMSA**	dimercaptosuccinic acid
AXR	abdominal X-ray		**DPL**	diagnostic peritoneal lavage
BBB	bundle branch block		**DSA**	digital subtraction angiography
BCG	bacille Calmette–Guérin		**DTPA**	diethylenetriamine-pentaacetic acid
BP	blood pressure		**DU**	duodenal ulcer
BTS	Blood Transfusion Service		**DVT**	deep venous thrombosis
CABG	coronary artery bypass graft		**ECG**	electrocardiogram
CAPD	continuous ambulatory peritoneal dialysis		**EEG**	electroencephalogram
CBD	common bile duct		**EMD**	electro-mechanical dissociation
CCF	congestive cardiac failure		**EMG**	electromyography
CCU	Coronary Care Unit		**EMSU**	early morning specimen of urine
CDH	congenital dislocation of the hip			

ePTFE	expanded polytetrafluoroethylene		**ITP**	idiopathic thrombocytopenic purpura
ERCP	endoscopic retrograde cholangiopancreatography		**ITU**	Intensive Therapy Unit
ESR	erythrocyte sedimentation rate		**IVC**	inferior vena cava
EUA	examination under anaesthesia		**IVDSA**	intravenous digital subtraction angiography
FBC	full blood count		**IVU**	intravenous urography
FDPs	fibrin degradation products		**JVP**	jugular venous pressure
FEV₁	forced expiratory volume (1 second)		**KCCT**	kaolin cephalin clotting time
FFP	fresh frozen plasma		**KUB**	kidney ureter bladder (plain X-ray)
FNAC	fine needle aspiration cytology		**LA**	left atrium
FOBs	faecal occult bloods		**LAD**	left axis deviation
GA	general anaesthetic		**LBBB**	left bundle branch block
GCS	Glasgow coma scale		**LE**	lupus erythematosus
GI	gastrointestinal		**LDH**	lactate dehydrogenase
GORD	gastro-oesophageal reflux disease		**LFTs**	liver function tests
GU	genitourinary		**LH**	luteinizing hormone
GVH	graft-versus-host disease		**LHRH**	luteinizing hormone releasing hormone
HBsAg	hepatitis B surface antigen		**LIF**	left iliac fossa
HBV	hepatitis B virus		**LP**	lumbar puncture
HCG	human chorionic gonadotrophin		**LV**	left ventricle
5HIAA	5-hydroxyindoleacetic acid		**LVF**	left ventricular failure
HIV	human immunodeficiency virus		**MEN**	multiple endocrine neoplasia
HLA	human leukocyte antigen		**MI**	myocardial infarction
HRT	hormone replacement therapy		**MLC**	mixed lymphocyte culture
HSV	highly selective vagotomy		**MRI**	magnetic resonance imaging
HVA	homovanillic acid		**MSSU**	midstream specimen of urine
ICP	intracranial pressure		**MTP**	metatarsophalangeal
IGTN	ingrowing toenail		**NG**	nasogastric
IHD	ischaemic heart disease		**NMR**	nuclear magnetic resonance
INR	International Normalized Ratio		**NSAID**	non-steroidal anti-inflammatory drug
			OA	osteoarthritis

OGD	oesophago-gastro-duodenoscopy		**RUQ**	right upper quadrant
PA	pulmonary artery		**RV**	right ventricle
PAP	prostatic acid phosphatase		**RVF**	right ventricular failure
PCA	patient-controlled analgesia		**SBE**	subacute bacterial endocarditis
PCV	packed cell volume		**SLE**	systemic lupus erythematosus
PDA	patent ductus arteriosus		**SVC**	superior vena cava
PDS	polydioxanone		**TB**	tuberculosis
PE	pulmonary embolus		**TED**	thromboembolic deterrent
PEEP	positive end-expiratory pressure		**TENS**	transcutaneous electrical nerve stimulation
PET	positron emission tomography		**TFTs**	thyroid function tests
PND	paroxysmal nocturnal dyspnoea		**TIA**	transient ischaemic attack
PR	per rectum		**TNM**	tumour, node, metastasis
PSA	prostate-specific antigen		**TPN**	total parenteral nutrition
PTA	percutaneous transluminal angioplasty		**TSH**	thyroid stimulating hormone
PTFE	polytetrafluoroethylene		**TURP**	transurethral resection of the prostate
PTH	parathyroid hormone		**U&Es**	urea and electrolytes
PT	prothrombin time		**UC**	ulcerative colitis
PTC	percutaneous transhepatic cholangiography		**UO**	urine output
PTT	partial thromboplastin time		**URTI**	upper respiratory tract infection
PUJO	pelvi-ureteric junction obstruction		**USS**	ultrasound scan
PUO	pyrexia of unknown origin		**UTI**	urinary tract infection
PV	per vaginam		**VDRL**	venereal disease research laboratory
PVD	peripheral vascular disease		**VF**	ventricular fibrillation
RA	rheumatoid arthritis		**VMA**	vanillylmandelic acid
RAD	right axis deviation		**V/Q**	ventilation/perfusion ratio
RBBB	right bundle branch block		**VSD**	ventricular septal defect
RIF	right iliac fossa		**WCC**	white cell count
RTA	road traffic accident		**WLE**	wide local excision
			ZN	Ziehl–Neelsen

TERMS AND DEFINITIONS

Students starting a surgical firm will be introduced to a number of terms and definitions which, it is often taken for granted, they will have heard before. As a useful reminder, these are listed below.

TERMS

Angio- Relating to (blood) vessels, e.g. angiogram – contrast imaging of an artery; cholangiogram – contrast imaging of the bile ducts.

Antegrade Going in the direction of flow, e.g. antegrade pyelogram – injection of contrast medium under imaging control into the renal pelvis percutaneously to delineate a distal obstruction.

Chole- Related to the biliary tree or bile, e.g. cholelithiasis – gallstones; cholecystectomy – removal of the gall bladder; choledochoscopy – examination of the bile ducts with an instrument.

-cele A cavity containing gas or fluid, e.g. hydrocele – collection of fluid between the layers of the tunica vaginalis of the testes; lymphocele – a localized collection of lymph; galactocele – a cavity containing milk in a lactating breast.

-docho- Related to ducts, e.g. choledochoscopy – examination of the bile ducts with an instrument; mammadochectomy – removal of the lactiferous ducts of the breast (for duct ectasia).

-ectasia Related to dilatation of the ducts, e.g. mammary duct ectasia – abnormal dilatation of the lactiferous ducts with periductal inflammation; sialectasia – dilatation of salivary gland ducts.

-ectomy Cutting something out, e.g. appendicectomy, gastrectomy, parotidectomy.

-gram An imaging technique using radio-opaque contrast medium, e.g. angiogram – visualization of the arterial tree; venogram – visualization of veins, e.g. to look for deep vein thrombosis; cholangiogram – to visualize the bile ducts.

Lith- Stone, e.g. pyelolithotomy – removal of a stone from the renal pelvis by opening the renal pelvis; cholelithiasis – gallstones.

-oscopy The inspection of a cavity, tube or organ with an instrument, e.g. cystoscopy – inspection of the bladder; laparoscopy – inspection of the abdominal cavity; colonoscopy – inspection of the colon; endoscopy – general term for inspection of internal organs.

-ostomy Opening something into another cavity or to the outside, e.g. colostomy – an opening of the colon onto the skin; gastroenterostomy – an opening of the stomach into the small bowel.

-otomy Making an opening in something, e.g. laparotomy – exploring the abdomen; cystotomy – opening the bladder.

Per- Going through a structure, e.g. percutaneous – going through the skin.

-plasty Refashioning something to alter function, e.g. pyloroplasty – to relieve pyloric obstruction; ileocystoplasty – to enlarge the bladder with a piece of ileum; angioplasty – to widen an obstruction in an artery.

Pyelo- Relating to the pelvis of the kidney, e.g. pyelogram – contrast imaging showing the renal pelvis; pyelonephritis – inflammation of kidney and renal pelvis.

Retrograde Going in a reverse direction against flow, e.g. endoscopic retrograde cholangiopancreatogram (ERCP) – retrograde injection of contrast medium up the common bile duct via cannulation of the papilla of Vater via a duodenoscope; retrograde pyelogram – injection of contrast medium in a reversed direction up the ureter to delineate the ureter and renal pelvis.

Trans- Going across a structure, e.g. percutaneous transluminal angioplasty – going through the skin and across an obstructed lumen in an artery to widen it and improve distal blood flow.

SOME IMPORTANT DEFINITIONS

Abscess A localized collection of pus.

Aneurysm An abnormal dilatation of an artery.

Cyst A fluid-filled cavity.

Fistula An abnormal communication between two epithelial surfaces (endothelial in the case of an arteriovenous fistula), e.g. colovesical fistula – between the sigmoid colon and the bladder, occurring usually as a complication of diverticulitis, carcinoma, or Crohn's disease.

Gangrene Death of tissue.

Sinus A blind-ending track communicating with an epithelial surface, e.g. pilonidal sinus where the 'sharp' end of hairs burrow into the skin.

Ulcer A break in the continuity of an epithelial surface.

Varix An abnormal dilatation of a vein.

BIOCHEMICAL VALUES

Venous blood: adult reference values

Analyte	Reference values
Acid phosphatase (unstable enzyme)	0.1–0.4 IU/L
Alanine aminotransferase (ALT) (glutamic-pyruvic transaminase (GPT))	10–40 IU/L
Alkaline phosphatase	40–100 IU/L
Amylase	50–300 IU/L
α_1-Antitrypsin	2–4 g/L
Ascorbic acid – serum	23–57 µmol/L 0.4–1.0 mg/dL
Ascorbic acid – leucocytes	1420–2270 µmol/L 25–40 mg/dL
Aspartate aminotransferase (AST) (glutamic-oxaloacetic transaminase (GOT))	10–35 IU/L
Bilirubin (total)	2–17 µmol/L
Caeruloplasmin	1–2.7 µmol/L
Calcium (total)	2.12–2.62 mmol/L
Carbon dioxide (total)	24–30 mmol/L
Chloride	95–105 mmol/L
Cholesterol (fasting)	3.6–6.7 mmol/L
Copper	11–24 µmol/L
Creatinine	55–150 µmol/L
Creatinine clearance	90–130 mL/min
Creatine kinase (CK) – males	30–200 IU/L
Creatine kinase (CK) – females	30–150 IU/L
Ethanol – marked intoxication	65–87 mmol/L
Ethanol – coma	109 mmol/L
Ferritin – males	6–186 µg/mL
Ferritin – females	3–162 µg/mL
α-Fetoprotein	2–6 units/mL
γ-Glutamyl transferase (γ-GT) – males	10–55 IU/L
(γ-GT) – females	5–35 IU/L
Glucose (fasting)	3.9–5.8 mmol/L
Immunoglobulins (Ig): IgA	0.5–4.0 g/L (40–300 IU/L)
Immunoglobulins (Ig): IgG	5.0–13.0 g/L (60–160 IU/L)
Immunoglobulins (Ig): IgM – males	0.3–2.2 g/L (40–270 IU/L)
Immunoglobulins (Ig): IgM – females	0.4–2.5 g/L (50–300 IU/L)
Iron – males	14–32 µmol/L
Iron – females	10–28 µmol/L
Iron binding capacity (total)	45–72 µmol/L
Iron binding capacity (saturation)	14–47%
Lactate	0.4–1.4 mmol/L
Lactate dehydrogenase (LDH)	100–300 IU/L
Lead	0.5–1.9 µmol/L
Magnesium	0.75–1.0 mmol/L
5′ Nucleotidase	1–11 IU/L
Osmolality	285–295 mOsm/kg
Phosphatase, *see* acid and alkaline	
Phosphate	0.8–1.4 mmol/L
Potassium	3.3–4.7 mmol/L
Proteins – total	62–82 g/L
Proteins – albumin	36–47 g/L
Proteins – globulins	24–37 g/L
Proteins – electrophoresis (% of total)	
albumin 52–68	
globulin α_1 4.2–7.2	
α_2 6.8–12	
β 9.3–15	
γ13–23	
Sodium	132–144 mmol/L
Triglyceride (fasting)	0.6–1.7 mmol/L
Urate – males	0.12–0.42 mmol
Urate – females	0.12–0.36 mmol/L
Urea	2.5–6.6 mmol/L

HAEMATOLOGICAL VALUES

Analyte	Reference values
Bleeding time (Ivy)	Up to 11 min
Body fluid (total)	50% (obese)–70% (lean) of body weight
Intracellular	30–40% of body weight
Extracellular	20–30% of body weight
Blood volume	
Red cell mass, men	30 ± 5 mL/kg
Red cell mass, women	25 ± 5 mL/kg
Plasma volume (both sexes)	45 ± 5 mL/kg
Erythrocyte sedimentation rate (Westergren)	0–6 mm in 1 h normal
	7–20 mm in 1 h doubtful
	>20 mm in 1 h abnormal
Fibrinogen	1.5–4.0 g/L
Folate – serum	2–20 µg/L
Folate – red cell	>100 µg/L
Haemoglobin – men	13–18 g/dL
Haemoglobin – women	11.5–16.5 g/dL
Haptoglobin	0.3–2.0 g/L
Leucocytes – adults	$4.0–11.0 \times 10^9$/L
Differential white cell count	
Neutrophil granulocytes	$2.5–7.5 \times 10^9$/L
Lymphocytes	$1.0–3.5 \times 10^9$/L
Monocytes	$0.2–0.8 \times 10^9$/L
Eosinophil granulocytes	$0.04–0.4 \times 10^9$/L
Basophil granulocytes	$0.01–0.1 \times 10^9$/L
Mean corpuscular haemoglobin (MCH)	27–32 pg
Mean corpuscular haemoglobin	30–35 g/dL concentration (MCHC)
Mean corpuscular volume (MCV)	78–98 ft
Packed cell volume (PCV) or haematocrit	
Men	0.40–0.54
Women	0.35–0.47
Platelets	$150–400 \times 10^9$/L
Prothrombin time	11–15 s
Red cell count – men	$4.5–6.5 \times 10^{12}$/L
Red cell count – women	$3.8–5.8 \times 10^{12}$/L
Red cell life span (mean)	120 days
Red cell life span $T^1/_2(^{51}Cr)$	25–35 days
Reticulocytes (adults)	$10–100 \times 10^9$/L
Vitamin B_{12} (in serum as cyanocobalamin)	160–925 ng/L

EMERGENCIES

Introduction to surgery

The practice of surgery today involves not only technical skills but a whole range of other skills, such as communication skills, delivery of informed consent, breaking bad news and bereavement counselling. Surgical practice must be evidence-based and surgeons must conduct regular audits as well as being aware of their accountability in patient care.

EVIDENCE-BASED MEDICINE

Evidence-based medicine is the conscientious, explicit and judicious use of current best evidence in making decisions about the care of individual patients. Evidence-based medicine combines the individual doctor's expertise and the best available external evidence when making decisions about the patient's healthcare.

Evidence-based medicine is a lifelong process which involves:

- Asking clinical questions
- Tracking down the best evidence
- Assessing the evidence
- Applying the results in practice
- Evaluating subsequent performance.

Evidence-based medicine has the following advantages:

- It offers an objective way to determine and maintain consistently high quality and safety standards in medical practice
- It helps speed up the process of transferring clinical research findings into clinical practice
- It has the potential to significantly reduce the cost of delivery of healthcare.

External evidence includes research from basic medical sciences, patient-centred clinical research, randomized trials and meta-analyses. Patient-centred clinical research looks at the accuracy and appropriateness of diagnostic tests, the use of prognostic indicators and the effectiveness and safety of treatments. External clinical evidence may invalidate previously accepted tests and treatments, replacing them with new ones that are more accurate, effective and safe. Without the current best evidence, surgical practice risks becoming out of date, to the detriment of patient care.

Evidence may be available from individual randomized trials or via meta-analysis of several trials such as those published in the Cochrane Database of Systematic Reviews.

CLINICAL GOVERNANCE IN SURGICAL PRACTICE

Clinical governance is – a framework through which healthcare organizations are accountable for continually improving the quality of their services and safeguarding high standards of care by creating an environment in which excellence in clinical care will flourish.

The purpose of clinical governance is to ensure a systematic approach to maintaining and improving the quality of patient care. It embodies three main areas:

1. Recognizable high standards of care
2. Transparent responsibility and accountability for those standards
3. A drive for improvement through constant monitoring of standards.

Clinical governance covers organizational systems and processes for monitoring and improving services including:

● Education and training
● Clinical audit
● Clinical risk management
● Clinical effectiveness
● Research and development
● Openness.

Effective clinical governance addresses those structures, systems and processes that ensure quality and accountability thus ensuring proper management of an organization's operations and delivery of service in an open and transparent setting. In so doing, it ensures continual improvement of patient care with a commitment to quality and the prevention of clinical errors.

CLINICAL AUDIT

Clinical audit is a continuous cycle of quality improvement that seeks to improve patient care and service delivery through systematic review of care against explicit criteria and the implementation of change. The clinical audit process is known as the audit cycle. This involves observation of existing practice, the setting of standards, comparison between observed and set standards, implementation of

Figure 1.1 The audit cycle.

change and re-audit of clinical practice (Fig. 1.1). The main components of the audit cycle are:

- Choose a topic
- Review current standards or agree standards
- Accurate collection of data on current practice
- Use of data to compare with standards
- A system for implementing change to make improvement
- Re-audit to ensure practice has improved.

Benefits of undertaking clinical audit:

- Improvements in clinical practice benefiting patient care and service delivery
- Meeting evidence-based best practice
- Minimizing error
- Developing local guidelines/protocols
- Reducing adverse clinical incidents, complaints and claims.

Clinical audit is used to compare current practice with evidence of good practice. It basically asks the question, 'are we actually doing what we think we are doing?'. Clinical audit can:

- identify major risk, resource and service development implications
- reinforce implementation of evidence-based practice
- influence improvements to individual patient care
- provide assurance on the quality of care.

When considering topics to audit, the following may be a useful guide; high-risk practice, cost-effectiveness, patient concerns, local concerns, conforming to international guidelines, new treatments or procedures.

Types of audit vary from basic clinical audit, e.g. morbidity/mortality, to national audit, e.g. National Confidential Enquiry into Patient Outcome and Death (NCEPOD). Whatever the subject audited, the following are essential requirements:

- Accurate high quality data collection
- Recognition of variation in case mix
- Clearly defined outcome measures
- Appropriate statistical analysis
- A system for introducing change
- Re-evaluation of the system after change.

How does *audit* differ from *research*?

- Research:
  — aims to establish best practice
  — aims to generate new knowledge
  — is theory driven
  — may involve a completely new treatment.
- Audit:
  — aims to evaluate how close actual practice is to best practice
  — aims to improve service delivery
  — is practice based
  — never involves a completely new treatment.

CONSENT

Informed consent is required for all invasive procedures. Consent should be obtained by the person who is actually going to carry out the procedure or certainly by somebody who is suitably trained and qualified and has sufficient knowledge of the proposed treatment. It is probably best that consent for major procedures is obtained either by the consultant or with the consultant present. It is good practice that consent should be obtained for any procedure that can have a complication.

For consent to be valid, the patient must have the capacity to:

1. Be able to comprehend and retain the information relevant to the decision in question
2. Believe that information
3. Weigh that information in the balance to arrive at a decision.

Consent should be informed, i.e. the patient should be given the full information about:

- The procedure
- The reasons for carrying it out
- Any alternative treatments
- Benefits of the procedure
- Adverse effects or complications
- The outcome without any treatment.

Consent must be voluntary, i.e. not the result of coercion by medical staff, relatives or friends.

Minors between the ages of 16 and 18 are presumed to have capacity to consent in English law. If a doctor feels that a child under 16 has the intelligence and maturity to comprehend the risks and benefits of an intervention (Gillick competence), the patient may consent against parental wishes. Children under 16 who are not Gillick competent may not withhold or give consent; parents must act on their behalf. Patients over 16 with fluctuating capacity (e.g. under the influence of drugs affecting mental state) should be given the opportunity to consent when lucid, if their medical condition can wait until then. Otherwise, doctors may consent on their behalf.

Consent may be verbal or written. Consent forms provide some evidence that the process of consent has taken place, but are not themselves legal documents that prove that consent is valid.

Risks of operation may be general or specific to the operation. The general risks include the risks of anaesthesia and the risks of any operation, e.g. haemorrhage, wound infection, deep vein thrombosis. Examples of specific complications are recurrence after inguinal hernia repair, recurrent laryngeal nerve palsy after thyroid surgery, facial nerve palsy after superficial parotidectomy.

It is generally accepted that complications should be explained to the patient when they arise at a rate of 1% or greater. However, any devastating complication which may occur and has an incidence of less than 1% should be explained to the patient, e.g. paraplegia after aortic cross clamping.

The degree of information to be conferred to a patient continues to evolve through debate in English law. Consent issues challenged by a claimant are tested in English law against the elements of negligence. Rulings have been led by legal precedent. In Sidaway vs. Bethlem Royal Hospital (1985), a patient undergoing cervical cord decompression was not warned against a 1–2% risk of spinal cord injury, which she subsequently suffered. Although she claimed she would not have undergone surgery if she had been warned, a responsible body of surgical opinion would also not have warned a patient of the risk and therefore, the court ruled for the doctor of the basis of the Bolam test.

Since then, in Chester vs. Afshar (2004), surgery for back pain resulted in cauda equina syndrome, the possibility of which the patient was not informed prior to surgery. The judges ruled that failure to inform had violated her right to choose. She may, however, have still opted for this surgery, therefore it is debated that it is difficult to establish causation if the failure to inform may not have changed the outcome, i.e. the patients choice for surgery.

Any move away from Bolam towards a Bolitho-style ruling by the English courts has not yet led to a deviation from the 'prudent doctor test' where it is a matter of clinical judgement by the doctor as to the degree of information to be given to the patient. However, in an Australian case (Rogers vs. Whitaker, 1992), a patient underwent surgery to her blind right eye but suffered a 1:14 000 complication of sympathetic ophthalmia leading to blindness in her functional left eye. She successfully claimed, as the court ruled that the doctor had failed to answer her questions with proper care and skill, and if the risk had been disclosed, the plaintiff would not have had the operation. This approach to disclosure of all relevant information is called the 'prudent patient test'.

MEDICO-LEGAL ISSUES

When a patient pursues a claim of negligence against an individual or trust, they must establish three elements:

1. The doctor owes a duty of care to that individual
2. A breach of that duty has occurred that falls below the required standard
3. That this breach of duty was responsible for the harm that has resulted in the claim (causation). Causation may be accepted on a balance of probability of >50% that the actions of the defendant caused the harm.

Breach of duty has historically been tested against the Bolam principle (Bolam *vs.* Friern Hospital Management Committee 1957), where the doctor is not guilty if he has acted in accordance with a practice accepted as proper and responsible by a responsible body of medical men skilled in that particular art. Although there may be a body of professional opinion opposing the view, as long as it can be considered acceptable practice to a group of doctors of similar standing, then the action may not form a breach of duty.

More recently, the case of Bolitho *vs.* City & Hackney Health Authority (1997) led to the House of Lords deciding that if professional opinion called in support of a defence case was not capable of withstanding logical analysis, then the court would be entitled to hold that the body of opinion was not reasonable or responsible. This means that a court can overrule a body of professionals supporting a defendant through the Bolam principle, if it feels that their argument does not follow logical reasoning.

With the exception of minors, patients have 3 years from the time of injury, or recovery from mental illness if present at the time of injury, to bring a case to court. There can therefore be a considerable time lag prior to representation in court. It is therefore vital to maintain high standards of thorough and contemporaneous note-keeping.

Civil Procedure Rules require a Letter of Claim to be sent to the defendant, and a response drawn. Particulars of Claim and Negligence then are prepared by the plaintiff, which are defended with any statements as a formal defence. If the case is to proceed, then the Court will hear expert opinions on each area of disagreement. If no agreement is formed, the case will go to trial.

Compensation may be awarded by the courts as 'general' damages for pain and suffering and 'special' damages for actual amounts such as claim expenses, need for care, loss of income, etc.

BREAKING BAD NEWS

Breaking bad news to patients and their relatives is almost a daily occurrence. Most medical schools provide tutorials on 'breaking bad news' as part of the course and much experience may be obtained in role-play in such tutorials. However, there is no substitute for the real thing and it is appropriate for a medical student to sit in when bad news is actually being broken to relatives or patients. A doctor who is explaining the bad news should always check with the patient or the relatives that it is appropriate for a medical student to be present at the time. It is understandable that some patients' relatives may find this obtrusive.

When we think of the nature of breaking bad news, we usually think in terms of explaining to someone that they have an inoperable condition. However, for some patients' relatives, it is merely bad news that the patient actually requires surgery or that as a result of curative surgery, the patient, e.g. needs a permanent colostomy. Usually, however, breaking bad news involves explaining inoperable and incurable cancer and the need to face death. A problem then arises about how much the patient needs to know, and occasionally, in some cases, whether the patient actually needs to know at all. The answer to the latter is that the patient should always be told. Unless the patient is fully aware of the facts, it is difficult to deal with subsequent management, particularly explaining palliative treatment, e.g. radiotherapy or the fact that the patient requires hospice care.

Occasionally, relatives request that the patient is not told. This is not appropriate and should be explained to the relatives, particularly the fact that if the patient finds out by other means (and the patient surely will, maybe even through a careless word on a ward round), then trust is lost between patient and relative and patient and doctor. It is well recognized that most patients are told less than they would actually like to know. Occasionally, even the medical profession will rationalize reasons for not wanting to tell the patient, e.g. the patient would not want to know. In fact, most patients are intelligent and shrewd and when you actually sit down to explain the bad news to them you will realize that they have already half suspected it and many will thank you for being honest with them. Always remember that patients have many affairs that they wish to put in order, and also explaining to them honestly about life expectancy will enable them to decide if further unpleasant palliative therapy is worthwhile.

It is always difficult to know how and what to tell the patient. It is probably best not to do this on a busy ward round but to take time to go back to the bed with the nurse who is looking after the patient, sit down and take time to explain. There is a balance to explaining bad news which is somewhere between giving a long explanation skirting round the problem without actually indicating how bad the problem is and the brusque honesty approach ('you have got incurable cancer and less then 3 months to live'). Do not leave the bedside immediately after giving bad news and worse still, do not indicate that somebody else will come back shortly and re-explain what you have already said. It is best to wait a while to give patients a chance to ask any questions. If they do not have any at the time, then indicate that you will go back later when they have had a chance to let the bad news sink in and when they may have thought of some questions that they wish to ask. It is important to allow sufficient time to talk to patients and to talk to them sensitively and also indicate that you are prepared to talk to members of the family and explain things fully to them. Some patients would be grateful if members of the family are there when bad news is broken.

Accepting terminal illness often takes time and involves a number of well-defined stages, although not all these may occur in a particular patient. These include:

- shock and numbness
- denial

- anger
- grief
- acceptance.

It is important that every member of the team knows exactly what has been explained to the patient and also that the family doctor is aware. Over the days following the breaking of bad news, the patient and relatives may often have numerous questions and time must be taken to sit down and provide the answers.

DEATH AND THE CERTIFICATION OF DEATH

When you are qualified, you will be required to diagnose death. The patient is pulseless, apnoeic, and has fixed, dilated pupils. Auscultation reveals no heart sounds or breath sounds. If the patient is on a ventilator, brain death may be diagnosed even although the heart is still beating. The preconditions and the criteria for testing for brain death are explained in Chapter 18. Do not forget that after death, organs and tissue may be donated for transplantation purposes. Any solid organ and tissues may be removed from a ventilated brain-dead patient but remember that kidneys may be removed within 30 min of death and other tissues such as cornea, bone, skin and heart valves may be removed within 24 h of death.

Certification of death is important and should be carried out as soon as possible after death. This is not the same as certifying (or diagnosing) death, but is the official documentation of the patient's cause of death that must be delivered, usually by the next of kin, to the Registrar of Births and Deaths within 5 days of the death. In practice, death certification should normally be carried out on the day after death to allow the patient's relatives to make the funeral arrangements as soon as possible. Only a doctor who has seen the patient within 14 days prior to the death can legally fill in the certificate. In some cases, e.g. where the patient has died postoperatively, or after an emergency admission, or accident, the Coroner must be informed. If in any doubt, it is always best to ring the Coroner and discuss the case. If the Coroner decides to take the case, his department will deal with the certification of death.

BEREAVEMENT COUNSELLING

Explaining the death of loved ones to their relatives is never easy. It is best that the medical student attends a course in bereavement counselling and also, during attachments to both medical and surgical firms, accompanies the houseman or consultant who is explaining the death to relatives. The circumstances of death may cause different emotional reactions in relatives: some react with shock, others with anger and guilt, the latter being common emotions. Anger may be directed towards the deceased, other family members or the medical profession involved in the patient's care. Support offered to the family both during the patient's illness and at the time of the patient's death not only helps them to cope better but may also reduce the likelihood of future problems. Religious beliefs and cultural background may influence reactions and some individuals may resort to alcohol, drugs or denial, as a way of coping with loss. In such cases, help of bereavement counsellors should be sought.

APPROACH TO THE PATIENT

Most patients are quite happy to be seen and examined by medical students. Their usual attitude is: 'Doctors have to learn, don't they?'. Some patients, however, resent being seen by students; some understandably because they are shy and embarrassed by their condition, but others because they do not feel they should be treated as 'guinea-pigs'. The latter are almost certainly those who in subsequent years will complain that doctors have failed to make the correct diagnosis, and one wonders exactly how they consider that medical students should learn.

Bedside manner is extremely important. It is important to establish rapport with patients so that they can trust you. Before approaching any patient on the ward, always ask the nurse in charge of the ward if you can see the patient. It may be that the patient is not well enough to be seen and examined repeatedly by students. When approaching the patient, introduce yourself with a handshake and let the patient know who you are: 'My name is John Smith. I am a medical student. Would you mind if I talk to you and examine you?'. Always attend the ward at a sensible time and try to avoid disturbing the patients during their rest period. Always examine the patient with a colleague or a nurse present (chaperone). Do not carry out intimate examinations such as rectal or vaginal examinations except under strict supervision.

In the outpatient clinic, there will usually be notices displayed that students may be present during the consultation. Patients are told that if they do not wish to see students then they should inform the nurse in charge of the outpatient clinic. It is our practice always to ask the accompanying nurse to check with the patients whether they mind seeing students before they are brought into the consultation room. Always take plenty of time to take a history from the patient. Never rush or you may miss important points in the history. Always wash your hands both before and after examining a patient.

TAKING A HISTORY

Always allow yourself plenty of time to take a full history. Develop a method of taking it, trying not to write and talk to the patient at the same time. Although as students you will not normally write the patient's history in the notes, you should get used to recording it so that you know exactly how to record it in the notes when you become a qualified doctor. Initially you should record the following:

- Full name
- Address
- Sex
- Age
- Ethnic group
- Marital status
- Occupation.

Make sure that you record the date of the examination. You will need this so that you can record subsequent progress.

The remainder of the history should be taken in the following order:

1. *The presenting complaint.* Ask what symptoms the patient is complaining of. If there is more than one complaint, list them in the order in which they are most troublesome to the patient.

2. *The history of the presenting complaint.* Record the full details of the main complaint or complaints. Allow the patient to give a full record of complaints relating to a particular system and then ask any remaining questions that you may have about the abnormal system. For example, if the patient complains of indigestion, nausea and vomiting, make sure that as part of the history of the presenting complaint, which clearly relates to the alimentary tract, that you ask all other questions in this section about the alimentary tract, e.g. bowel habit, abdominal distension, jaundice.

3. *Systematic enquiry.* Once you are satisfied that you have obtained the full history of the presenting complaint and have asked all pertinent questions about the abnormal system, then you should ask direct questions about other systems. These are laid out below.
   — *Alimentary system.* Appetite. Change in diet. Change in weight. Nausea. Difficulty in swallowing. Regurgitation. Heartburn. Flatulence. Indigestion. Vomiting. Character of the vomit, e.g. coffee grounds, blood, bile, faeculent. Abdominal pain. Abdominal distension. Change in bowel habit. Characteristics of the stool. Rectal bleeding. Change of skin colour, e.g. pallor of anaemia, jaundice.
   — *Respiratory system.* Cough. Sputum – character of sputum, e.g. purulent, haemoptysis. Dyspnoea. Wheezing. Hoarseness. Chest pain.
   — *Cardiovascular system.* Chest pain. Dyspnoea. Paroxysmal nocturnal dyspnoea. Orthopnoea. Palpitations. Ankle swelling. Cough. Dizziness. Intermittent claudication. Rest pain. Temperature or colour changes of hands and feet. Oedema.
   — *Nervous system.* Blackouts. Fits, loss of consciousness. Fainting attacks. Tremor. Weakness of limbs. Paraesthesia. Disturbances of smell, vision or hearing. Headaches. Change of behaviour.
   — *Musculoskeletal system.* Pain in joints. Swelling of joints. Limitation of movement. Muscle pain. Muscle weakness. Disturbance of gait.
   — *Genitourinary system.* Frequency of micturition. Hesitancy. Poor stream. Dysuria. Colour of urine, e.g. haematuria. Thirst. Polyuria. Symptoms of uraemia – headache, drowsiness, fits, vomiting, peripheral oedema. Loin pain. Date of menarche or menopause. Menstruation. Dysmenorrhoea. Previous pregnancies and their complications. Breast symptoms – pain, lumps. Impotence. Dyspareunia.

4. *Past medical history.* Previous illnesses, operations or accidents. Diabetes. Rheumatic fever. Tuberculosis. Asthma. Hypertension. Sexually transmitted disease.

5. *Family history.* Cause of death of close relatives, e.g. parents, brothers and sisters. Enquire particularly about cardiovascular disease and malignancy. Check for familial illnesses, e.g. adult polycystic kidney disease.

6. *Social history.* Occupation – check fully the details of the occupation and make sure you understand exactly what the patient does. Housing. Travel

abroad. Leisure activities. Marital status. Sexual habits. Smoking. Drinking. Eating habits.

7. *Drug history*. Check the patient's present medication. Make particular enquiries about steroids, anticoagulants and contraceptive pill. Drug abuse. Ask about allergies, especially to antibiotics. Ask specifically 'does any drug bring you out in a rash?'.

EXAMINATION OF A LUMP

HISTORY

1. When did the patient first notice the lump?
2. What brought the lump to the patient's notice, e.g. pain?
3. Is the lump symptomatic?
4. Has there been any change in size?
5. Does the lump ever disappear, e.g. a hernia may disappear on lying down or a sebaceous cyst may discharge and settle down only to fill up again at a later date?
6. Are there any other lumps on the body of similar nature, e.g. lipomas or neurofibromata may be multiple?
7. Does the patient know of any cause for the lump, e.g. trauma?

EXAMINATION

- *Site*: describe this in exact anatomical terms. It is best to measure it from a fixed bony point.
- *Shape*: e.g. is it spherical, does it have an irregular outline?
- *Size*: measure this accurately using a tape measure.
- *Surface*: is it smooth or irregular?
- *Edge*: is the edge of the lump clearly defined or indistinct?
- *Colour of overlying skin*: e.g. red and inflamed suggesting an inflammatory lesion.
- *Temperature*: is the skin overlying the lump hot or of normal temperature?
- *Tenderness*: is the lump tender?
- *Composition*: is the mass solid, fluid or gas? Check for consistence, fluctuation, fluid thrill, translucency, pulsation, compressibility and bruits.

Consistency. A lump may vary from soft to bony hard. A simple scale of consistence is suggested: soft, e.g. subcutaneous lipoma; firm, e.g. Hodgkin's lymph node; hard, e.g. carcinoma of the breast; stony hard, e.g. ivory osteoma of skull.

Fluctuation. Demonstration of this sign indicates a fluid-filled cavity. Pressure on one side of a fluid-filled cavity causes the other surface to protrude because an increase in pressure within a cavity is transmitted equally and at right angles to all parts of its wall. The test should be carried out in two planes at right angles to each other.

Fluid thrill. This detects the presence of free fluid in a cavity. A percussion wave can be conducted across the fluid. Tap one side of the lump and feel the transmitted vibration at the opposite extremity. This is a classical sign of ascites and to prevent a thrill being transmitted through the abdominal wall, a second person should place the edge of a hand along the abdomen, midway between the percussing and palpating hands.

Translucency. If a swelling transilluminates then it must contain clear fluid. Use a bright torch in a darkened room. Lumps that classically transilluminate brilliantly are hydroceles and cystic hygroma in children.

Resonance. Solid and fluid-filled lumps are dull to percussion. Gas-filled swellings are resonant, e.g. distended obstructed bowel.

Pulsatility. Rest your hand on every lump and make sure that it does not pulsate. If a pulse is present, distinguish between transmitted pulsation through a lump and an expansile pulsatile lump, i.e. an aneurysm. To do this, place a finger of either hand on opposite sides of the lump. If the fingers are pushed up and down in the same plane, it is a transmitted pulsation. If they are pushed upwards and apart, it is a true expansile pulsation, i.e. aneurysm.

Compressibility. Try to empty a lump by gentle pressure and see if it refills spontaneously. This is the sign of compressibility, e.g. strawberry naevus, saphenovarix.

Bruit. Listen over the lump. A systolic bruit may be heard over an aneurysm or a vascular goitre associated with thyrotoxicosis. A continuous machinery bruit may be heard over an arteriovenous fistula.

Reducibility. This is a property of herniae. The lump may be gently compressed and reduced to the cavity in which it is normally contained. It will reappear by coughing or gravity (standing up).

Relation to surrounding structures. Assess the mobility of the lump. Is it attached to the skin or is it attached to deep structures? Is it within the peritoneal cavity or the abdominal wall? Tensing the abdominal muscles by raising the head and shoulders will allow you to distinguish.

Regional lymph nodes. Always remember to palpate the regional lymph nodes.

Surrounding tissues and extremities. If the lump is on a limb, make sure that it is not interfering with the normal function of the limb, such as pressure on a nerve or interference with distal circulation, e.g. a popliteal artery aneurysm associated with distal ischaemia, or pressure on the common peroneal nerve.

GENERAL EXAMINATION

Always remember to examine the whole of the patient, e.g. a lump in the breast may not only be associated with axillary lymphadenopathy but may be associated with a pleural effusion, and a malignant melanoma on the leg may be associated with hepatomegaly.

EXAMINATION OF AN ULCER

DEFINITION

An ulcer is a break in the continuity of an epithelial surface. Many ulcers are occult in the GI tract and unfortunately many of these tend to be malignant. However, ulcers on the skin and in the oral cavity are easily noticed by the patient.

HISTORY

1. When did the patient first notice the ulcer?
2. What first made the patient notice the ulcer, e.g. was it painful or did it start as a different sort of lesion and then become ulcerated, e.g. malignant melanoma?
3. What are the symptoms of the ulcer?
4. Has the ulcer changed since it first appeared, e.g. has there been a chronic venous ulcer on the leg which has previously healed and then broken down again?
5. Has the patient ever had any other ulcers?
6. Is there any obvious cause for the ulcer, e.g. trauma?

EXAMINATION

Record accurately the site and size of the ulcer. Check for colour, tenderness, increased temperature, base, edge, depth, discharge, surrounding tissues. Check the state of the local lymph nodes and carry out a general examination.

Base. Usually slough or granulation tissue. Some ulcers have a characteristic base, e.g. ischaemic ulcers often contain no granulation tissue but may contain black necrotic tissue, or tendons or bone may be seen in the base of the ulcer. Syphilitic ulcers have a classic slough that looks like a wash leather.

Edge. Classically, five types are described. These are shown in Figure 1.2 together with their usual aetiologies.

Depth. Record this accurately in millimetres.

Discharge. This may be serous, sanguineous or purulent. It may be necessary to remove slough from the base of an ulcer to accurately assess it.

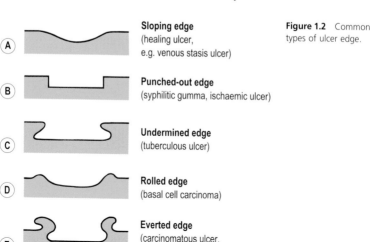

(A) Sloping edge
(healing ulcer,
e.g. venous stasis ulcer)

(B) Punched-out edge
(syphilitic gumma, ischaemic ulcer)

(C) Undermined edge
(tuberculous ulcer)

(D) Rolled edge
(basal cell carcinoma)

(E) Everted edge
(carcinomatous ulcer,
e.g. squamous cell carcinoma)

Figure 1.2 Common types of ulcer edge.

Surrounding tissues. Are the surrounding tissues pink and healthy? Is the innervation normal, e.g. neuropathic ulcer associated with diabetes? Are there black satellite nodules around the ulcer, e.g. malignant melanoma?

Examine the local lymph nodes.

Carry out a general examination.

CLASSIFICATION OF DISEASE

When initially starting your surgical training, your knowledge will be limited. You will, therefore, find it difficult to reach a diagnosis. In order to do this you should go through a broad classification of the aetiology of disease as shown in Table 1.1. This is sometimes known as the 'surgical sieve'. Ask yourself, is this lesion congenital (usually easy to decide) or is it acquired? If it is acquired, then go through the 'sieve' and try and decide which classification it belongs to. As you learn more pathology and more surgery, you will still find this classification suitable when trying to reach a differential diagnosis. It is a good idea when you are first learning, with every disease, lump or ulcer you meet, to sit down and go through the 'surgical sieve' and decide which of these groups it belongs to.

TABLE 1.1 Classification of disease ('surgical sieve')

Congenital

Acquired

Traumatic
Inflammatory:
- physical stimuli
- chemical stimuli
- infection
Neoplastic:
- benign
- malignant
Degenerative
Vascular
Endocrine/metabolic
Autoimmune
Iatrogenic
Psychogenic

CHAPTER 2

An introduction to surgical techniques and practical procedures

This chapter will describe various techniques which are part of the 'stock-in-trade' of the surgeon and therefore the student training in surgery. It will also describe some practical procedures with which the surgical trainee should be familiar.

SURGICAL INCISION

When choosing an incision, the following points should be considered:

- *Access*: the incision must be appropriately placed, large enough and capable of extension
- *Orientation*: if possible in the lines of skin tension (Langer's lines) or skin creases. This leads to minimal distortion and better healing
- *Healing potential of tissues*
- *Anatomy of underlying structures*, e.g. the avoidance of nerves
- *Good cosmetic result*
- *Abdominal incision*: the common abdominal incisions are shown in Figure 2.1 and the indications for such incisions are indicated on the diagram. Paramedian incisions are rarely used nowadays but are included as their scars are still seen on the abdominal wall of the older patient.

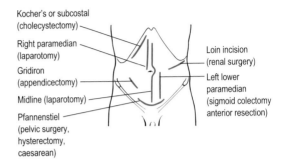

Figure 2.1 Abdominal incisions.

Kocher's or subcostal (cholecystectomy)

Right paramedian (laparotomy)

Gridiron (appendicectomy)

Midline (laparotomy)

Pfannenstiel (pelvic surgery, hysterectomy, caesarean)

Loin incision (renal surgery)

Left lower paramedian (sigmoid colectomy anterior resection)

SUTURES

Students are usually introduced to suturing in a Clinical Skills Laboratory and during their A&E attachment. There is a wide range of suture materials, broadly divided into absorbable and non-absorbable, natural and synthetic, braided and monofilament.

Absorbable

These are plain catgut (natural monofilament); chromic catgut (natural monofilament); polyglycolic acid (synthetic braided – Dexon); polyglactin (synthetic braided – Vicryl); polydioxanone (PDS – synthetic monofilament). The strength of absorbable sutures declines according to the material, catgut being the quickest to lose strength. (Catgut sutures are no longer available in the UK because of their theoretical potential for transmitting spongiform encephalopathy and the fact that there are adequate supplies of acceptable alternative synthetic sutures.)

Non-absorbable

These include silk (natural braided); linen (natural braided); wire (stainless steel, usually monofilament); nylon (synthetic monofilament – Ethilon); polypropylene (synthetic monofilament – Prolene); expanded polytetrafluoroethylene (ePTFE – expanded monofilament). Non-absorbable sutures retain strength indefinitely and are used where strength is needed until repair is completed naturally, e.g. abdominal incisions and hernia repair. Non-absorbable sutures are often used for skin closure – synthetic monofilament used in subcuticular fashion giving the best cosmetic result.

Natural sutures

These are catgut, silk, linen, but their use is declining. Catgut is cheap but of variable strength. Silk handles well but, as with linen, it excites a strong inflammatory reaction.

Synthetic sutures

Types include Dexon, Vicryl, PDS, nylon, polypropylene and ePTFE. They are more expensive than natural sutures, but cause little tissue reaction. The degree of strength and absorbability can be controlled in manufacture.

Monofilament

These include catgut, polydioxanone, wire, polypropylene and nylon. They are smooth and pass easily through tissues and cause less tissue reaction. The disadvantage is that they are stiff, slippery and difficult to knot.

Braided (polyfilament)

These include polyglycolic acid, polyglactin, silk, nylon and linen. They handle well, but interstices harbour bacteria.

Wire

This is useful for closing the sternum in cardiac procedures and for orthopaedic procedures. It is strong, inert, but subject to breakage and handles poorly.

Gauge

Gauge (G) is the calibre of the suture and is expressed in numbers. Originally, the finest gauge was '1' and the heaviest '4' but with the development of finer sutures a scale of '0s' was developed, the more 0s, the finer the suture, e.g. '0', '00' (2/0), '000' (3/0). The finest suture is 10/0, used in eye surgery. The gauge used depends on the strength required, number of sutures, type of suture material being used and cosmetic requirements.

Needles

Needles are cutting or round-bodied. They come in a variety of shapes and lengths and may be straight or curved. Cutting needles are usually triangular in cross-section, and are useful for skin, tendon, and breast tissue. Round-bodied needles are oval or round in cross-section. Round-bodied needles are useful for GI tract and vascular anastomoses.

Methods of suturing

Sutures may be interrupted, continuous, vertical mattress, horizontal mattress or subcuticular. The choice depends on the site and nature of the operation and surgeon's preference. Interrupted sutures may be used if there is a risk of infection, where some individual sutures may be removed to allow drainage. Subcuticular sutures may be used to give good cosmetic results, especially when using synthetic monofilament. Synthetic absorbable subcuticular sutures (e.g. Vicryl) may be used in children to avoid the trauma of suture removal.

Removal of sutures

The timing is a balance between strength of healing and a good cosmetic result. Some areas are better vascularized, under less tension, and therefore heal quicker than others. The following is a rough guide for the time of removal for different areas: face and neck (3–4 days); scalp (5–7 days); limbs (5–7 days); hands and feet (10–14 days); abdomen (8–10 days).

Alternatives to sutures

Alternatives include clips and staples. Michel clips appose the skin edges but do not penetrate the skin, and cosmetic results are good. Preloaded disposable staples have largely replaced Michel clips. Cosmetic results are excellent. Stapling devices are also available for GI anastomoses. Simple wounds in children can be

closed with adhesive strips (Steri-Strips). Scalp lacerations in children can be
closed using hairs adjacent to the wound edges as 'sutures'. The hairs are
knotted across the wound.

DRAINS

Drains are used prophylactically to drain anticipated collections, e.g. haematomas,
bile leaks, urine leaks, or therapeutically to remove collections of pus, blood or
other body fluids. Most drains consist of latex-based material or silicone. Red
rubber tube drains are still used occasionally. Red rubber and latex drains form
better tracks than silicone by exciting more tissue reaction. Drainage may be open
or closed, suction or non-suction.

Open drainage
This is drainage by capillary action or gravity into dressings or stoma bags.
Drainage may depend on position of patient. Sepsis is commoner with open drains.

Closed drainage
This is drainage into a bag or bottle attached to the drain. Usually, it is a suction
system although it may be passive, working on the syphon system. Sepsis is less
common with closed systems.

Suction drains
These help collapse down potential spaces as well as draining blood and other
fluids. They are usually closed systems and therefore the risk of sepsis is less. Sump
drains are open drains used in connection with suction. Sump drains contain an air
inlet lumen to prevent blockage with soft tissue. Sepsis is a risk with sump drains.

Non-suction drains
These are used mainly intraperitoneally to drain gastrointestinal and biliary
anastomoses. They are usually left for up to 5 days. They are usually rubber, PVC
or silastic. If prolonged drainage is necessary and there is need for a tract to be
established, rubber drains should be used as they stimulate fibrosis.

Complications of drains
● Sepsis: commoner with open drains
● Failure: especially suction drains which draw fat or omentum into the side holes
● Pressure or suction necrosis of the bowel leading to leakage of the intestinal
  contents with peritonitis
● Rarely, erosion into a vessel with haemorrhage.

STOMAS (-OSTOMIES)

Colostomy
A permanent colostomy usually opens onto the anterior abdominal wall in
the left iliac fossa (LIF). It is flush with the skin and the contents of the bag are
usually formed faeces. It is most commonly created following an operation for
abdominoperineal resection of the rectum. A temporary colostomy in this position
is usually consequent on a Hartmann's procedure. Colostomies may occasionally be

seen in the upper abdomen, either to the right or left of the midline, when they are defunctioning colostomies fashioned in the transverse colon to protect a distal anastomosis, although defunctioning ileostomies are preferred nowadays.

Ileostomy

An ileostomy is usually in the right iliac fossa (RIF). It is *not* flush with the skin but overhangs as a 'spout' for about 2.5 cm. This is so that the liquid small bowel content, rich in pancreatic enzymes, does not come into contact with the skin of the abdominal wall, resulting in tryptic digestion of the skin. The contents of the bag are fluid and are of the consistency of porridge. An ileostomy usually results from total colectomy with excision of the rectum (panproctocolectomy) for ulcerative colitis. Defunctioning loop ileostomies are used to protect distal anastomoses.

Urostomy (ileal bladder)

A urostomy is usually in the RIF. It is a blind-ended loop of ileum and looks not dissimilar to an ileostomy, i.e. it is not flush with the skin edge but looks like a 'spout'. The ureters have been transplanted into the ileal loop. Urine drains from the ileal loop. It is usually created following total cystectomy for carcinoma of the bladder.

Mucous fistula

In some operations it may be necessary to bring out both ends of bowel, e.g. ischaemic bowel to assess viability. One end will be the functioning draining stoma (either ileostomy or colostomy) and the other end will be the functionless stoma termed a mucous fistula.

LOCAL ANAESTHESIA

Techniques with local anaesthetics include topical (surface) anaesthesia, local infiltration, regional nerve block, spinal or epidural anaesthesia. Only local anaesthetic infiltration will be described here since regional nerve blocks, spinal and epidural anaesthesia are the province of the anaesthetist.

Many minor surgical procedures are carried out under local anaesthetic. Some require very small amounts, while others may reach the maximum safe dose, e.g. repair of an inguinal hernia. Local anaesthetics reversibly block nerve conduction by inactivating sodium channels, blocking electrical depolarization. Smaller nerve fibres are more sensitive than larger so that pain and temperature sensation are lost first, followed by proprioception, touch and pressure and motor impulses. This explains why the patient may feel pressure but no pain, and loss of motor function occurs later.

Types of local anaesthetic

Three main types of local anaesthetic are available: lidocaine, bupivacaine and prilocaine – lidocaine being the most widely used.

Lidocaine. Rapid onset, short duration. Comes in three strengths: 0.5% (5 mg/mL), 1% (10 mg/mL), 2% (20 mg/mL). The upper dose limit for lidocaine is 3 mg/kg (plain), 7 mg/kg (with 1:200 000 adrenaline).

Bupivacaine. Slower onset, longer duration. Comes in two strengths: 0.25% (2.5 mg/mL), 0.5% (5 mg/mL). Upper dose limit is 2 mg/kg (both plain and with adrenaline).

Prilocaine. Rapid onset, shorter duration than lidocaine. Comes as 1% solution (10 mg/mL). Upper dose limit is 6 mg/kg.

Local anaesthetics may be mixed with 1 in 200 000 adrenaline. Adrenaline is included as a vasoconstrictor. It diminishes local blood flow, slows the rate of absorption of the local anaesthetic and prolongs its local effect. Adrenaline should be used in low concentration, e.g. 1 in 200 000 (5 μg/mL). The total dose of adrenaline should not exceed 500 μg.

> ⚠ **Adrenaline must not be used where there are 'end' arteries, i.e. never on the digits or penis. It is also inadvisable to use it on other extremities, i.e. the nose, nipple or lobe of the ear. Addition of adrenaline does not increase the safe dose of bupivacaine and there is little point in using it for infiltration with bupivacaine except to reduce bleeding. The total dose of adrenaline should not exceed 500 μg. Local anaesthetic techniques should only be performed where adequate resuscitation facilities are available. Local anaesthetics should not be injected into inflamed or infected tissues where they are largely ineffective and may be responsible for further spread of infection.**

Complications
- Injection site: pain, haematoma, direct nerve trauma (with delayed recovery of sensation), infection
- With adrenaline: ischaemic necrosis (digits and penis)
- Systemic effects: idiosyncratic or allergic reactions (rare)
- Toxicity.

Toxicity
This may be due to excess dosage, inadvertent intravenous infection, or premature release of a Bier's block (intravenous regional anaesthesia) cuff. Toxic effects include: lightheadedness, tinnitus, circumoral and tongue numbness, nausea, vomiting, visual disturbances, fits, CNS depression leading to coma, arrhythmias, cardiovascular collapse.

TOURNIQUETS

Tourniquets are used in limbs where a bloodless field is required or to limit blood loss. They can also be used for a Biers Block (i.v. local anaesthetic for the manipulation of upper limb fractures). The principles of use of tourniquets include:

- Empty the limb of blood (this can be performed by elevation, Esmarch bandage or rubber 'sleeve-like' appliances which both aim to empty the limb of blood)
- The tourniquet is placed at the proximal end of the limb (layers of crepe bandage are used underneath the cuff to protect the skin)

- For upper limb surgery an inflation pressure of 200 mmHg (or 50–75 mmHg above patient's systolic blood pressure) and for lower limb surgery 250–350 mmHg (100–150 mmHg above patient's systolic blood pressure).
- One hour is the recommended inflation time for upper extremity surgery and 1.5–2 h for lower extremity surgery. The tourniquet should be deflated for 10 min after the maximum recommended time, after which the tourniquet may be re-inflated for another full period.

Complications of tourniquet use include:

- Nerve injury – associated with pressure
- Emboli – use of tourniquet may lead to formation of a DVT and PE
- Sickle crisis – in susceptible patients the build up of potassium, lactate, etc. may precipitate a sickle crisis
- Compartment syndrome – prolonged ischaemia may lead to reperfusion injury and swelling of muscles
- Post-tourniquet syndrome – consists of non-pitting oedema, sensory loss, muscle weakness and stiffness. This may last up to a month
- Burns – can occur if alcohol containing skin preparations get under the tourniquet
- Raised core temperature and increased plasma viscosity – these events are known to occur after tourniquet use but their clinical significance is uncertain
- Increased postoperative pain.

Important safety points for tourniquet use include:

- Correct size with adequate padding
- Keep duration of inflation to a minimum (2 h is considered the absolute maximum)
- Use minimum pressure needed to achieve desired effect
- Time the period accurately of tourniquet inflation
- Avoid multiple inflation and deflation
- Contraindicated in patients with a history of DVT and/or PE, peripheral vascular disease and sickle cell disease.

DIATHERMY

Surgical diathermy is an invaluable tool in providing haemostasis but can also be used to cut tissues. It involves high frequency alternating current (AC). There are a number of important points to understand regarding surgical diathermy:

- Diathermy used in surgery is very high frequency (400 kHz–10 MHz) and uses high current intensity (as high as 500 milliamps (mA) can be used). However, home electricity is capable of inducing VF (as much as 100 mA is sufficient); this is due to the much lower frequency of around 50–60 Hz.
- Monopolar. This is the most common type of diathermy. An AC is produced and passed to an electrode with a small surface area (the diathermy tip). Current is passed to the tissues as heat. The current passes through the body tissue and completes the circuit by returning to a much larger surface plate, i.e. the indifferent electrode plate which is usually placed on the patient's thigh (Fig. 2.2A).

Figure 2.2 (A) Monopolar diathermy. Current passes through the fine instrument tip (a), through the patient (b) and returns via the large indifferent electrode (c). (B) Bipolar diathermy. Current passes between the tips of the forceps (a) and coagulates tissue grasped between the tips. It does not pass through the patient.

Good contact is essential. Current recommendations to improve contact include shaving hair from the skin where the plate is placed and using disposable self-adhesive diathermy plates. Monopolar diathermy is most widely used for operative haemostasis but there is wide dispersion of coagulating and heating effects, which makes it unsuitable for use near nerves and other delicate structures.

- Bipolar. There is no need for a plate and uses much less power. The two active electrodes are the tips of a pair of forceps. Current flows between the tips of the forceps and thus only affects the tissues between them (Fig. 2.2B). Bipolar diathermy is used for finer surgery where greater precision is required. There is minimal tissue damage around the point of coagulation and therefore safety in relation to nearby nerves and blood vessels.

- Coagulation. This involves sealing blood vessels. The AC output is pulsed and haemostasis occurs by a combination of cellular dehydration and protein denaturation.
- Cutting. In this form, the AC output is continuous and forms an arc between the diathermy and the tissue. The heat generated is sufficient to cause water to explode into steam. A combination of cutting and coagulation is often referred to as 'blend'. Cutting diathermy is mainly used for dividing large muscle masses, e.g. thoracotomy and transverse abdominal incisions.
- Fulguration. A form of coagulation in which a higher voltage is used that creates sparks which arc from the diathermy to the tissues and create charring of the tissue.

Complications of diathermy include:

- Electrocution. Very low risk with modern equipment.
- Explosion. Rare can occur with pooling of alcohol based skin preparations or with colonic gases.
- Burns. Most common problem. Can occur with faulty application of the patient plate. Patient is earthed by touching a metal object (e.g. drip stand), faulty insulation on the diathermy wires, accidental activation and accidentally touching another metal object while activating diathermy (e.g. retractor).
- Interference with pacemakers. Diathermy activation may result in no pacing or the pacemaker may revert to a fixed rate. Bipolar diathermy is considered safe to use. If monopolar diathermy must be used, then the patient plate should be sited as far away as possible from the pacemaker.
- Channelling. The use of diathermy in tissues with narrow channels or pedicles can lead to the current being 'channelled' through a short surface area and thus high heat production. Examples of this would be in a child's penis during circumcision or along the spermatic cord with operations on the testicle. Bipolar diathermy is safe to use.
- Direct coupling. The active diathermy comes into contact with another metal instrument (e.g. camera) that is touching tissues (e.g. bowel) and results in a burn.
- Capacitance coupling. Very rare with modern ports. Occurred when ports had a plastic portion to anchor them into the abdomen. When a current is applied through an insulated instrument within a metal tube (e.g. port), some electrical charge is transferred to the cannula. If the port is entirely metal, then there is no problem as the charge will dissipate through the abdominal wall over a large area of contact. If a plastic collar is present, then this will prevent discharge and potentially lead to burns on adjacent tissue. Diathermy injury during laparoscopic surgery may also occur with accidental activation, faulty insulation of equipment and retained heat in the instrument.

LASER

Laser stands for **L**ight **A**mplification **S**timulated **E**mission of **R**adiation. Lasers work by energy being directed at a lasing medium. This excites atoms into a higher energy state. Photons are emitted as electrons fall from the excited to a ground state. These photons are amplified by being reflected between two mirrors. A small amount of laser light is allowed to emerge and this forms the laser beam. This beam vaporizes tissues and coagulates small vessels. A number of lasing mediums are used, usually gaseous (e.g. carbon dioxide, argon) but crystals are also used (neodymium, yttrium, aluminium and garnet – NdYAG). The lasing medium determines the wavelength and the wavelength determines the depth of absorption and thus clinical effect. Lasers are used in a number of surgical specialities such as destroying tumours of the GIT (e.g. oesophageal) urinary bladder and female genital tract. They are used in ophthalmology to destroy thickened lens capsules with cataracts. They are classified according to the degree of danger in their use (class I to class IV).

Potential risks involved with lasers include:

- Risks to patient – burning of normal tissue can lead to perforation, e.g. in the oesophagus
- Risk to operator – the laser can damage the eyes or skin.

A number of safety measures should therefore be adhered to:

- Appropriate local personnel. A laser safety officer and laser protection advisor should be nominated to draft safety protocols and ensure that they are followed
- All lasers should be labelled with their hazard category
- All personnel using or involved in the use of lasers should wear eye protection
- An appropriate environment with minimal reflective surfaces should be provided for laser use.

LAPAROSCOPIC SURGERY

Laparoscopy has been in use by gynaecologists for many years in diagnosing pelvic disorders and for sterilization by tubal ligation. It is now being used more widely in other branches of surgery, particularly for minimally invasive surgery. Laparoscopy may be either diagnostic or therapeutic.

Diagnostic laparoscopy: For biopsy of lesions, staging of cancers, e.g. gastric and pancreatic; and increasing diagnostic accuracy in the acute abdomen.

Therapeutic laparoscopy: Widely practiced, the most common operation being cholecystectomy. Other procedures include appendicectomy, inguinal hernia repair, division of adhesions, colonic resection, Nissen fundoplication for gastro-oesophageal reflux disease, nephrectomy, splenectomy. Laparoscopic operations may need to be converted to 'open' surgery if difficulties are encountered, e.g. gross adhesions, poor visualization of the operation site, slow progress with the operation, uncontrollable haemorrhage.

Technique

Usually performed under general anaesthesia. A pneumoperitoneum is created by introducing carbon dioxide under controlled pressure. This may be done by direct visualization of the peritoneal space by an open cut down technique made below the umbilicus (Hassan technique). The use of a Veress (insufflation) needle is still popular but it requires gas to be insufflated without confirmation of the correct location of the needle tip. The first port is inserted at the umbilicus for the telescope and camera. To perform procedures, additional puncture sites are required (secondary ports). Trocars are inserted at these sites under direct laparoscopic vision to prevent injury to the viscera. Various instruments are then introduced through these port sites. Basically, these instruments may be divided into those for visualization, grasping, retraction, dissection, ligation/suturing and retrieval.

Instruments introduced through port sites include scissors, diathermy hooks, clip applicators. Some operations are described as 'laparoscopic assisted', where the major dissection is performed laparoscopically and subsequently a small incision made in the abdomen to deliver the specimen. 'Hand assisted' laparoscopy requires a small incision to insert the operator's hand to assist with dissection and delivery of the specimen. Retrieval bags may be introduced into the peritoneal cavity to aid the delivery of specimens, the aim being to prevent the spread of infection, seeding of tumours, or to prevent disruption of the specimen when it is pulled out through an abdominal incision. The operation is performed by the operator with one or more assistants who control the camera or manipulate the ports, the progress of the operation being observed on video monitors.

Complications

These include:

- Dangers of pneumoperitoneum; needle/trocar injury to bowel or blood vessels; compression of venous return predisposing to DVT and PE; subcutaneous emphysema; shoulder tip pain (irritant effect of carbon dioxide producing carbonic acid locally and irritating the diaphragm with referred pain to the shoulder tip); pneumothorax (rare); pneumomediastinum (rare)
- Inadvertent injury to other structures either by dissection or diathermy or inappropriate application of clips, e.g. damage to the bile duct in cholecystectomy; uncontrollable haemorrhage
- Complications related to duration of anaesthesia, which may be longer for laparoscopic procedures than for open procedures. The diaphragm is splinted by abdominal inflation and this may result in cardiorespiratory complications
- Herniation at port sites with possible subsequent strangulation.

VENOUS ACCESS

Venous access may be required for simple venepuncture or insertion of a cannula. Suitable sites are veins on the back of the hand or the antecubital fossa. The foot veins may also be used if there are no suitable veins in the arm. Injections should not be given into veins in the antecubital fossa however, in case of accidental puncture of the brachial artery, which is immediately deep to the veins separated from them only by the bicipital aponeurosis. In children and patients with needle phobia, EMLA cream may be applied and left for 45–60 min to anaesthetize the skin. It should be wiped off before cannulating. The following steps are required in the procedure:

- Choose the site
- Place a tourniquet or sphygmomanometer (inflated to just below diastolic pressure) above the site
- Swab with alcohol

- Advance cannula until flashback of blood
- Release tourniquet or sphygmomanometer
- Withdraw needle leaving cannula in vein
- Connect infusion.

When removing the needle or cannula, raise the arm and compress the site for about 1 min to prevent bruising.

If no other site is available for venous access in an emergency, a venous cut-down may be required. This should only be used if it is not possible to gain venous access elsewhere. A cut-down is usually carried out at the ankle where there is a constant vein, i.e. the great saphenous vein lying immediately anterior to the medial malleolus. The steps in the procedure are as follows:

- Prepare skin and drape
- Infiltrate with local anaesthetic
- Make an incision over the vein
- Dissect the vein from other structures, e.g. the saphenous nerve in association with the great saphenous vein at the ankle
- Ligate the distal end of the vein and put a suture sling around the proximal end
- Make an incision in the vein
- Insert a large bore cannula into the vein and ligate proximally to secure cannula in vein
- Attach infusion
- Close wound and apply dressing.

CENTRAL VENOUS CATHETERIZATION – INTERNAL JUGULAR VEIN

Indications for internal jugular vein cannulation include the determination and monitoring of central venous pressure and establishing a route for intravenous therapeutic agents. Complications include pneumothorax, carotid artery damage and haematoma. A clotting screen should be checked before starting the procedure.

The following are the steps in the procedure:

- Patient is prepared with head tilt 15° down and head turned to the opposite side
- Infiltrate the skin with local anaesthetic at the level of the thyroid cartilage (three fingers breadth above the medial end of the clavicle) lateral to the carotid artery pulse
- Site of entry is at the apex of the triangle formed by the two heads of sternocleidomastoid and the clavicle
- Using an 18G 'finder' needle, enter the apex of the triangle keeping lateral to the pulse of the carotid artery. (Most CVP lines are inserted under ultrasound guidance.)
- Insert the needle at 30° angle and aim for the ipsilateral nipple
- Once in the vessel, remove the syringe, hold the thumb over the needle to avoid air embolism
- Insert guidewire
- Make a small nick in the skin where the guidewire enters

- Advance dilator over guidewire
- Remove dilator
- Place catheter over guidewire
- Remove guidewire and aspirate blood and flush all three ports of cannula
- Suture to skin
- Arrange CXR to check position.

BLOOD GAS SAMPLING

Vessels of choice are the radial artery (immediately lateral to the tendon of flexor carpi radialis just above the wrist), the brachial artery (immediately medial to the biceps tendon at the elbow) or the femoral artery at the mid-inguinal point (halfway between the anterior superior iliac spine and the pubic symphysis). For radial artery cannulation, always check the patency of the ulnar artery (Allen test).

The following are the steps in the procedure:

- Swab site the alcohol
- Use a 2 mL heparinized syringe (usually pre-filled syringes are available)
- Expel air from syringe
- Advance at 60–90° into the artery (it may help to rest the wrist on a bag of saline). The artery may have been transfixed so it may be necessary to withdraw the needle slowly until blood fills the syringe
- Obtain 2 mL of blood and cap the syringe immediately
- Compress puncture site for 3–5 min
- Empty syringe of any air bubbles and send to laboratory immediately for analysis. If there is any delay, place the syringe on ice.

URINARY CATHETERIZATION (MALE)

A Foley catheter is inserted into the bladder. For adults a 12–14F gauge should be used. For children an 8–10F gauge should be used.

The following are the steps in the procedure:

- Wash hands, put on sterile gloves and arrange contents of catheter pack on sterile tray
- Position patient flat
- Drape with sterile towels with penis exposed
- Grasp penis with sterile swab, retract foreskin and clean the urethral opening and glans with antiseptic solution
- Squeeze lignocaine gel into urethra and allow time for it to work
- Remove catheter from pack and insert fully into bladder to ensure balloon is in bladder. *Do not use force*
- Check that there is urine flow from catheter
- Inflate balloon with sterile water 5–10 mL
- Withdraw catheter to lodge against bladder neck
- Remember to replace foreskin to avoid paraphimosis
- Attach drainage bag.

Investigative procedures

This chapter describes various investigative procedures commonly used in surgery. The procedures are described briefly, together with their indications and possible complications.

CONVENTIONAL RADIOLOGY

Radiographs penetrate differentially through tissues of the body, resulting in different exposure of the silver salts in the radiograph film. On a plain radiograph, gas and fat absorb few X-rays and consequently appear dark, while bone and calcified defects are poorly penetrated and appear white or radio-opaque.

- A *plain* radiograph is one where no contrast medium is administered to the patient, e.g. routine CXR.
- A *contrast* study involves administration of a contrast medium, which outlines or delineates the structure under study, e.g. barium in GI studies or iodinated benzoic acid derivatives in arteriography.

PLAIN FILMS

Chest X-ray (CXR)
- Always check the name of the film and the right and left markers.
- Make sure the whole chest and diaphragm are clearly on the film. You may need to count the ribs to exclude a cervical rib.
- Check that the trachea is central.
- Check the mediastinal width.
- Check cardiothoracic ratio. Maximum width of heart divided by maximum 'bony' (rib-to-rib) diameter of chest should be <50% in normal adults.
- Check vascular pattern, e.g. reduced in recent pulmonary embolus, distension of upper lobe veins in pulmonary venous hypertension.

- Check lung fields, e.g. lobar collapse, pneumonic consolidation, bronchial carcinoma, pneumothorax.
- Check bony thoracic cage, e.g. fractures, secondary deposits, notching (coarctation of aorta).
- Check soft tissues, e.g. surgical emphysema, mastectomy.
- Check for free air under the diaphragm on erect chest X-ray.

Abdominal X-ray (AXR)

Check for the following:

- Dilated hollow viscus with or without air/fluid levels, e.g. small and large bowel obstruction
- Free intraperitoneal gas (check position in which film was taken, e.g. air under the diaphragm with perforated hollow viscus)
- Abnormal gas patterns, e.g. air in biliary tree with cholecystoduodenal fistula and gallstone ileus, bladder with colovesical fistula
- Calcified calculi – kidney, ureter, bladder, gallbladder; 10% of gallbladder stones are radio-opaque and 85% of renal stones are radio-opaque
- Foreign bodies, e.g. swallowed keys, etc.; trauma, e.g. bullet wounds; carelessness, e.g. swabs
- Abnormal calcification, e.g. arteriosclerotic vessels, pancreatic calcification seen with chronic pancreatitis (rarely carcinoma of the pancreas calcifies), uterine fibroids
- Retroperitoneum, e.g. absence of psoas shadows with retroperitoneal haemorrhage, retroperitoneal gas with retroperitoneal perforation of a viscus
- Bones, e.g. bony metastases, fractures, osteoarthritis (plain radiographs of the limbs and skulls are dealt with in Chapters 4, 17 and 18).

CONTRAST STUDIES

Gastrointestinal tract

Barium meal. This investigation is used less commonly now in view of the increased use of endoscopy. Barium suspension is given orally together with sodium bicarbonate tablets to give a barium/air double-contrast study. The progress of barium is checked by screening, image intensification being used to show a moving image on a TV monitor. Areas of interest are noted and radiographs taken. The patient should not have any solid food overnight but sips of water are allowed prior to the investigation. A study is useful for diagnosis of pharyngeal lesions, e.g. pharyngeal pouch; oesophageal lesions, e.g. carcinoma, reflux, achalasia; stomach, e.g. ulcers and carcinoma; duodenum, e.g. duodenal ulcer and pyloric stenosis.

Barium enema. Barium suspension is administered rectally. Rectal and lower sigmoid lesions should have first been excluded by sigmoidoscopy. Air is usually insufflated to give a double-contrast picture. Buscopan, an anticholinergic agent, may be given intravenously (i.v.) to relax the bowel during the investigation.

Strict bowel preparation is required prior to barium enema. A laxative should be administered the evening prior to the enema and the occasional rectal washout is required if there is evidence of residual faecal loading. Barium enema should not be performed within 7 days of a rectal biopsy because of the risk of perforation. The study is useful for diagnosis of bowel carcinomas, polyps, diverticular disease and inflammatory bowel disease. Fine mucosal abnormalities may be missed on barium enema and colonoscopy should now be considered the first-line investigation for large bowel lesions.

Barium follow-through or small bowel enema. Barium may be swallowed and followed through the small bowel into the colon. Alternatively, a duodenal tube may be positioned under radiographic control and barium injected into the duodenum and followed through the small bowel (a small bowel enema). This is useful for the diagnosis of Crohn's disease and small bowel tumours.

Barium should be avoided in the following situations:

- If there is a significant risk of peritoneal leakage, e.g. assessing the integrity of an anastomosis. Barium causes an intense peritoneal irritation and adhesion formation, and water-soluble contrast media should be used in preference when checking an anastomosis, e.g. Gastrografin.
- In bowel obstruction, as the barium may rest at the site of a partial obstruction, solidify and cause a partial obstruction to become complete.

Biliary tree

Ultrasound. Ultrasound is now the first-line test for diagnosis of gallstones. It will also show a dilated biliary tree but will rarely pick up stones in the common bile duct due to the fact that the lower end of the common bile duct is likely to be obscured by gas from the transverse colon.

Magnetic resonance cholangiopancreatography (MRCP). MRCP is now the initial imaging test of choice for biliary tree abnormalities, e.g. obstruction. It is a non-invasive method of imaging the biliary and pancreatic ducts. The technique does not require intravenous contrast material and uses specialized MRI sequences (i.e. heavily T2-weighted) to make the fluid in the ducts appear bright, while the surrounding organs and tissues are suppressed and appear dark. Heavily T2-weighted images give excellent anatomical detail. MRCP may be used as a screening examination in patients with a low or intermediate probability of choledocholithiasis, failed or incomplete ERCP, demonstrating variations in ductal anatomy, demonstrating postoperative anatomy (e.g. biliary-enteric anastomoses, sclerosing cholangitis), complications of chronic pancreatitis (e.g. ductal dilatation, strictures).

Endoscopic retrograde cholangiopancreatography (ERCP). Contrast medium is injected retrogradely through the ampulla of Vater via a side-viewing duodenoscope. The technique is described more fully in the section on endoscopy, below.

Percutaneous transhepatic cholangiography (PTC). This is used for diagnosis of obstructive jaundice. A long fine needle (22G Chiba) is passed percutaneously into the liver until a duct is pierced, witnessed by the aspiration of bile. Contrast is then injected to outline the biliary tree. Jaundiced patients may have clotting defects, e.g. abnormal prothrombin time (PT), and therefore a clotting screen should be carried out prior to this investigation. Vitamin K or fresh frozen plasma (FFP) should be administered i.v. if the PT is abnormal. Complications include haemorrhage, bile peritonitis, cholangitis and septicaemia. This technique however, has been largely superseded by MRCP.

Operative cholangiogram. At operation for cholecystectomy, the ducts should be checked for stones. Contrast is injected via a cannula inserted into the common bile duct via the stump of the cystic duct and radiographs are carried out or the image intensifier used. The diameter of the ducts, presence of filling defects and failure of contrast to pass into the duodenum are significant.

T-tube cholangiogram. If the common bile duct has been explored to exclude or remove stones, a latex T-tube is usually inserted. The horizontal bar of the T is in the duct and the vertical bar is brought out through the skin. Contrast is injected down the T-tube 8–10 days postoperatively to check for any residual stones, biliary leakage or stenosis prior to removal of the tube. There should be free flow of contrast medium into the duodenum and no filling defects.

Urinary tract

Intravenous urography (IVU). Intravenous contrast is administered, which is excreted by the kidneys and eventually delineates the renal pelvis, ureters and bladder. A plain film is taken first so that any opacities seen can be compared with the films after contrast is given. It is useful for the diagnosis of obstruction, tumours, infection, congenital abnormalities and trauma. The only contraindication is allergy to the contrast medium. Caution must be exercised in diabetes mellitus, renal failure, multiple myeloma and cardiac failure.

Cystography. The patient is catheterized and the bladder filled with contrast medium. Bladder leaks, tumours, vesicoureteral reflux, and diverticulae can be diagnosed. A post-micturition film will diagnose residual urine. This technique has largely been superseded by ultrasonography.

Urethrography. A water soluble contrast medium is injected per urethram. Ruptures of the urethra, strictures or tumours may be seen.

Retrograde pyelography. This is carried out via cystoscopy by passing a ureteric catheter into each ureteric orifice. Clear views of the ureter and pelvicalyceal system are obtained. This test is used in patients with impaired renal function with poor concentration of contrast or if incomplete filling of the collecting structures is seen on IVU. The ureteric catheter may be left *in situ* to allow drainage of an obstructed system and for renal function tests to normalize prior to operative procedures.

Antegrade pyelography. The pelvicalyceal system of the kidney is punctured with a fine 22G needle. Contrast is injected and allows accurate assessment of the ureter and pelvicalyceal system, as well as assessing drainage.

Vascular system

Arteriography. Contrast medium is injected directly into the lumen of an artery. The catheter is usually introduced via the Seldinger wire technique into a suitable and easily accessible artery. The femoral artery at the groin is the usual portal of entry, although the brachial and axillary may be used. A careful history of allergies to contrast media needs to be ascertained. A clotting screen should be carried out prior to vascular radiology. With a catheter *in situ*, water soluble contrast medium is injected directly into the artery and images recorded in rapid sequences. Stenosis, thrombosis, embolism or aneurysm can be demonstrated. Complications include haemorrhage at the puncture site, dislodgement of atheromatous plaques, embolism, thrombosis.

Digital subtraction angiography (DSA). DSA is now commonly used. Vascular images may be obtained with lower concentrations of contrast medium. The digital images are processed by subtracting unnecessary background, e.g. bones, and enhancing contrast between the tissues. Where high resolution is not needed, the contrast can be given intravenously into a fast-flowing vein, e.g. via a central line or into the femoral vein, and the arteries imaged when the contrast reaches them. These studies are known as intravenous digital subtraction angiography (IVDSA) or digital intravenous angiography (DIVA).

Venography. Contrast is injected into a superficial vein, i.e. a vein on the dorsum of the foot in the lower limb, and a tourniquet is placed around the ankle to direct the contrast into the deep veins. Lower limb venography is used to confirm or exclude DVT or to investigate deep venous insufficiency, i.e. it would demonstrate the site of incompetent perforating veins. This technique has been largely superseded by Doppler ultrasound.

ULTRASONOGRAPHY

Ultrasound works on the principle that the ultrasound emitted as a pulse from a transducer travels at constant velocity into tissue and is reflected by varying amounts from different tissue interfaces and travels back to the receiver at the same speed. The transducer is a piezoelectric crystal that both transmits and receives the ultrasound. The time required for the pulse to travel to the interface and back can be used to determine the depth of that interface. An image of the slice of the body is obtained by directing a narrow beam of high-energy sound waves into the body and recording the manner in which the sound is reflected by different structures. Sound is transmitted well through any fluid but poorly or not at all through air or bone. Returning echoes are electronically converted into a video image on a monitor, the resulting picture being a wedge-shaped slice of the area of interest.

Advantages
- It does not employ ionizing radiation and therefore produces no biological injury in the tissues.
- Any plane can be employed to examine the region of interest.

- It is less expensive than CT or MRI.
- It can be used at the bedside if the patient is too ill to be moved.

Dimensions of organs or lesions can be measured and the volume of the bladder and the left ventricle can also be assessed. Stones cause marked changes in acoustic impedance with almost complete reflection of ultrasound, showing echogenic foci with fan-shaped acoustic shadowing.

Very little preparation is necessary. For pelvic ultrasound the bladder should be full, providing a fluid-filled non-reflective medium for the ultrasound to reach the pelvic organs. The patient should be starved for biliary ultrasound to allow the gallbladder to fill with bile and to minimize gas shadows.

Ultrasound is non-invasive, painless, safe and cheap in comparison with CT and MRI, although it does not produce as sharp an image.

Ultrasound may be used for the following:

- Assessment of abdominal masses
- Distinguishing solid from cystic lesions, e.g. Renal carcinoma from a renal cyst
- Assessment of liver secondaries
- Detecting stones in the gallbladder or urinary bladder
- Measuring the size of lesions, e.g. The diameter of an abdominal aortic aneurysm or the width of a dilated bile duct
- Guided biopsy, e.g. biopsy of liver secondary or other mass
- Guided drainage, e.g. of localized collections of fluid or subphrenic or pelvis abscesses.

Disadvantages

Although limitations are few, lesions of the lower end of the common bile duct and head of the pancreas may be obscured by bowel gas. Bone completely reflects ultrasound and the method is therefore useless for studying organs encased by bone, e.g. brain and spinal cord.

DOPPLER ULTRASOUND

Doppler ultrasound is used in vascular monitoring to study blood flow. A beam of ultrasound is directed at a vessel using a special probe. Ultrasound is reflected from the red cells, which cause a frequency shift related to their velocity. The shift can be heard as a noise or recorded as a waveform or sonogram. The faster the flow of red cells past the probe the higher the sound pitch. The Doppler probe is coupled to the skin with acoustic gel and angled towards the direction of arterial flow. Stenoses and occlusions cause diminished signals distal to a proximal obstruction.

Uses of Doppler ultrasound

Measurement of systolic pressure in peripheral arteries. A sphygmomanometer cuff is applied to occlude the artery. The probe is placed over the artery (dorsalis pedis, posterior tibial in the case of the lower limb), the tourniquet released and the pressure recorded when a signal is picked up. This pressure is compared with a normal brachial pressure, i.e. the ankle/brachial pressure index. The normal value is 1.0–1.2.

Other methods include analysis of waveforms to assess stenoses and occlusions.

Duplex scanning

This combines real-time B-mode imaging with a pulsed Doppler spectral analysis of flow velocity pattern. Blood vessels are identified by their characteristic B-mode images with prominent wall echoes and dark sonar-lucent lumina. Calcified plaques show bright echoes with acoustic shadowing behind. The pulsed Doppler beam is placed in the centre of the identified vessel and the spectral analysis allows classification of the degree of stenosis. Duplex scanning may be applied to analyse carotid disease, lower extremity arterial disease, intestinal arteries, renal arteries, and venous thromboses. Colour coding of flow direction may give further information.

COMPUTERIZED TOMOGRAPHY (CT)

CT produces cross-sectional images of the body, taking a series of transverse slices through the body. Sensitive X-ray detectors measure the X-ray attenuation through the patient in a large number of different directions, and a fast digital computer then uses the measurements to compute an image. These images are displayed on a screen and subsequently recorded on film. CT scanning may be used in conjunction with contrast medium enhancement. This may be given i.v. to show, for example, hepatic tumours, renal parenchyma and collecting system, aorta and IVC. It may enhance brain lesions when the blood–brain barrier is breached. Contrast may also be given by mouth or enema to outline the GI tract.

A new generation of spiral CT scanners is in use. The patient passes quickly through the scanner and a volume of data is obtained and analysed. Scanning is performed in a single breath-hold, decreasing motion artefact and allowing accurate timing of intravascular contrast enhancement. Images are superior to conventional CT. Specific applications include CT angiography and imaging of pulmonary emboli.

Advantages

CT has many uses but is the investigation of choice in head injuries. It is also useful for studying the retroperitoneum, pancreas, mediastinum, and lungs. It can be used for staging tumours, e.g. lymphomas, and can be used for guided biopsy.

CT angiography. Scan is performed simultaneously with high speed contrast media injection. It may be used for visualizing vessels anywhere in the body. Specific uses include:

- Examination of the pulmonary arteries in suspected pulmonary embolism
- Visualizing blood flow in the renal arteries in suspected renal artery stenosis
- Assessment of prospective kidney donors to visualize the arterial anatomy of the kidney

- Identification of aortic aneurysms
- Identification of aortic dissection
- Identification of deep vein thrombosis.

CT urography. Multidetector CT urography is a single examination that allows evaluation of potential urinary tract calculi, renal parenchymal masses and both benign and malignant urothelial lesions. Upper tract urothelial malignancies, including small lesions <5 mm in diameter can be detected with high sensitivity. It is useful in the assessment of haematuria and also trauma to the urinary tract,

MAGNETIC RESONANCE IMAGING (MRI)

MRI is also known as nuclear magnetic resonance (NMR). MRI is based on the fact that certain atomic nuclei placed in a magnetic field and acted on by a suitable radiofrequency pulse undergo changes in their energy states, which result in the emission of measurable radio signals. The signals are then manipulated in a computer to provide sectional radiographic images. No ionizing radiation is involved. The procedure is non-invasive and can be carried out as an outpatient procedure. It is relatively time consuming, with extensive studies taking in excess of 1 h. MRI gives high soft tissue contrast and the body can be imaged in coronal, sagittal or transverse planes.

Advantages

The technique is particularly useful for studies of the CNS (lipids have a high hydrogen content), soft tissues of the pelvis, soft tissue tumours, and orthopaedic problems. Magnetic resonance angiography is also being increasingly used to assess the heart, renal arteries, and peripheral vessels. Magnetic resonance cholangiopancreatography (MRCP) can also be used to image the biliary tract.

Disadvantages

These include high cost, limited availability, low patient throughput, poor detail of bone and calcified tissues, and image artefacts from respiratory and cardiac movement and bowel peristalsis. The patient is in the 'tube' for long periods and it is difficult to monitor the ill patient. Contraindications include patients with cardiac pacemakers, and cranial surgery with metal clips.

POSITRON EMISSION TOMOGRAPHY (PET)

PET is an imaging technology which produces a 3-dimensional image or picture of functional processes within the body. The system detects a pair of gamma rays emitted by a positron-emitting radionuclide which is introduced into the body on a biologically active molecule, usually a sugar. The most common form of tracer used is FDG, a glucose analogue. The concentrations of tracer image then give tissue metabolic activity in terms of glucose intake. Images of the tracer concentration in 3-dimensional space within the body are then reconstructed by computer analysis. PET scans are increasingly read alongside CT scans, a combination giving both anatomic and metabolic information. Modern PET scanners are integrated with high-end multi-detector row CT scanner. PET scanning is advantageous in the management of malignancy, as it can often detect tumours before structural changes are seen on CT or MRI. Its extreme sensitivity makes it possible to detect cancers at their earliest stages and to outline their exact locations. It is useful in follow-up looking for cancer recurrence and monitoring the effectives of chemotherapy and other treatments. It is also useful in neurological diseases such as Alzheimer's disease.

Advantages

Advantages of PET scanning include more detailed diagnostic information not available from other investigations such as CT or MRI, shorter time for definitive diagnosis, earlier detection of disease with the need for less invasive diagnostic procedures, precise staging of disease and improved monitoring of recurrences and more effective assessment of results of chemotherapy. Its ability to distinguish between benign and malignant tumours can result in the avoidance of unnecessary surgery.

Disadvantages

These include high cost and limited availability. The radioactive component used in PET scanning means that there is only a limited number of times a patient can undergo this procedure.

MAMMOGRAPHY

A mammogram is a soft tissue radiograph of the breast. The tissues constituting the breast have a very low inherent contrast. Soft tissue mammography depends on the fact that tumour tissue is denser than breast tissue, particularly in the older patient (age 40+), where glandular tissue has been replaced by fat. The study is uncomfortable and somewhat undignified for the patient, since compression of the breast is essential in order to 'spread' the breast over the film cassette, immobilize the breast and reduce the radiation dose. A radiolucent, translucent compression plate is used. Two projections are usually taken – superoinferior and mediolateral. For screening programmes, two projections are used on the first attendance and one projection only on follow-up, unless the patient is symptomatic, and then two projections are used. Careful viewing of the film under high intensity light with magnification is essential. An infiltrating radio-opaque mass is suggestive of malignancy but fine-stippled calcification (like salt grains scattered on the film) strongly suggests the diagnosis. Mammography is used for the following:

● To assess palpable lumps
● To exclude lumps in other symptomatic patients, e.g. painful breasts
● Screening.

If a non-palpable lump is picked up on mammography, preoperative localization with wires is undertaken via mammography. The wire is left in the breast and acts as a guide to the surgeon to the location of the radiological abnormality. When the specimen of breast tissue has been removed it is submitted to radiography to confirm that the abnormal area has in fact been excised.

RADIOISOTOPE SCANNING

A suitable tracer agent is given intravenously or orally. The tracer agent is a substance taken up by the target tissue. This substance is combined with a radioactive label, the most commonly used being technetium-99m (^{99m}Tc). A gamma camera is placed over the area of interest and simultaneously collects and counts the level of radioactivity. Dynamic imaging involves measuring the changing level of radioactivity over a period of time and storing this in a computer for later analysis. Renal blood flow measurement is an example of dynamic imaging. The following are applications of radioisotope scanning which are used in clinical practice.

Bone scans

Phosphates labelled with technetium are tracer agents. The tracer is taken up in areas of increased bone deposition and resorption. Uptake occurs in sites of infection, secondary tumour and acute arthritis. Indications for bone scanning include suspected bony secondaries, suspected osteomyelitis, abnormal biochemical profiles suggesting bone disease, e.g. raised calcium or alkaline phosphatase.

Renal scans

Two isotopes are commonly used, i.e. mercaptoacetyltriglycine (MAG3) and dimercaptosuccinic acid (DMSA). MAG3 is excreted dynamically through the kidney while DMSA remains in cortical tissue. They are useful in assessing asymmetrical renal function. Dynamic computer analysis allows assessment of renal blood flow as well as excretory activity. Practical applications include investigation of renal artery stenosis, and also differentiating acute tubular necrosis (ATN), renal ischaemia and obstruction in transplanted kidneys.

Lung scanning

This is important in the diagnosis of pulmonary embolism (PE), although it is being somewhat superseded by CT pulmonary angiography. Emboli obliterate areas of pulmonary arterial circulation but ventilation remains intact. A ventilation/perfusion scan (V/Q scan) is usually carried out. The perfusion scan involves the injection of radioactive particles small enough to temporarily block a small number of pulmonary capillaries. Technetium-labelled albumen microspheres are usually used. A ventilation scan using an inert radioactive gas, e.g. xenon, is performed simultaneously. The scans are compared. Areas that are ventilated and not perfused suggest embolism. Areas that are perfused but not ventilated suggest consolidation or collapse.

Scanning for infection

Ultrasonography or CT scanning will locate a collection of pus but in equivocal cases, white cell scanning may help. The patient is bled and the white cells separated. These are then labelled with indium-111 (^{111}In) and reinjected. The body is then scanned and areas of interest noted. The test is useful in patients with pyrexia of unknown origin or septicaemia, where other methods have failed to locate an area of sepsis.

Screening for GI bleeding

The patient's own red cells are labelled with technetium and reinjected. The abdomen is scanned at intervals over the next 24 h. The investigation reveals only the general area of bleeding, e.g. stomach, right or left colon, rather than the exact site.

ENDOSCOPY

Endoscopy implies examination of part of the body through an instrument. This may be through a natural orifice, e.g. oesophagoscopy or sigmoidoscopy, or through a surgically created hole, e.g. laparoscopy or arthroscopy. Endoscopy may be carried out with a rigid instrument, e.g. oesophagoscopy or sigmoidoscopy, the latter two being the most commonly used rigid endoscopy instruments. More recently, fibreoptic instruments have become more sophisticated and more widely used, e.g. gastroscopy, colonoscopy.

USE OF ENDOSCOPES

Rigid endoscopes

Sigmoidoscope. This is probably the most commonly used rigid endoscope. It is 25 or 30 cm long. Examination is usually carried out in the left lateral position. The position of a lesion is usually indicated by measuring its distance in centimetres from the anal verge. Biopsies may be taken with long forceps inserted through the scope.

Oesophagoscopy. This has largely been superseded by the flexible instrument. The rigid one, however, remains useful for removing large foreign bodies from the oesophagus.

Cystoscopy. The rigid instrument has been widely used for many years but has now been largely superseded by the flexible scope. The rigid instrument remains useful for retrograde ureteric catheterization. Transurethral resection of the prostate has been carried out for many years via the rigid cystoscope.

Laparoscopy. This technique was widely used by gynaecologists but is now being more widely used by the general surgeon, particularly for minimally invasive surgery. A cannula is introduced into the peritoneal cavity and the peritoneal cavity distended with carbon dioxide gas. It is useful not only for diagnosis and biopsy but invasive procedures are now being carried out through it, e.g. cholecystectomy, appendicectomy.

Flexible endoscopes

Gastroscope (oesophago-gastro-duodenoscope). This is used with intravenous sedation and a pharyngeal local anaesthetic spray. A clear view can be obtained of the oesophagus, stomach, duodenum, and with a side viewing scope the ampulla of Vater may be clearly seen. It is used for the identification and biopsy of lesions; tracing sources of GI haemorrhage; injection of oesophageal varices; lasering of bleeding lesions; dilatation of oesophageal strictures; cannulation of the ampulla of

Vater for ERCP. With the technique of ERCP a diathermy wire can be used down the gastroscope for dividing the sphincter of Oddi and allowing stones to pass out into the GI tract.

Colonoscopy. It is possible to inspect the whole of the colon after adequate bowel preparation. Biopsies can be carried out. Polyps can be removed by a wire snare or diathermy. Routine follow-up of patients having had previous carcinomas resected or ulcerative colitis can be carried out, avoiding the need for repeated barium enemas.

Bronchoscopy. Narrow fibreoptic bronchoscopes can be passed under local anaesthetic. They are mainly used for diagnostic purposes but can also be used postoperatively for removing mucus plugs that have caused segmental collapse.

Other flexible scopes. These include cystoscopes, sigmoidoscopes, choledochoscopes (for inspecting the common bile duct at open surgery to assess for stones, tumours, etc.), and arterioscopes, which will show areas of stenosis, embolus and allow inspection of arterial anastomoses for patency.

ADVANTAGES AND DISADVANTAGES OF ENDOSCOPY

Advantages

- Usually well tolerated. No need for general anaesthetic and therefore can be used on the elderly and unfit patient
- Any lesion can be directly visualized and biopsy taken under direct view
- Flexible endoscopy is safer than rigid endoscopy.

Disadvantages

- Perforation of a hollow viscus
- Tissue samples are usually small due to the size of the biopsy channel
- Sterility of the instrument is paramount to offset the risk of HIV or hepatitis B.

Complications

The main complications include perforation, haemorrhage at the site of biopsy or operative procedure and pulmonary aspiration. Cardiovascular complications may be related to the medication.

TISSUE DIAGNOSIS

Biopsy

This is removal of a piece of tissue from the living to provide a diagnosis. *Incisional biopsy* is the surgical removal of a piece of accessible tissue. *Excisional biopsy* is the complete removal of a discrete lesion without a wide margin and without it being considered curative of the disease.

Lesions may be biopsied as follows:

- direct vision, e.g. skin lesion
- forceps via an endoscope, e.g. sigmoidoscopic biopsy of a rectal lesion

- percutaneously using a Tru-Cut punch needle, e.g. breast lesions
- percutaneously by guided needle under ultrasound or CT control
- laparoscopically
- by open surgical excision, e.g. lymph node biopsy.

Cytology

Specimens obtained by scraping or fine-needle aspiration are spread on a slide and stained. The earliest example of this technique was cervical smears stained by the Papanicolaou technique.

Cytological diagnosis requires a skilled pathologist. The method must be both specific and sensitive. False positives and false negatives may occur. Cytological diagnosis is useful in the following situations in general surgery:

- Aspiration of ascites or pleural effusions
- Aspiration of solid masses, e.g. breast, thyroid, pancreas or lymph nodes.

INTERVENTIONAL RADIOLOGY

Interventional radiology has increased markedly over the past two decades and has probably been most marked in the areas of vascular radiology, urological radiology and the treatment of obstructive jaundice. The areas listed below have seen advances in interventional radiology.

Tissue diagnosis

- Automated Tru-Cut needle biopsy under ultrasound or CT control, e.g. liver biopsy
- Fine-needle aspiration cytology (FNAC). A 22G needle can usually be safely passed through most organs to aspirate the suspicious lesion under ultrasound or CT control, e.g. lesions in the head of the pancreas.

Biliary tract

In obstructive jaundice caused by malignant compression, either intrinsic (cholangiocarcinoma) or extrinsic (nodes at porta hepatis), the site can be accurately located by PTC and treated by stenting. A guide wire is passed through the stenosis and the stenosis dilated, following which a stent is passed over the guide wire to lie across the stenosis. This procedure may also be carried out at ERCP and is likely to be associated with fewer complications by the latter method.

Urinary tract

The renal pelvis can be punctured by percutaneous insertion of a needle under ultrasound or CT control. The tract can be dilated to allow tubes to be inserted and this allows for removal of stones from the renal pelvis or the insertion of nephrostomy tubes to drain the kidney prior to definitive treatment of a distal obstruction. The procedure is known as percutaneous nephrostomy.

Vascular system

Percutaneous transluminal angioplasty (PTA). Arteriography is carried out by the Seldinger technique. A flexible guide wire is then passed across the stenosis.

A catheter with a rigid plastic inflatable balloon is then placed along the guide wire to lie within the stenosis and its position is checked under the image intensifier. The balloon is inflated to dilate the stenosis. Measurement of pressures above and below the site of the dilatation is used to assess the success of the procedure. The complications include arterial rupture, embolism, thrombosis or dissection. It is also possible to insert percutaneously a stent across the dilated stenosis in an attempt to prevent restenosis. A vascular surgeon should always be available to deal with any complications that may arise.

Thrombolysis. This is used very rarely nowadays. Acute-on-chronic ischaemia of a limb without gross neurological deficit may be treated with thrombolytic therapy. Systemic thrombolysis carries dangers of haemorrhage, e.g. GI or cerebral, and local thrombolysis is safer. Arteriography is carried out to confirm the diagnosis. The tip of a catheter is then placed within the clot and a thrombolytic agent, e.g. streptokinase, urokinase or tissue plasminogen activator, is infused directly into the clot. Radiographs are repeated at 8–12-h intervals to check progress. At each radiograph the catheter is advanced further into the dissolving clot. When the clot is cleared any stenoses demonstrated radiologically may be submitted to angioplasty if suitable.

Embolization. This is suitable for highly vascular tissues, e.g. arteriovenous malformations, or to treat lesions not amenable to surgery, e.g. liver metastases or extensive renal carcinoma. The main arterial supply is identified via arteriography and a catheter placed within it. An occlusive material is then injected. Suitable agents include gelatin foam or minute steel coils. Embolization is being increasingly used to arrest haemorrhage following trauma or from the GI tract.

Prevention of pulmonary emboli. Recurrent pulmonary emboli in the presence of adequate anticoagulation is an indication for interrupting the IVC. It is possible to insert a filter in the cava percutaneously via the internal jugular vein or femoral vein. A commonly used filter is the Greenfield, which is shaped like a shuttlecock and is held closed with a special introducing catheter. This catheter is inserted through a sheath in the femoral vein. It is positioned in the inferior vena cava below the renal veins and released. The feet of the filter hook into the vein wall to prevent it becoming dislodged.

Shock and trauma

SHOCK

> Shock is defined as an abnormality of the circulation that causes inadequate organ perfusion and oxygenation. Five types of shock may be encountered in surgical practice: hypovolaemic, septic, cardiogenic, neurogenic and anaphylactic.

HYPOVOLAEMIC SHOCK

> This is due to decreased circulating blood volume.

Causes
These include:

- haemorrhage, e.g. trauma, haematemesis, ruptured aortic aneurysm
- dehydration, e.g. severe vomiting or diarrhoea, third space loss in inflammatory conditions
- burns resulting in massive loss of serum.

Classification
The blood volume of a 70 kg man is approximately 5 L or 80 mL/kg. Hypovolaemic shock can be divided into four categories, depending on the amount lost:

I.   <750 mL or <15%
II. 750–1500 mL or 15–30%
III. 1500–2000 mL or 30–40%
IV. >2000 mL or >40%.

Symptoms and signs
The symptoms and signs relate to the amount of blood lost:

I.   Minimal symptoms
II. Tachycardia >100, tachypnoea, decreased pulse pressure, pale, sweaty, cold peripheries
III. Classic symptoms of shock – tachycardia >120, hypotension, tachypnoea, pallor, cold peripheries, decreased conscious level, oliguria

IV. Immediate threat to life – tachycardia >140, hypotension (unobtainable diastolic), pallor, cold peripheries, unconscious (>50%), anuria.

Treatment
Shock is a surgical emergency and needs rapid treatment.

1. Ensure an adequate airway. Deliver 100% oxygen by mask. If comatose, intubate.
2. Keep the patient recumbent and elevate the foot of the bed.
3. Establish vascular access with two large-bore intravenous catheters – ideally in the antecubital fossa. If the cause of shock is haemorrhage, take blood for cross-matching. Also take blood for haemoglobin, haematocrit and U&Es. Restore circulating volume with crystalloid initially and with plasma expanders or blood as indicated.
4. Compression of any obvious external haemorrhage, i.e. stab wound to the groin.
5. Insert a central venous line to monitor CVP and to assess the response to fluid administration.
6. Insert a urinary catheter to monitor urinary output.
7. Establish basic observations of temperature, pulse, BP, respiratory rate and level of consciousness and urinary output.
8. The underlying cause of the shock should be ascertained and definitive treatment planned. Failure of resuscitation may be due to persistent massive haemorrhage. Surgical intervention is often necessary.

SEPTIC SHOCK

> Septic shock is part of the systemic inflammatory response syndrome (SIRS). Sepsis is defined as SIRS with a confirmed source of infection. Septic shock is defined as hypotension and hypoperfusion despite adequate fluid resuscitation. Septic shock is uncommon in trauma unless there has been a delay in presentation.

Causes
Septic shock is due to the release of a number of pro-inflammatory mediators such as IL-1, IL-6, TNF-α, PAF and the eicosanoids; and as a result of bacterial endotoxins (lipopolysaccharides). Septic shock is usually due to Gram-negative organisms such as *E. coli*, *Klebsiella* and *pseudomonas*, although peptidoglycans and teichoic acids in Gram-positive bacteria can also have similar effects. The pathophysiology underlying shock in septic patients includes:

- peripheral vasodilation
- ↑ vascular permeability (third space loss)
- peripheral arteriovenous shunting
- myocardial depression due to toxic effects on heart
- uncoupling of oxidative phosphorylation and anaerobic respiration leading to severe metabolic acidosis.

Symptoms and signs

There may be an obvious source of infection, together with a predisposing condition. The patient may be confused and restless; initially the skin is hot and flushed and the pulse characteristically 'bounding'. Vasoconstriction and the classic signs of shock may develop later.

Treatment

This is urgent and involves resuscitation, identification of the source of sepsis, appropriate antibiotic therapy and any necessary surgery to eradicate the focus of infection.

1. Ensure adequate airway and ventilation.
2. Restore circulating volume with plasma expanders while monitoring the venous pressure and urine output.
3. Obtain FBC, U&E, LFTs, clotting screen, ABG, serum lactate, cultures of blood, sputum, urine and any drainage fluid.
4. Commence intravenous antibiotics. This will depend on a number of factors. These include:
   — *Site of sepsis* – from the patient history and clinical examination, a best guess site of sepsis can usually be ascertained, i.e. GI, respiratory, urinary and secondary to intravascular lines.
   — *Previous antibiotics* – a patient who develops septic shock after prophylactic antibiotics is likely to have infection from a resistant organism and thus use of a different antibiotic is essential.
   — *Length of time in hospital* – organisms in the community and nosocomial organisms differ greatly; a patient admitted from the community with septic shock from a respiratory infection will require different antibiotics to a patient from ITU who has been in hospital for 4 weeks.
   — *Local resistance* – depending on whether the patient is ward-based or on ITU, the likely infecting organism and likely antibiotic resistance will differ. This is also true from hospital to hospital. In these situations it is best to consult the on-call microbiologist. They will be able to give advice on the likely organisms responsible and on the most appropriate antibiotic therapy.
5. Carry out appropriate surgical intervention, e.g. drainage of abscess, peritoneal lavage.
6. Further supportive measures may be required, e.g. inotropic agents, ventilation.

Complications

Sepsis and septic shock can progress to MODS (multi-organ dysfunction syndrome) and MOFS (multi-organ failure syndrome). Patients with MODS often present with sequential failure of organs, lung – liver – intestine – kidney; this may present as ARDS, abnormal LFTs, ileus and renal failure. With continued illness, organ dysfunction progresses to organ failure. Mortality with one-organ failure is around 30%. This rises to 100% with four-organ failure.

CARDIOGENIC SHOCK

> Cardiogenic shock or 'pump failure' is due to a loss of myocardial contractility.

Causes
These can be divided into cardiac compressive, cardiac obstructive or functional. All lead to problems with myocardial function and an inadequate cardiac output.

- Compressive – external forces compress the heart and great vessels leading to impairment of diastolic filling, a decrease in stroke volume and consequent hypotension. Causes include cardiac tamponade, positive pressure ventilation, tension pneumothorax and abdominal compartment syndrome.
- Obstructive – occurs when intravascular obstruction, excessive stiffness of arterial walls and microvascular blockage places an undue stress on the heart. It may be right- or left-sided. Tension pneumothorax is the commonest traumatic cause but other causes include valvular stenosis, PE and ARDS.
- Functional – the heart itself is not functioning efficiently. This may be due to arrhythmias or impaired muscle function after contusion or infarction.

Symptoms and signs
The traumatic causes will be discussed later in the chapter. Cardiac causes may present with chest pain and collapse. There may be a past history of cardiac problems or presence of risk factors, i.e. diabetes. Patients may be dyspnoeic with signs of pulmonary oedema. The patient may also display the classic signs of shock, i.e. pale, clammy, tachycardia, hypotension. Pulmonary embolism may present similarly (→ Ch. 5).

Investigations
Urgent investigations include portable CXR, FBC, U&E, cardiac enzymes, D-dimers, ABGs, ECG, CXR.

Treatment
1. ABC – high flow oxygen administration and i.v. access
2. Place patient in most comfortable position, i.e. sat up with pulmonary oedema
3. Pain relief, e.g. diamorphine
4. Drugs – consider aspirin (if MI), furosemide (if pulmonary oedema), inotropic agents
5. Correct arrhythmias
6. Correct U&Es and acid–base abnormalities
7. Cardiac monitoring (preferably on CCU)
8. CVP monitoring – avoid fluid overload
9. Consider angioplasty for MI in the postop setting as thrombolytic therapy is contraindicated
10. Surgery for valvular abnormalities
11. Consider aortic balloon pump in extreme circumstances.

NEUROGENIC SHOCK

Neurogenic shock is due to impaired descending sympathetic pathways in the spinal cord; this results in loss of vasomotor tone and sympathetic innervation to the heart. This leads to pooling of blood in the lower limbs. Although neurogenic shock can occur with spinal injury, it is *not* synonymous with spinal shock; this refers to the flaccidity and areflexia seen after a spinal injury. Neurogenic shock also occurs from certain nervous stimuli, i.e. fright – this leads to a sudden dilation of the splanchnic vessels and a bradycardia – the transient hypotension may lead to collapse.

Symptoms and signs
The classic sign of neurogenic shock in the trauma patient include:

- Bradycardia – due to loss of sympathetic tone
- Hypotension – there is no narrowed pulse pressure
- No vasoconstriction of peripheries.

Treatment
In the trauma patient shock should never be assumed to be neurogenic; hypovolaemia is by far the most common cause of hypotension and patients with spinal injury often have concurrent thoracic or abdominal injuries. Management includes:

- ABC
- Maintain spinal immobilization
- Vasopressors may be needed to maintain blood pressure
- Atropine – if significant bradycardias occur.

In the non-trauma setting neurogenic shock is self-limiting.

ANAPHYLACTIC SHOCK

Anaphylactic shock is a type I hypersensitivity reaction occurring in response to a previously sensitized antigen. Shock occurs as a result of vasodilation and increased vascular permeability. In surgical practice this may follow administration of drugs or radiological dyes. In the community it may follow wasp or bee stings or ingestion of certain foods, i.e. peanuts.

Symptoms and signs
Generalized urticaria, wheezing, laryngeal oedema, hypotension, loss of consciousness.

Treatment
1. ABC
2. Remove the cause
3. Give i.v. fluids, i.e. normal saline
4. 1 mL of 1:1000 adrenaline i.m. (can be repeated every 10 min)
5. Chlorpheniramine 10 mg i.v.
6. Hydrocortisone 100 mg i.v.

> ⚠ The importance of an adequate drug and sensitivity history cannot be overemphasized. Always make sure before giving parenteral injections that resuscitation equipment and drugs are available.

TRAUMA

Trauma is the main cause of death in people under the age of 35 years. It constitutes up to 20% of surgical admissions. Mortality can be greatly reduced by appropriate handling of the injured in the following three settings:

1. Emergency medical teams capable of going to the scene of an accident and providing the necessary first aid
2. A transportation system capable of rapid transport to a specified trauma centre
3. A trauma centre with trained personnel who are capable of rapidly assessing the injuries with facilities capable of handling a large number of trauma cases with trained teams.

INITIAL ASSESSMENT OF THE TRAUMA PATIENT

Pre-hospital care. In the pre-hospital phase, the same priorities exist in terms of ABCs; there is particular emphasis on airway control, control of external bleeding and immobilization. The key is to limit time on the scene and to transfer the patient to the nearest appropriate hospital. Communication with the hospital to allow mobilization of the trauma team is vital.

Major incident triage. Triage is the process of defining the most serious injuries in a mass casualty situation and attempting to have the greatest benefit with the given resources. Multiple casualties implies a number of wounded patients but not sufficient to exceed the ability of the hospital to offer care. Mass casualties implies that the number of injured will exceed the facility's ability to treat all patients and those with the greatest chance of survival are treated first. In the military, colour categories are applied to the wounded and indicate immediate, urgent or delayed treatment, dead or expectant.

Trauma scoring systems. Scoring systems in trauma can be divided into physiological scores and are based on a patient's response to injury (e.g. GCS and Revised Trauma Score); anatomical scores based on the injury that has occurred (e.g. Injury Severity Score and Liver Injury Scale); and outcome systems based on the result after recovery (e.g. GCS). Scoring systems are useful for a number of reasons such as facilitating triage, organizing trauma systems and to allow accurate comparisons between populations and treatment methods.

Initial assessment and resuscitation. This should follow ATLS (Advanced Trauma Life Support) guidelines. Initial assessment is divided into a primary survey where patients are assessed and their treatment priorities established based on their injuries, vital signs and mechanism of injury. This is followed by a secondary survey, which does not begin until the primary survey is completed, resuscitation is well established and the patient has normal vital signs.

Primary survey

This process constitutes the ABCDE protocol of ATLS and aims to rapidly identify immediately life-threatening injuries in a sequence in which the most rapidly fatal conditions are diagnosed first (i.e. airway obstruction will be fatal before splenic injury). The ABCDE of the primary survey is below.

> **⚠ ABCDE of emergency management:**
>
> - **A = Airway and cervical spine control** – Ensure a clear airway. The mouth and upper airway should be inspected for foreign bodies; these should be removed. In an unconscious patient the initial airway management may be a simple chin lift or jaw thrust; if this is unsuccessful in maintaining an airway then an oral (Guedel) or nasopharyngeal airway can be used. If these fail to maintain the airway then intubation will be necessary. In patients with severe maxillofacial trauma a surgical airway such as jet insufflation (needle cricothyroidotomy) or surgical cricothyroidotomy may be needed. Emergency tracheostomy has no role as an emergency airway manoeuvre.
> - **B = Breathing** – Check for chest movements, asymmetry of movements, respiratory rate, abrasions or bruising over the chest, cyanosis, use of accessory muscles, distension of neck veins. Examine the chest for pain, crepitations (indicating subcutaneous emphysema), auscultation, percussion and palpation of the trachea. Needle decompression may be needed for tension pneumothorax and a chest drain may be required for pneumothorax or haemothorax.
> - **C = Circulation and haemorrhage control** – i.v. access should be gained with two large bore cannula (12–14G) in the antecubital fossa. Two litres (L) of Hartmann's solution should be rapidly infused. Alternative sites for vascular access include central veins, i.e. subclavian or femoral (internal jugular can be difficult to use due to the presence of C-spine collars), cut-down onto the long saphenous vein and intraosseous infusion (children only). Obvious haemorrhage can be treated with compression dressings. Tourniquets are not indicated.
> - **D = Disability** – In the primary survey a rapid assessment of neurological status is made. This includes assessment of pupillary size and level of consciousness. The level of consciousness can be remembered by the mnemonic AVPU:
>   - A = Alert
>   - V = responds to Vocal stimuli
>   - P = responds to Painful stimuli
>   - U = Unresponsive.
> - **E = Exposure and environmental control** – The patient should be fully undressed and examined from head to toe (secondary survey). The patient's temperature must be monitored and hypothermia prevented by covering with warming blankets and the use of warmed i.v. fluids.

During the primary survey and in tandem with examining the patient, certain adjuncts are used, including ECG, pulse oximetry, BP and respiratory rate, insertion of NG tube and urinary catheter (as required); also the patient is provided with adequate analgesia.

Secondary survey

The secondary survey is a head-to-toe evaluation of the trauma patient, i.e. a complete history and physical examination, including a reassessment of all vital signs. Each area of the body should be completely examined. A full neurological examination is carried out including a GCS (Glasgow Coma Score) determination (Table 4.1).

History

This is obtained from the patient (if possible), ambulance staff or other witnesses. Ascertain the time of the accident, the type of accident, the conscious level of the patient at the time of the accident and any change since; any blood loss, details of drugs administered at the scene of accident, previous medical history including drugs and allergies, details of food, alcohol and drug intake. In road-traffic accidents (RTAs), details of the patient's position in the car, speed, use of

TABLE 4.1 Glasgow Coma Scale (GCS)

Responses	Score
Eye-opening response	
Spontaneous	4
To voice	3
To pain	2
None	1
Best verbal response	
Orientated	5
Confused	4
Inappropriate speech	3
Incomprehensible speech	2
None	1
Best motor response	
Obeys commands	6
Localizes pain	5
Withdraws to pain	4
Flexion to pain	3
Extension to pain	2
None	1
Total	3–15

A score of 3 indicates a severe injury with a poor prognosis. A score of 13–15 indicates minor injury with a good prognosis.

airbags/seat belts and degree of damage to the car should be obtained. A mnemonic to help remember this is to take an AMPLE history:

- **A**llergies
- **M**edications
- **P**revious illnesses
- **L**ast meal
- **E**vents surrounding injury.

Examination
An initial rapid preliminary examination will have been made during the primary survey. A full examination is carried out during the secondary survey looking for head injuries, maxillofacial injuries, cervical spine injuries, chest injuries, abdominal and perineal injuries, musculoskeletal injuries, and neurological trauma. Typical injuries include:

- Frontal impact – injuries to diaphragm, cervical spine, flail chest, myocardial contusion, pneumothorax, TRA, ruptured liver and spleen, possible dislocation of hip or knee
- Side impact – injuries to cervical spine, flail chest, pneumothorax, TRA, diaphragmatic tear, ruptured liver, ruptured spleen, ruptured kidney, fractured pelvis or acetabulum
- Rear impact – cervical spine injury
- Pedestrian – head injury, TRA, abdominal visceral injury, fractured lower limb and pelvis
- Fall from a height – calcaneal fracture, tibial plateau fracture, pelvic or acetabular fracture, lumbar spine compression fracture, TRA, pneumothorax, head injury.

Investigations
The timing of the investigations depends on the clinical state of the patient. These include: blood grouping and cross-match, FBC, U&E, amylase, LFT, glucose, β-HCG (in women of child-bearing age) arterial blood gas. X-rays in the primary survey include chest and pelvis X-ray. FAST (**F**ocused **A**bdominal **S**onography for **T**rauma) is an imaging modality often performed during the primary survey to identify an abdominal source of bleeding in a hypotensive patient. All other X-rays, CT, contrast studies, etc. are obtained depending on the stability of the patient and the presence of other injuries. As a rule, these would be obtained as part of the secondary survey. Examples include: spinal X-rays in suspected spinal injury, CT head in patients with head trauma (can often include cervical spine views), CT abdomen and chest in suspected abdominal/thoracic trauma in patients who are haemodynamically stable. Urethrography/cystography in patients with suspected urethral or bladder injury.

HEAD INJURY (→ Ch. 18)

Primary brain damage occurring at the time of injury cannot be repaired. Management should be aimed at preventing secondary injury.

Management

The management of specific head injury is dealt with in the section on Neurosurgery (→ Ch. 18) but the basic principles are outlined here as far as trauma management is concerned.

Treat hypoxia, hypercapnia, hypovolaemic shock, and anaemia to prevent further neurological deterioration. Primary neurological management is identification and rapid treatment of localized lesions and intracranial haemorrhage, cerebral debridement and prevention of raised ICP.

Hypotension in adults is not due to intracranial blood loss. However, in children, significant blood loss can occur in head injuries and can be responsible for hypotension. The scalp should be examined for lacerations and boggy wounds. Observation should be made for bleeding and CSF leakage from the ear and nose. The cranial nerves should be checked and the limbs examined. Assessment of head injured patients include skull X-rays and CT scan; indications for these are detailed in Chapter 18.

> ⚠ **Immediate management depends on severity. The presence of abnormal pupillary reflexes, asymmetrical motor signs or deteriorating level of consciousness is an immediate indication for treatment.**

Immediate measures:

- ABC
- Intubation
- Ventilate with 100% oxygen and maintain normovolaemia – prevention of secondary brain injury
- Intravenous mannitol can be given to produce a diuresis and reduce cerebral oedema
- Maintain normovolaemia
- Monitor ABGs and maintain normocapnia
- Immediate transfer to theatre for burr holes and evacuation of haematoma.

Less urgent management is required where there are focal lesions without brainstem compression and with an unconscious patient without focal neurological signs.

THORACIC TRAUMA

> Blunt and penetrating thoracic trauma are responsible for 25% of deaths due to trauma, but less than 20% of patients require thoracotomy for the treatment of their injuries.

Management
Most patients with thoracic trauma can be managed as follows:

1. Adequate resuscitation
2. Respiratory support
3. Chest drain.

Thoracic injuries can be divided into those that are immediately life-threatening and those that are potentially life-threatening.
    Immediately life-threatening injuries can be remembered by '**ATOM FC**':

● **A**irway obstruction
● **T**ension pneumothorax
● **O**pen pneumothorax
● **M**assive haemothorax
● **F**lail chest
● **C**ardiac tamponade.

Potentially life-threatening injuries can be remembered by '**ATOM PD**':

● **A**ortic disruption
● **T**racheobronchial injury
● **O**esophageal injury
● **M**yocardial contusion
● **P**ulmonary contusion and **P**neumothorax
● **D**iaphragmatic rupture.

Airway obstruction
Usually as a result of foreign bodies (e.g. blood, teeth or loss of muscular control of the tongue). More unusual causes include laryngeal trauma and posterior dislocation of the sternoclavicular joint.

Symptoms and signs
These include tachypnoea, altered level of consciousness (agitated with hypoxia and obtunded with hypercapnia), use of accessory muscles and abnormal sounds such as gurgling, snoring or stridor.

Management
Initial manoeuvres include chin lift and jaw thrust; adjuncts to this include oropharyngeal (Guedel) or nasopharyngeal airways. If a patient's airway is not improved by these methods, then a definitive airway (tube present in trachea with the cuff inflated and secured with tape) in the form of orotracheal intubation is required. In circumstances of severe facial trauma, glottic oedema, bleeding or inability to intubate then a surgical airway is needed – this can be via jet insufflation or a surgical cricothyroidotomy.

Airway techniques
Guedel airway. Size is judged on the distance from the corner of the patient's mouth to the angle of the mandible, inserted upside down and rotated to lie in the patient's throat over the tongue.

Nasopharyngeal airway. Placed in the patients nostril, size is judged by comparing the tube to the patients little finger.

Jet insufflation. Surgically prepare the neck and infiltrate local anaesthetic, then insert a large bore cannula through the cricopharyngeal membrane (this can be confirmed by aspirating air into a syringe attached to the cannula once in the correct position). The plastic cannula is then advanced into the trachea, oxygen tubing is attached to the cannula with a side hole and 15 L O_2 is delivered. The side hole is occluded for 1 s and left open for 4 s. This will allow 30–40 min of ventilation before the CO_2 rises to high.

Surgical cricothyroidotomy. Surgically prepare the neck and infiltrate local anaesthetic, then make a transverse incision in the cricothyroid membrane. This is then dilated (using the handle of the scalpel or a clip) and a size 5.0 to 7.0 tracheostomy tube is inserted.

Tension pneumothorax

Injury results in the formation of a 'one-way' valve – air enters the pleural cavity but is unable to escape, therefore pressure (or tension) in the chest rises, causing distortion of the vena cava and trachea.

Symptoms and signs

Tachypnoea, use of accessory muscles, cyanosis, hypotension (due to kinking of vena cava and decreased venous return), deviated trachea (*away* from the affected side), distended neck veins (variable sign), hyper-resonant percussion and absent breath sounds.

Management

This is a clinical diagnosis. Immediate management is the placement of a wide bore cannula in the 2nd intercostal space in the mid-clavicular line. A chest drain must then replace this as the tension pneumothorax has been converted to a simple pneumothorax.

Open (sucking) pneumothorax

Produced by injuries that cause large defects of the chest wall, i.e. gunshot wound. The injury leads to intrathoracic and atmospheric pressure equalizing. If the defect is >⅔ the diameter of the trachea, then air will preferentially enter the defect and bypass the lungs – and thus produce hypoxia.

Symptoms and signs

Tachypnoea, use of accessory muscles, cyanosis, obvious chest wound.

Management

Immediate management is the placement of a dressing secured on three sides to create a 'flutter-valve' (securing on four sides will produce a tension pneumothorax). A chest drain distant from the injury must then be placed.

Haemothorax and massive haemothorax

Most often due to penetrating injury to the hilar or systemic vessels. Can occur with blunt injury with rib fractures and damage to intercostals vessels – a massive haemothorax is defined as immediate evacuation of 1.5 L at insertion of a chest drain or >200 mL every hour after drain insertion. It produces hypoxia by the pressure effect of the additional volume in the thorax compressing the lung but also by hypovolaemia.

Symptoms and signs
Signs of shock, tachypnoea, using accessory muscles, cyanosis, dull percussion note and absent breath sounds.

Management
Obtain i.v. access prior to insertion of chest drain as rapid infusion of fluids may be needed. If blood loss from the chest drain in massive, it should be clamped in an attempt to re-tamponade the bleeding. Thoracotomy if >1.5 L immediately or >200 mL/h is lost.

Flail chest
Occurs when more than two adjacent ribs are fractured in two or more places. This results in a segment of the chest moving paradoxically with respiration (in with inspiration and out with expiration). Contrary to belief, it is not the paradoxical chest movement that causes respiratory problems but the lung contusion underlying the rib injury.

Symptoms and signs
Pain, bruising, tachypnoea, paradoxical respiratory movement (often not present acutely due to muscle splinting).

Management
Analgesia, high flow oxygen, judicious fluid replacement (at risk of pulmonary oedema due to the lung contusion), regular ABGs to identify patients at risk of respiratory failure and the need for artificial ventilation. Rarely surgical fixation of the rib fractures is needed.

Cardiac tamponade
Usually occurs as a result of penetrating trauma, blood within the pericardium compresses the heart leading to cardiogenic shock.

Symptoms and signs
Becks triad (distended neck veins, hypotension, muffled heart sounds), pulsus paradoxus, Kussmaul's sign (↑ JVP with inspiration), small complexes on ECG, EMD and on a FAST scan (see later).

Management
Needle pericardiocentesis or a pericardial window (performed at laparotomy) can be immediately life-saving; thoracotomy is the definitive treatment with repair of the injury.

Procedure
Needle pericardiocentesis

This is both therapeutic and diagnostic, removal of as little as 20 mL of blood can lead to improvement in symptoms. Surgically prepare the chest and infiltrate local anaesthetic, then insert a 16–18-gauge needle 2 cm below the xiphisternum and advanced upwards towards the tip of the left scapula. The procedure should be performed with ECG monitoring. If the needle is advanced too far then there will be ECG changes such as ST elevation, etc. Once all the blood has been aspirated then a catheter with a 3-way tap can be left in case of reaccumulation.

Aortic disruption (traumatic rupture of the aorta – TRA)

This is due to deceleration injuries such as in RTAs or a fall from a great height; the body rapidly decelerates but the organs continue to move. It particularly affects sites where a mobile part of an organ meets a relatively fixed point (i.e. renal pedicle, duodenum at the ligament of Treitz and the aorta). The commonest point of deceleration injury in the aorta is in the ascending aorta just proximal to the innominate artery and at the point of attachment of the ligamentum arteriosum. Tears in the ascending aorta often have associated cardiac damage and rarely reach hospital; tears at the ligamentum arteriosum may be contained by adventitia and allow the patient to reach hospital (typically young males).

Symptoms and signs

These are variable. The patient may have no signs or be moribund with signs of massive haemothorax. Other signs include upper extremity ↑ BP with diminished pulses in the lower limbs, diminished pulses in the upper limbs (due to occlusion of vessels along the aortic arch) and neurological compromise from spinal ischaemia.

Investigations

- CXR (signs include widened mediastinum, fractured 1st or 2nd rib, obliterated aortic knuckle, pleural cap – small amount of blood in the pleural cavity, deviated trachea to the right, elevation of right bronchus and right deviation of NG tube)
- Arch aortogram
- CT (comparable with aortogram)
- Trans-oesophageal echo.

Management

Surgical repair with resection of damaged segment and replacing with a graft, endovascular repair.

Tracheobronchial injury

Larynx

Rare, usually due to direct trauma.

Symptoms and signs. May present late, these include hoarseness, stridor, subcutaneous emphysema and fracture crepitus.

Management. Intubation.

Trachea
Usually injured by penetrating trauma.

Symptoms and signs. Include noisy breathing and visible bubbles in the neck wound.

Management. Surgical repair.

Bronchi
Rare, usually fatal at the scene, occurs due to severe deceleration injury; it is usually within 2.5 cm of the carina.

Symptoms and signs. Haemoptysis, subcutaneous emphysema, tension pneumothorax, large air leak after placement of a chest drain.

Investigations. Bronchoscopy is diagnostic.

Management. May require further chest drain if large air leak, intubation of opposite bronchus if acutely hypoxic followed by surgical repair.

Oesophageal injury
Can occur with penetrating or blunt injury. Penetrating injury is more common. Cervical oesophageal injuries present in a similar manner to tracheal injuries. With blunt injury, blows to the oesophagus can result in traumatic rupture (similar to Boerhaave's syndrome); this most commonly occurs in the lower left posterolateral oesophagus.

Symptoms and signs
Haemo/pneumothorax with no rib fractures, pain and shock out of proportion to the apparent injury, particulate matter in the chest drain.

Management
Give i.v. antibiotics, surgical repair (in early diagnosis), with late diagnosed injuries the management is via antibiotics, chest drainage and oesophageal diversion.

Myocardial contusion
Blunt injury. Difficult to diagnose. May result in a number of ECG abnormalities such as multiple ectopics, sinus tachycardia, atrial fibrillation or raised ST segments (similar to an MI).

Management
Cardiac monitor and treat arrhythmias as and when they arise.

Pulmonary contusion
Common injury in blunt trauma. Analogous to a soft tissue bruise, with haemorrhage and oedema into the lung parenchyma. This impairs gas exchange and leads to respiratory failure (especially in the elderly and in those with coexistent lung disease).

Management
As for flail chest.

Pneumothorax (→ Ch. 9)

May occur with blunt or penetrating injury. A laceration of the lung parenchyma occurs and air enters the pleural space; this results in loss of the negative intrapleural pressure and the lung collapses. The collapsed segment of lung leads to V/Q mismatching and hypoxia.

Symptoms and signs

Tachypnoea, use of accessory muscles, cyanosis, decreased breath sounds, resonant percussion note.

Management

Chest drain.

Diaphragmatic rupture

Can occur with blunt or penetrating trauma. Blunt trauma usually results in tears of the left posterolateral hemi-diaphragm. Penetrating injury may be missed and present many years later with visceral herniation.

Symptoms and signs

Respiratory compromise, hypoxia and CXR appearance (bowel in chest cavity, 'fluffy' hemidiaphragm, NG tube in chest).

Investigations

- CT
- Thoracoscopy
- Laparoscopy.

Management

Surgical repair.

Miscellaneous thoracic injuries

Rib fractures

Common injury following blunt trauma. Rib fractures can lead to:

- Pneumothorax (rib fragments lacerate lung parenchyma)
- Haemothorax (rib fragments lacerate intercostal vessels)
- Pain: impairs ventilation which may lead to atelectasis and pneumonia.

Rib fractures can indicate other potential injuries:

- Fractures of ribs 1–3: head injury, spinal injury, great vessel injury
- Fractures of ribs 10–12: hepatosplenic injury.

Symptoms and signs. Pain, crepitus, visible deformity, respiratory compromise, CXR (fractures are not always visible).

Management
1. Analgesia – oral, i.v., intercostal block with LA, epidural
2. Chest drain (if associated with pneumo/haemothorax)
3. Chest physiotherapy
4. Frequent ABGs in the elderly or patients with co-existent lung disease to assess impending respiratory failure.

Sternal fractures
Blunt injury. Usually occurs at the manubriosternal junction. Associated with myocardial and pulmonary contusions.

Management. Cardiac monitoring and analgesia. ABG assessment if pulmonary contusion suspected.

Scapular fractures. Considerable force is required, therefore suspect associated injuries. Fractures are divided into:

● Body – sling and analgesia
● Neck – may need ORIF (**O**pen **R**eduction and **I**nternal **F**ixation) if displaced glenoid
● Glenoid – ORIF if loss of joint congruity
● Acromion – ORIF only if gross displacement.

Pulmonary haematoma
Produced by bleeding intra-parenchymal bleeding, mechanism of injury is similar to a contusion but respiratory dysfunction is less. A traumatic pneumatocoele (cavity in the pulmonary substance) may develop after resolution of a haematoma.

Symptoms and signs. May be some respiratory signs, CXR may appear more dramatic with a sharp demarcated edge to the opacity.

Management. Conservative, the haematoma will resolve over 2–3 weeks.

Air embolism
A rare event that occurs with penetrating trauma when a fistula is formed between the bronchus and a pulmonary vein. When breathing normally, the pressure is higher in the vein than bronchus – this results in haemoptysis. However, if the patient performs a Valsalva type respiration, i.e. grunts or is intubated, then pressure is higher in the bronchus and air will enter the pulmonary vein.

Symptoms and signs. Haemoptysis. After air has entered the circulation presentation includes the development of focal neurological signs, sudden cardiovascular collapse after intubation and froth when an ABG is obtained.

Management. Immediate thoracotomy, clamp the hilum of the injured lung and repair the laceration. If air is seen in the coronary vessels the ascending aorta can be occluded for a few seconds to push out the air.

Procedure

Chest drain insertion

The drain is placed in the 5th intercostal space in the anterior axillary line, this area is sometimes referred to as the 'triangle of safety' – an area bordered by the lateral edge of pec major the anterior edge of lat dorsi, a line from the nipple level (i.e. 5th intercostal) and an apex in the axilla. Surgically prepare and drape the chest; infiltrate local anaesthetic down to the pleura. Make a 2–3 cm horizontal incision and, with blunt dissection, open the wound over the *top* of the rib. Puncture the pleura and then enlarge the hole with your finger and sweep away any organs or adhesions. Then, using a suitable clamp to hold the tip of the drain (either 34 or 36F), insert it through the hole and direct it up and posteriorly. Connect to an underwater seal and suture in place; look for fogging of the tube and 'swinging' of the drain to confirm correct position. Obtain a chest X-ray.

Emergency thoracotomy

Indications for emergency thoracotomy include witnessed arrest and a thoracic injury (especially from penetrating trauma) and severe post-injury hypotension as a result of cardiac tamponade, air embolism or thoracic bleeding. Surgically prepare the chest and fully abduct the patients arm (if time, place a rolled sheet between the scapula). Make an incision in the 4th intercostal space from the sternal border to the midaxillary line. Once into the pleura open the full length of the wound with mayo scissors and insert a rib retractor. Objectives at this stage include: releasing cardiac tamponade, controlling intrathoracic bleeding, controlling air embolism, perform open cardiac massage and clamping the descending aorta to control infra-diaphragmatic bleeding.

ABDOMINAL TRAUMA

Abdominal trauma may be blunt (direct, deceleration and rotational forces are applied) or penetrating. Injury to an abdominal viscus should be suspected in any blunt injury to the thorax or abdomen or in penetrating injuries anywhere between the nipple and perineum. Obtain information about the injury from the patient, relatives and ambulance personnel.

The abdominal cavity can be divided into peritoneal and retroperitoneal cavities. The peritoneum can be further divided into 'Intrathoracic', Abdominal and Pelvic:

- 'Intrathoracic' abdomen – from the diaphragm to the costal margins, it contains the liver, spleen, stomach and transverse colon (remember that the diaphragm can rise to the 4th intercostal space in expiration)
- Abdominal – small and large bowel, distended bladder, pregnant uterus
- Pelvic – sigmoid colon, rectum, small bowel, bladder, uterus and ovaries.

Organs in the retroperitoneum include:

- kidneys and ureter
- duodenum – except the first 2.5 cm (1 inch) of the first part.
- pancreas
- caecum and ascending colon
- ⅔ of descending colon
- lower rectum
- aorta and IVC.

Penetrating trauma

Causes of penetrating trauma include stab wounds and gunshot wounds. The most commonly injured organs are the liver and small bowel. Significant injury is much greater with gunshot wounds (80%) compared with stab wounds (30%).

Management

Initial management is via ATLS protocols, however, note specific points to remember:

1. Look for the wound – wounds on the back are easy to miss.
2. Look for the exit wound in gunshot wounds (GSW), it may indicate likely injuries. Remember abdominal GSWs may traverse the thorax and vice versa.
3. High velocity GSWs injure widely along their path (cavitation).
4. Low velocity GSWs injure along their path only.
5. **ALL** penetrating trauma secondary to GSWs should be explored via a laparotomy due to high risk of injury.
6. Penetrating injury secondary to knife wounds in the absence of haemodynamic instability, signs of peritonism, evisceration or free air under the diaphragm on CXR can be managed expectantly. Alternatively, a diagnostic laparoscopy can be performed to confirm peritoneal breach (the majority of stab wounds do not breach the peritoneum and those that do, do not always injure any organs).

Blunt trauma

Abdominal injury due to blunt trauma may result from direct injury, deceleration or rotational forces. Blunt trauma is more common in the UK and results from RTAs, falls and pedestrian/vehicle accidents. The most commonly injured organs are the spleen and liver.

Symptoms and signs

Skin abrasions, bruising, seat belt imprints (particularly with lap belts), fractures of ribs 10–12, abdominal tenderness or rigidity (peritonism), distension, absent bowel sounds, shock, haematuria.

Investigations in abdominal trauma

1. CXR – part of the ATLS protocol, may show free air in a stable patient with penetrating trauma who is able to sit upright.
2. AXR – not part of the ATLS protocol and unlikely to add a great deal to patients with blunt or penetrating trauma.
3. Ultrasound – this can be done in the A&E department and is known as FAST scanning (**F**ocused **A**bdominal **S**onography for **T**rauma). It simply aims to look for fluid in three areas of the abdomen (perihepatic, perisplenic and pelvic), and for a cardiac tamponade (pericardial). Detects a minimum of around 200 mL of fluid; must be interpreted with clinical findings. A positive FAST scan is *not* an absolute indication for laparotomy.
4. CT – sensitive and specific for the injured organ, also allows an assessment of severity. Not suitable for unstable patients.

5. DPL, **D**iagnostic **P**eritoneal **L**avage – rarely needed with the availability of
FAST scans. Basically entails placing a catheter into the abdomen; if frank blood
is aspirated then it is a positive test, if not, a litre of fluid is run in and then
drained off; this then sent for analysis. A positive test is indicated by >100 000
RBCs/µL, bile or faecal matter.

Indications for laparotomy include:

● Hypotension refractory to resuscitation
● Peritonitis
● Air under the diaphragm on CXR
● Evisceration
● All gunshot wounds
● Positive investigations, i.e. CT.

Specific organ injuries

Stomach
Usually secondary to penetrating trauma.

Symptoms and signs. Peritonitis, air under the diaphragm, bloody NG aspirate.

Management. Debridement and primary closure; with severe injuries resection may
be necessary.

Complications. Fistula, abscess.

Duodenum
The majority of injuries are penetrating. In blunt trauma, duodenal injury
classically occurs with severe frontal impacts, e.g. hitting handlebars of a motorbike
(usually involves the third part of the duodenum).

Symptoms and signs. Bloody NG aspirate, retroperitoneal air, raised amylase (with
associated pancreatic injury).

Management. Depends on the severity but may include:

● simple closure ± tube duodenostomy decompression
● ± omental or serosal patching
● ± gastroenterostomy
● duodenal diverticulization (with pancreaticoduodenal injuries); this consists of:
   — repair injury
   — oversew duodenal stump and tube duodenostomy
   — gastrojejunostomy
   — T-tube in CBD
● Whipple's procedure in severe pancreaticoduodenal injuries.

Complications. Fistula, abscess.

Pancreas
Secondary to blunt trauma, typically an epigastric blow; the pancreas is compressed
against the vertebral column.

Symptoms and signs. Difficult to diagnose; classically presents with severe abdominal pain that decreases over 1–2 h and then increases in severity.

Investigations
- Serum amylase – may be raised in pancreatic injury
- DPL – raised amylase
- CT.

Management. Distal pancreatectomy; Whipple's procedure in severe injuries with proximal duct injury, injury involving the CBD or ampulla, and devascularizing injuries.

Complications. Fistula.

Liver

Most commonly injured intra-abdominal organ. Injury does not always need operative intervention. In general, management is based on CT appearances. However, transfusion of >3 units of blood and the patient is still shocked is an indication for laparotomy. Indications for non-operative management include:

- haemodynamically stable
- no persistent or increase in abdominal pain
- <4 units transfusion
- CT –<500 mL blood in the peritoneum, parenchymal laceration or intrahepatic haematoma.

Symptoms and signs. Few, other than haemodynamic instability in severe injuries; suspect with RUQ bruising/abrasions or broken right 10–12th ribs, right shoulder tip pain.

Management

Non-operative. With no signs of peritonitis and no haemodynamic instability, the injury can often be managed non-operatively. CT scan can be a useful guide to the severity of injury but in the main it is the absence of hypotension or tachycardia that dictates non-operative management. Other points to consider include persistent or increased abdominal pain or the transfusion of >3 units of blood. Frequent checks of haemoglobin and haematocrit, clinical examination and invasive monitoring (i.e. CVP) will identify patients failing non-operative management.

Radiological. If CT demonstrates extravasation, indicating arterial bleeding, an option is to perform angiography and embolization. This can also be performed after operative packing if bleeding continues.

Operative. Operative intervention with liver trauma includes the following alone or in combination:

- Packing the liver with gauze rolls to compress the injured segment (this can be helped by mobilizing the injured lobe); the packs can be left for 48 h but antibiotics should be given
- Diathermy to superficial bleeding

- Deep liver sutures
- Hepatotomy and vascular ligation (i.e. open laceration more to suture bleeding vessels)
- Resect injured lobe – if a lobe is shattered, it may be better to resect
- If exsanguinating, then Pringle's manoeuvre can be performed – compression of the structures of the free edge of the lesser omentum (can be left for approximately 45 min).

Complications. These include re-bleeding, bile leaks, jaundice, coagulopathy, hypoglycaemia, ischaemic segments, infection/abscess and haemobilia.

Spleen

Most commonly injured in blunt trauma.

Symptoms and signs. Left upper quadrant (LUQ) bruising or abrasions, lower rib fractures, shoulder tip pain (Kehr's sign); LUQ mass (Balance's sign), displacement of gastric bubble on CXR. Following resuscitation, indications for non-operative management include:

- haemodynamically stable
- <2 units transfused
- stable serial Hb estimation
- no increase in size of splenic haematoma on serial USS
- no deterioration of condition on close observation
- needs observation for 7–10 days, as there is a risk of delayed rupture of a splenic haematoma.

Management

Non-operative. The patient must be haemodynamically stable, have <2 units transfused, have no evidence of other intra-abdominal organ injury, no evidence of active bleeding on CT or evidence of shattered spleen or hilar injury (both mandate operative intervention). The patient should have frequent checks of haemoglobin and haematocrit. Clinical examination and invasive monitoring (i.e. CVP) will identify patients failing non-operative management.

Radiological. As with liver injury, certain splenic injuries can be managed via angiography and embolization.

Operative. Operative management depends on the severity of injury but may include the following, either alone or in combination:

- Packing
- Diathermy
- Topical haemostatics, e.g. Surgicel
- Wrapping in a mesh bag to tamponade bleed
- Suture lacerations
- Ligation of splenic vessels – decreased function with arterial ligation but preferred to splenectomy
- Partial splenectomy for polar injuries.

Complications. These include LUQ haematoma (may progress to abscess), pleural effusion, pseudoaneurysm of the splenic artery, arteriovenous fistula between the artery and vein, pancreatic injury/fistula and overwhelming post-splenectomy sepsis (OPSI, → Ch. 14). With splenic haematomas that were treated non-operatively, there is a small risk of delayed rupture, which can occur days or weeks later. It is prudent to monitor these patients with a repeat USS to identify an enlarging haematoma.

Small bowel

Commonly injured in penetrating trauma. In blunt trauma, injuries may occur due to:

- crushing between abdominal wall and vertebra
- sudden increase in intraluminal pressure, i.e. blast injuries
- deceleration injuries causing tears at fixed points, e.g. ligament of Treitz, ileocaecal area. Note: CT scan can miss small bowel injuries in as many as 30% of cases.

Symptoms and signs. Peritonism, air under diaphragm, absent bowel sounds, particulate matter on DPL.

Management. Simple closure; resection and anastomosis; resection and ileostomy (in delayed injuries, gross peritoneal contamination or haemodynamic instability).

Complications. Anastomotic leak, obstruction, abscess, fistula.

Colorectal

Injuries are usually a result of penetrating trauma. Less than 5% are due to blunt trauma but indicates a significant force. Rectal injuries are also rare. They may be associated with pelvic fractures, penetrating trauma in the buttock and perineum. May also occur with sexual misadventures! Rectal injuries can be divided into extraperitoneal and intraperitoneal.

Symptoms and signs. Peritonism, absent bowel sounds, faecal matter on DPL, blood on PR.

Investigations
- EUA
- Sigmoidoscopy (rigid or flexible)
- CT.

Management. With colonic injuries, primary repair or resection and anastomosis can be performed in the absence of complicating factors such as hypotension, more than two organs injured, significant faecal soiling and >6 h since injury. These latter patients should be treated by resection and end colostomy (Hartmann's procedure). In rectal injuries, a primary repair should be carried out for intraperitoneal injuries and extraperitoneal injuries that can be mobilized intraperitoneally or repaired transrectally. In more extensive injury, or with a delay in presentation, then a proximal loop colostomy can be performed.

Complications. With colonic injuries, these may include abscess, anastomotic leak and stoma-related problems. With rectal injuries, complications include abscess, fistulae, incontinence (urinary and faecal), structure and loss of sexual function.

URINARY TRAUMA

Upper urinary tract

Renal

The most commonly injured part of the genitourinary tract, the majority of injuries can be treated conservatively, i.e. contusion. However, more severe injury presenting as haemodynamic instability may require surgical intervention.

Symptoms and signs. Flank bruising/abrasion, fractured ribs or transverse processes of lumbar spine, haematuria (poor sign, 30% patients with severe trauma have no haematuria and many patients with serious abdominal trauma will have microscopic haematuria with no renal injury).

Investigations. IVU, CT.

Management. Depends on whether the patient is stable or unstable. In unstable patients, the choice is immediate surgery. Options include simple suture, partial nephrectomy or nephrectomy. In stable patients following suitable imaging, the majority of injuries can be managed conservatively.

Complications. Urinomas, abscess, bleeding, renal artery thrombosis, hypertension (late).

Ureteric

Ureteric injuries may occur with devascularization, deceleration and ureteric avulsion (usually at the PUJ and more common in children), penetrating trauma (usually affects the upper ureter) and iatrogenic injury.

Symptoms and signs. Haematuria is uncommon. If missed may present with ileus, ↑urea, urinoma, sepsis or urine in an abdominal drain.

Investigations. IVU

Management. If the patient is unstable, then the ureter can be left alone, stented or ligated and repaired later ± percutaneous nephrostomy. In stable patients, repair depends on the site of injury. From the PUJ to pelvic brim, the choice is to perform an end-to-end uretero-ureterostomy. With injuries below the pelvic brim, it is best to perform a uretero-neocystostomy (procedures such as Boari flap and psoas hitch may add more length). A ureteric stent should be used with all repairs.

Complications. Stricture, anastomotic leak and urinoma.

Lower urinary tract

Bladder

Injuries are usually the result of blunt trauma; they may be intraperitoneal (30%) (blunt trauma and full bladder) or extraperitoneal (70%) (pelvic fractures).

Symptoms and signs. Inability to void, haematuria, suprapubic pain, raised urea and creatinine and low sodium (with intraperitoneal injuries).

Investigations. USS, CT, retrograde cystography.

Management. Extraperitoneal injuries can be treated by urethral or suprapubic catheter drainage for 2 weeks and then a check cystogram for leaks. All intraperitoneal injuries should be repaired and are drained with a urethral and/or suprapubic (or both) catheter and a check cystogram performed in 2 weeks.

Complications. Fistula, abscess and urinary ascites (if undiagnosed).

Urethra

Urethral injuries may be posterior (membranous) or anterior (bulbar); the majority are due to blunt trauma. Posterior injuries occur above the urogenital diaphragm and are associated with pelvic fractures. Anterior urethral injuries are associated with a 'straddle' type injury.

Symptoms and signs. Blood at the urethral meatus; unable to void; high riding prostate on PR (posterior injury); sleeve haematoma of penis (if Buck's fascia intact); butterfly haematoma (if Buck's fascia is torn but Colles fascia is intact).

Investigations. Retrograde urethrogram.

Management. The management of urethral injuries can be divided into anterior and posterior secondary to blunt trauma and penetrating.

- Anterior – suprapubic catheter and leave for 2 weeks. If no extravasation at urethrogram then catheter removed; if extravasation will need end-to-end urethroplasty at approximately 6 weeks.
- Posterior – these are a little more complex. The initial options include suprapubic cystostomy or urethral re-alignment over a catheter. Following suprapubic cystostomy, a urethrogram is performed after 2 weeks; around 30% will be able to have the catheter removed. If the urethrogram shows obstruction of the urethra, then the patient will need a urethroplasty in 4 months. Urethral re-alignment is indicated if the patient has a rectal injury that will require operation, bladder neck injury or a major distraction. The catheter is left for 6 weeks and then removed.
- Penetrating – immediate surgery, repair and placement of a suprapubic cystostomy.

Complications. Stricture, impotence, incontinence, fistula and abscess.

LIMB TRAUMA

> Limb trauma involves injury to: soft tissues; blood vessels (→ Ch. 15); nerves; bones (→ Ch. 17). It can be life- or limb-threatening.

They can range from minor cuts to extensive deep contaminated wounds and crushed muscle. The types of injuries include:

- Incision – a cleanly cut wound, i.e. surgical
- Avulsion – implies tissue loss

- Degloving – form of laceration in which skin is sheared from the underlying fascia, usually by rotational forces, i.e. car tyre
- Contusion – crushing of the skin to split it
- Haematoma – like a contusion but skin is intact, may devitalize overlying skin if large enough; occasionally they need to be evacuated
- Abrasion – loss of superficial epithelium caused by friction
- Laceration – tearing of skin, the skin is stretched to its mechanical breaking point.

General principles of management:

1. Initial management is by ATLS protocols until immediate life-threatening injuries have been ruled out.
2. The injured limb should be examined for vascular compromise, nerve or tendon damage.
3. The patient should be taken to theatre and have thorough debridement of devitalized or necrotic tissue, cleansing and irrigation and removal of any foreign bodies (X-rays in two planes may be needed to locate some FBs).
4. If the wound is clean and <6–12 h old, then primary closure can be undertaken. If the wound is >12 h old, or grossly contaminated, then delayed primary closure should be performed. After 3–4 days if there is no oedema, erythema or pus, then the wound can be closed.
5. Antibiotics should be used in contaminated wounds or where dead tissue has been excised.
6. The tetanus status of the patient should be assessed. Some may require a booster dose. In cases of heavy contamination, i.e. farming injuries, they may require human anti-tetanus immunoglobulin.
7. Larger wounds that cannot be closed primarily, may need plastic surgical intervention or regular dressings to heal by secondary intention.

Vascular trauma (→ Ch. 15)

Skeletal trauma (→ Ch. 17)

Nerve injuries

Injuries to nerves can occur due to penetrating trauma or as a result of blunt injuries. Nerve injuries can be classified as follows:

Neurapraxia. A condition of transient physiological block without degeneration. There is continuity of the axons and the myelin sheaths remain intact. Function returns spontaneously in about 6 weeks.

Axonotmesis. Usually the result of compression or traction injuries causing disruption of the axons with intact myelin sheaths. The distal axons show degeneration but since the myelin sheaths are intact, return of function can be anticipated. The axons regenerate at the rate of about 1 mm/day. Return of function can be anticipated but may take many months.

Neurotmesis. This is division of the nerve in whole or in part which occurs after incised or lacerated wounds or may be a complication of a fracture. There is complete disruption of both the axon and the myelin sheath. Surgical repair is required. Residual neurological deficit is likely and neuroma may occur.

Symptoms and signs
These depend upon the site of injury to the nerve.

- **Upper trunk lesion of brachial plexus (Erb-Duchenne Palsy)** – injured by falls where the head is pulled away from the shoulder on the same side. Causes traction injury to C5–6 roots. Leads to paralysis of a range of muscles that leads to the classical 'waiters tip' position
- **Lower trunk lesion of brachial plexus (Klumpke's Palsy)** – upward traction of the arm, i.e. fall and grab to save themselves. Damages T1, leads to paralysis of intrinsic muscles of the hand causing a 'claw' deformity and an area of numbness on the inner forearm.
- **Long thoracic nerve** – can be damaged by blows to the posterior triangle of the neck. Leads to paralysis of serratus anterior and difficulty raising the arm above the head, also causes the classic 'winged scapula' deformity.
- **Axillary nerve** – damaged in fractures of the surgical neck of the humerus and anterior dislocations of the shoulder. Leads to loss of abduction (deltoid) and 'badge' patch loss of sensation over the shoulder.
- **Radial nerve** – damage to the radial nerve can occur at a variety of sites:
  - **Axilla:** secondary to fracture/dislocations of the proximal humerus. The patient will be unable to extend the elbow, wrist (wristdrop) or fingers. There is a variable area of sensory loss of the lateral aspect of the dorsum of the hand.
  - **Spiral groove:** secondary to mid-shaft fractures of the humerus. The triceps are preserved but the patient cannot flex the wrist (wristdrop) or fingers.
  - **Radial head:** fractures of the proximal radius and dislocations of the radial head lead to damage to the deep branch of the radial nerve. Supinator and extensor carpi radialis longus are unaffected and allow wrist extension.
  - **Wrist:** penetrating trauma at the wrist leads to damage to the superficial nerve and an area of sensory loss over the lateral aspect of the dorsum of the hand.
- **Ulnar nerve** – damage to the ulnar nerve can occur at the elbow or the wrist:
  - **Elbow:** secondary to fractures of the medial epicondyle or dislocations. Leads to a 'claw hand' deformity and loss of sensation in the medial one and a half fingers.
  - **Wrist:** penetrating trauma is the commonest cause. Results in a similar lesion but with a greater degree of clawing.
- **Median nerve** – damage to the median nerve can occur at the elbow or wrist:
  - **Elbow:** secondary to supracondylar fractures of the humerus, leads to loss of forearm pronation, weakness of wrist flexion and loss of sensation on the lateral palm and the radial three and a half digits.
  - **Wrist:** usually as a result of penetrating trauma, the thenar muscles are paralysed and opposition of the thumb is impossible. Sensory loss is as above.

- **Femoral nerve** – injury is rare, but may be damaged by penetrating groin wounds. The patient cannot extend the knee and there is sensory loss over the anteromedial aspect of the thigh, the medial side of the lower leg and the medial border of the foot as far as the ball of the big toe.
- **Sciatic nerve** – rare to have a complete injury; it may be damaged by penetrating wounds fractures of the pelvis and dislocations of the hip. It leads to loss of movement in all muscles below the knee and in the foot, the patient will have 'foot drop'. Sensation is lost below the knee apart from that supplied by the femoral nerve.
- **Common peroneal nerve** – injured relatively commonly, particularly by fractures of the neck of the fibula. Leads to foot drop and a loss of sensation to the dorsum of the foot and lower lateral leg.
- **Tibial nerve** – rarely injured due to its deep location. Penetrating trauma may lead to division and results in loss of plantar flexion and loss of sensation over the sole of the foot.
- **Obturator nerve** – occasionally injured by penetrating wounds or with anterior dislocation of the hip. Leads to loss of adductors and a small area of sensory loss over the medial thigh.

Investigations
Clinical. Nerve conduction.

Management
- Peripheral nerve injuries are frequently associated with limb trauma.
- A thorough inspection and examination of the limb should be carried out to establish the presence of a nerve lesion before any treatment is undertaken. This is important for medico-legal reasons.
- Nerve injuries associated with closed trauma do not usually require exploration. Physiotherapy will be needed to prevent contractures and muscle wasting while nerve recovery occurs.
- Penetrating injuries should be explored and nerve repair undertaken. Immediate surgical repair should be undertaken for digital nerves in clean wounds involving sharp lacerations. In contaminated wounds, repair may be delayed. It is wise to mark the nerve at the time of initial exploration with a suture to facilitate later identification. In extensive wounds with contusion and extensive tissue damage, e.g. gunshot wounds, nerve grafting may be necessary.

CHAPTER 5

Preoperative and postoperative care

PREOPERATIVE PREPARATION

> The purpose of preoperative evaluation is to identify the problems that may increase the operative risk and predispose to postoperative problems.

Assessment
1. *Full history*: present illness, past illnesses, bleeding tendencies, medication, allergies.
2. *Examination*: directed not only at the presenting complaint but also including a thorough examination of all systems, especially the cardiovascular and respiratory.
3. *Laboratory tests*: Hb, FBC and U&E for all but the most minor surgery.
4. *Radiographs*: CXR should be obtained in all patients with cancer, and cardiac, respiratory and renal disease. A routine preoperative CXR is unnecessary in young patients unless there are abnormalities on auscultation.
5. *ECG*: Obtain in all patients over the age of 40 and in those with a history of cardiac, respiratory or renal disease.

Principles of preoperative preparation
1. Correct any abnormalities that affect surgical risk.
2. Obtain informed consent. Explain all forms of possible treatment available for the condition. Explain the likely outcome without surgery. Explain the nature of the operation and the risks. Obtain the signature of the patient, parent or legal guardian. There is a special consent form for Jehovah's Witnesses.
3. Details of preparation:
   — nil by mouth for 4–6 h preoperatively
   — i.v. fluids
   — nasogastric aspiration

— bowel preparation

— medication planning, e.g. steroids, insulin, antihypertensives.

4. Laboratory investigations, e.g. blood sugar in diabetes, K^+ in renal failure.
5. Cross-match of blood if major operation with expected blood loss.
6. Physiotherapy – breathing exercises.
7. DVT prophylaxis, e.g. graded compression stockings (thromboembolic deterrent – TED), subcutaneous low molecular weight heparin, e.g. Clexane.
8. Anaesthetic premedication.

POSTOPERATIVE CARE

Monitor the patient's progress at least daily postoperatively and more frequently if indicated. Record in the notes at least daily.

1. *Detailed operation note* including intraoperative drugs; postoperative instructions should accompany the patient to the ward.
2. *Monitoring of vital signs.* Monitor BP, pulse and respiratory rate every 15 min until the patient is stable and thereafter hourly for 24 h. Monitor CVP after major surgery in the elderly and those with cardiac disease. Continuous ECG monitoring is advisable in those with cardiac disease or elderly patients undergoing major surgery.
3. *Early mobilization.* Patients requiring prolonged bed rest should be turned regularly from side to side to avoid pressure sores. Nurse on airbed. Protect sacrum and heels, especially in diabetics.
4. *Diet.* Nasogastric tubes are used in a number of abdominal operations. However, increasingly, these are taken out at the earliest opportunity to allow the patient to eat. If the patient is at high risk of ileus, then they may be retained for 24–48 h. In operations not involving the GI tract, the patient may drink when fully awake after a GA.
5. *Intravenous fluids.* Administer according to requirements – monitored by clinical examination, urine output and CVP.
6. *Intake/output chart.* Monitor closely to avoid dehydration or fluid overload.
7. *Urinary output.* If the patient is catheterized, monitoring is easy. If the urine output falls below 30 mL/h action is required. If the patient is not catheterized, inform the surgeon if urine has not been passed within 8 h postoperatively.
8. Medication:
   — Analgesics: the dose, frequency, and route of administration should be clearly indicated
   — Antibiotics as indicated
   — Routine medication as indicated; if the patient is 'nil by mouth', essential medication should be given parenterally.
9. Laboratory tests. After major procedures, the Hb, FBC and U&Es should be checked 24 h postoperatively and thereafter according to indications.
10. Radiographs and ECG. Carry out according to indications and not as routine. CXR may be necessary if pyrexia continues after 24 h postoperatively, if there is sputum production or chest signs.

PROGRESS

The following points should be noted:

- General condition, e.g. well, ill, improving, deteriorating; pain
- Vital signs, e.g. pyrexia, tachycardia
- Mobility
- Chest, e.g. clear, reduced air entry, consolidation
- Abdomen, e.g. distended, bowel sounds, tender
- Legs, e.g. DVT
- Wound, e.g. discharge, infection
- Intake/output
- Diet
- Results of any laboratory tests.

CONDITIONS AFFECTING SURGICAL RISK

GENERAL PROBLEMS IN SURGICAL PATIENTS

Age
Problems occur at the extremes of life. There are limits to cardiac, respiratory and renal reserves in the elderly. Fluid overload is tolerated poorly. Smaller doses of narcotics, sedatives and analgesics are required.

Obesity
This often results in poor wound healing and a higher incidence of respiratory problems. DVT and PE are more common. Pressure sores can develop. Delay elective surgery until the patient loses weight.

Compromised host
There is reduced response to trauma and infection, e.g. immunosuppressive drugs or uraemia. Malnutrition, e.g. vitamin deficiencies or liver disease, can also be a factor.

Allergies
Check for these preoperatively. Unsuspected reactions may occur. In severe cases, anaphylactic shock may result. Sensitivity to surgical dressings (e.g. Elastoplast) may occur.

Drugs
Current drugs should be monitored carefully, e.g. insulin and steroids. Diabetics may require conversion to sliding scale insulin (see below). Patients on steroids may need to continue their normal dose but with major surgery have additional steroid cover. Adjust anticoagulant therapy, e.g. conversion from warfarin to heparin over the perioperative period. Clopidogrel is contraindicated with regional anaesthesia (may cause epidural haematoma). Aspirin does not generally pose a problem in general surgical procedures. ACEI and ATII inhibitors should be stopped 24 h before surgery to prevent severe and refractive hypotension.

MEDICAL PROBLEMS IN SURGICAL PATIENTS

Cardiovascular

In elderly patients, the following are common: angina, cardiac failure, arrhythmias, valvular heart disease, hypertension, cerebrovascular disease, peripheral vascular disease. It is necessary to obtain a cardiology opinion, optimize medical treatment and assess operative risk. The decision to operate rests with the surgeon and anaesthetist.

MI and angina. Unstable angina and recent MI greatly increase the operative risk. Emergency surgery following recent MI has a mortality of 30%. Delay elective surgery for 6 months.

Cardiac failure. Treat prior to surgery. Stabilize at least 1 month prior to surgery. Digoxin. Diuretic. Check K^+ prior to surgery. Mild CCF well controlled with digoxin and diuretics carries little risk. CCF with dyspnoea on exertion, orthopnoea and PND carries a significant risk.

Arrhythmias. Uncontrolled AF may cause perioperative CCF. Digitalize adequately preoperatively. Some degrees of heart block require a prophylactic temporary transvenous pacemaker. Check digoxin levels in patients who have bradycardia. Arrhythmias developing during surgery may be due to hypoxia, hypercapnia or high or low K^+.

Valvular heart disease. May result in MI, CCF, arrhythmias, embolism or bacterial endocarditis in the perioperative period. Newly discovered murmurs require a cardiology opinion. Elective cases should be deferred until the murmur has been evaluated. Prophylactic antibiotics are important in the perioperative period and for patients with prosthetic valves. Check if patient is on anticoagulants.

Hypertension. Mild hypertension without renal or cardiac complications does not significantly affect surgical risk. Control BP at or below 160/95 mmHg. Defer and investigate elective cases with newly diagnosed hypertension. Check K^+ in patients on diuretics. Severe and poorly controlled hypertension should be adequately controlled prior to surgery.

Cerebrovascular disease. High risk of intraoperative CVA. Previous history of TIAs or stroke. Carotid bruits. Aspirin may be protective. Avoid intraoperative hypotension.

Peripheral vascular disease. Patients with peripheral ischaemia may develop arterial thrombosis if hypotensive. Take care to avoid pressure sores, which may not heal and lead to the need for amputation.

Respiratory disease

This is a major cause of postoperative morbidity and mortality in the elderly. COPD, asthma, and bronchiectasis are precipitating causes. Smoking, obesity, old age, general debility and cardiac disease are contributory. Preoperative investigations include CXR, lung function tests (e.g. FEV_1, peak expiratory flow rate, spirometry), sputum culture, ABG.

Perioperative management of respiratory disease
- Stop smoking. Preferably 4 weeks prior to surgery
- Preoperative chest physiotherapy and breathing exercises
- Drugs, e.g. bronchodilators, nebulized salbutamol, antibiotics
- Anaesthetic – local or spinal if possible
- Analgesia. Avoid narcotic analgesics that may lead to respiratory depression. Consider epidural pain relief
- Postoperative physiotherapy
- Early mobilization.

Renal disease

This should be managed jointly with a nephrologist. Symptoms of renal failure do not usually become apparent until 80–90% of renal function has been lost and there is little renal reserve.

Mild impairment of renal function. Mildly raised urea or creatinine. Refer to a nephrologist and delay elective surgery until a diagnosis has been reached and appropriate treatment instituted. Deterioration of renal function may occur after major surgery, especially if dehydration is allowed to occur. Adequate preoperative rehydration. Monitor CVP. Caution with nephrotoxic drugs, e.g. gentamicin.

Grossly impaired renal function (non-dialysis dependent). Inadequate management may precipitate end-stage renal failure. Problems include fluid overload, dehydration, hyperkalaemia, metabolic acidosis. Chronic anaemia occurs but patients are well adapted to this. Uraemia is immunosuppressive and prophylactic antibiotics are required. Uraemia alters platelet function and bleeding may be a problem.

Dialysis-dependent renal failure
Haemodialysis. Dialysis should take place 24 h prior to surgery to allow the effects of heparin to wear off. Check U&Es, creatinine, and HCO_3 post-dialysis. CXR to exclude pulmonary oedema. Check K^+ postoperatively as hyperkalaemia may occur following surgery under GA. If possible, delay postoperative dialysis for 24 h in view of risk of bleeding with heparin.

Continuous ambulatory peritoneal dialysis (CAPD). Check U&Es prior to surgery. If abdominal surgery, CAPD may need to be discontinued and patient instituted on haemodialysis via a central line until intra-abdominal healing has occurred.

Hepatic disease

There is a high incidence of morbidity and mortality with cirrhosis. Predisposing factors are anaemia, electrolyte disturbances, abnormal clotting, malnutrition, abnormal drug metabolism, ascites, portal hypertension. Defective synthesis of clotting factors in the liver and thrombocytopenia due to hypersplenism may result in excessive bleeding. The Child–Pugh score can be used to assess the 'hepatic reserve', the higher the score the greater the operative risk (measures albumin, bilirubin, prothrombin time and the presence and severity of ascites and encephalopathy).

Care must be taken to assess a past history of jaundice. This may be due to hepatitis, obstructive jaundice or haemolytic disease.

Hepatitis. Hepatitis A in the past carries little risk; hepatitis B and C may be carried permanently. Check HBsAg.

Obstructive jaundice. There is usually a clear history. Surgery will usually have been necessary to deal with the problem.

Haemolytic disease. May cause jaundice.

Perioperative management of patients with liver disease/obstructive jaundice
1. Full clinical examination
2. Hb, FBC, U&Es, Cr, LFTs, PT, glucose
3. Correct hypoglycaemia
4. Correct coagulation defect, e.g. vitamin K parenterally, but in severe disease FFP may be required. Platelet transfusion
5. Avoid saline infusions (risk of hypernatraemia)
6. Avoid hepatotoxic drugs
7. Avoid drugs metabolized by liver, e.g. opiates
8. Correct protein deficiency
9. Antibiotics.

The main postoperative problems are bleeding, infection, and poor wound healing.

Haematological disease

Anaemia. Mild anaemia, e.g. Hb >10 g/dL, imposes little risk. Anaemia may be related to the condition for which surgery is being undertaken, e.g. GI cancer. Hb <10 g/dL should be treated by preoperative iron therapy or transfusion. Unsuspected anaemia noted prior to elective surgery should be investigated and the operation deferred.

Polycythaemia. Hb >18 g/dL. PCV ↑. Risks of arterial and venous thrombosis. Venesect prior to surgery. Myelosuppressive drugs may be required.

Bleeding disorders

Inherited. Haemophilia is treated with cryoprecipitate preoperatively and until the danger of postoperative haemorrhage is over. Von Willebrand's disease is treated with FFP or cryoprecipitate.

Anticoagulant therapy. Warfarin – the patient may have a history of thromboembolic disease, valvular heart disease or prosthetic heart valves. Anticoagulation may need to be continued during surgery, albeit at a reduced level. The safest procedure is to discontinue warfarin 3–4 days preoperatively and start heparin i.v. This can be more readily adjusted and is more easily reversed (with i.v. protamine sulphate) if bleeding occurs. If a patient's INR needs to be reduced for urgent operation, then they may be given vitamin K (takes 4 h to work), FFP or in extreme cases, can be given prothrombin complex concentrate (Beriplex) that will reverse the warfarin in under 30 min.

Disseminated intravascular coagulation (DIC). Coagulation and fibrinolysis occur simultaneously. Surgically important causes precipitating the condition include

Gram-negative septicaemia, acute pancreatitis, malignancy, major surgery, e.g. ruptured aortic aneurysm. Clinical features include extensive bruising, oozing from drip and venepuncture sites, oozing from the wound, tracheostomy or bowel occurring in a severely ill patient. Diagnosis is confirmed by PT (prolonged); PTT (prolonged); thrombocytopenia; decreased fibrinogen level; raised FDPs. Treatment is by FFP, platelets and cryoprecipitate. Heparin i.v. may halt the coagulation element. Aggressive treatment of the underlying disease.

Clotting disorders

Acquired. Anti-phospholipid syndrome (associated with SLE; there is a higher risk of venous and arterial thrombosis. However, unless there is a history of thrombosis, no further intervention is required other than normal DVT prophylaxis) and malignant thrombosis associated with advanced malignancy (all patients are considered high risk for a DVT).

Inherited. These include antithrombin deficiency, protein C and protein S deficiency, Factor V Leiden and Prothrombin 20210A. These patients will require rigorous DVT prophylaxis, particularly if they have had a previous thrombosis.

Sickle cell anaemia.
These patients are at increased risk of surgical complications. Homozygote patients have 90–100% HbS. They may require transfusion if they are anaemic; or to decrease the amount of HbS. Heterozygote patients or those with the sickle cell trait have 20–40% HbS and are generally asymptomatic. Surgery and anaesthesia may lead to dehydration, hypoxia and vascular stasis. These may then lead to a sickle cell crisis with pain and ischaemia (even in trait patients). This can be avoided by adequate hydration, supplemental oxygen and avoiding blood stasis (e.g. pneumatic compression stockings and avoidance of the use of tourniquets).

Endocrine disease

Diabetes. This poses numerous risks and affects many systems. Complications include:

- Vasculopathy: heart – increased risk of MI; peripheral vascular disease (PVD) – risk of lower limb ischaemia with ulcers and gangrene; risk of stroke
- Nephropathy – risk of CRF
- Neuropathy – peripheral neuropathy with risk of pressure ulcers on heels and autonomic neuropathy with risk of cardiac arrest and gastric stasis with aspiration
- Retinopathy leading to blindness – problems with management of blind patient in unfamiliar surroundings; anticoagulation, if needed, may make retinal haemorrhage worse
- Increased incidence of infection.

The principles of management of diabetes in the perioperative period depend on whether patients are insulin dependent, on oral hypoglycaemics or controlled by diet.

Insulin-dependent
1. Admit 2 days preoperatively: CXR, ECG, FBC, U&Es, glucose, glycosylated Hb (HbA$_{1C}$)
2. Establish good diabetic control (glucose 4–10 mmol/L)

3. First on morning list. Check glucose
4. Dextrose/insulin/K^+ infusion
5. Check glucose intraoperatively and U&Es postoperatively
6. Monitor glucose regularly in early postoperative period
7. Continue infusion until full oral diet is established and then reinstitute normal insulin regime.

Oral hypoglycaemics
1. Review control
2. Major surgery: convert to insulin/glucose/K^+ infusion as above
3. Minor surgery: omit oral hypoglycaemic agent. Check blood sugar. If greater than 13 mmol/L give small dose of subcutaneous insulin.

Diabetics controlled by diet alone
1. Review control
2. If preoperative control is adequate, no other measure required other than routine check of blood sugar pre- and postoperatively.

Thyroid disease

Hypothyroidism. Patients should be euthyroid prior to elective surgery. Emergency surgery in a patient who is clinically hypothyroid presents a very high risk. Patients are at risk from MI, hypotension, hypothermia, hypoglycaemia and hyponatraemia (may cause convulsions) and coma (hypothyroid coma has a 50% mortality).

Hyperthyroidism. Patients should be euthyroid prior to elective surgery ($\rightarrow$ Ch. 11). Hyperthyroidism is associated with arrhythmias and hypertension. A thyroid crisis is associated with oversecretion and may be triggered by infection. This presents as hyperthermia, arrhythmias, cardiorespiratory failure and coma.

Adrenal disease

Adrenocortical insufficiency. This may be due to destruction of the adrenal gland by autoimmune disease, tumour, infection, infarction or the sudden withdrawal of steroid therapy. It should be considered in all patients with postoperative hypotension that is refractory to fluid replacement or inotropes with no obvious cause. Patients taking steroids, or who have taken steroids in the last 9 months, should have supplemental steroid cover. A guide to additional hydrocortisone cover is 25 mg i.v. hydrocortisone at induction for minor surgery; 25 mg i.v. hydrocortisone at induction; followed by 100 mg in the postoperative period for moderate surgery, and 100 mg hydrocortisone on induction followed by 100 mg 6-hourly for 48 h or until blood pressure is stable, in major surgery.

Cushing's syndrome. Patients have excess levels of glucocorticoids and are at risk of hypertension, hypokalaemia, hypernatraemia and diabetes. May be corrected by metyrapone which inhibits steroid synthesis. These patients are often obese, making surgery more challenging with poor wound healing and increased risk of respiratory complications.

AMERICAN SOCIETY OF ANESTHESIOLOGISTS' CLASSIFICATION OF PHYSICAL STATUS (ASA GRADING)

When an operation is planned and there are problems concerning the patient's fitness for anaesthetic, then the anaesthetist should be involved as soon as possible. The American Society of Anesthesiologists has produced a grading system that attempts to quantify the risks of anaesthetizing patients with various clinical conditions.

The ASA grading system for quantifying anaesthetic risk is as follows:

I. A healthy patient with no systemic disease process, e.g. a fit patient with an inguinal hernia.
II. A patient with mild to moderate systemic disease process caused either by the condition to be treated surgically or by other pathological process which does not limit the patient's activity in any way, e.g. mild diabetic, treated hypertensive.
III. A patient with a severe systemic disturbance from any cause and which imposes a definite functional limitation on the patient, e.g. severely limiting organic heart disease, severe diabetes with vascular complications, severe COPD.
IV. A patient with severe systemic disease which is a constant threat to life, e.g. severe unstable angina, advanced liver failure.
V. A moribund patient who is unlikely to survive 24 hours with or without surgery, e.g. ruptured aortic aneurysm in a patient with severe COPD.

POSTOPERATIVE COMPLICATIONS

All operations carry a risk of complications (a Classification is shown in Table 5.1). Complications may be divided as:

- General complications of any operation
- Specific complications of individual operations
- Timing of complication, e.g. immediate, early or late.

Specific complications and timing of complications are discussed in relation to specific operations and conditions in the various chapters in this book.

HAEMORRHAGE

Early postoperative

Inadequate haemostasis, unrecognized damage to blood vessels, defective vascular anastomosis, slipped ligature, massive blood transfusion without adequate clotting factors, use of intraoperative anticoagulants, e.g. in vascular surgery. Treatment depends on cause. Check clotting screen. Surgical re-exploration is usually required.

Secondary haemorrhage

Several days postoperatively. Related to infection, which erodes vessels. Treatment of the infection and appropriate surgery to deal with the bleeding.

TABLE 5.1 Postoperative complications

Haemorrhage	Early postoperative Secondary haemorrhage
Wound	Infection Bleeding Haematoma Seroma Suture sinus Breakdown: • burst abdomen • incisional hernia • anastomotic breakdown: peritonitis, abscess, fistula
Cardiovascular	Cardiac arrest MI Pulmonary oedema Arrhythmias DVT
Lung	Atelectasis Aspiration Pneumonia PE Pulmonary oedema Pneumothorax ARDS
Cerebral	Confusion: • sepsis • electrolyte/glucose • hypoxia • alcohol withdrawal Stroke
Urinary	Acute retention UTI Acute renal failure
Gastrointestinal	Paralytic ileus Mechanical obstruction Acute gastric dilatation Constipation
Other	Pressure sores

WOUND PROBLEMS

Infection

Incidence varies according to type of surgery and potential for contamination (→ Ch. 6). Factors leading to increased risk of wound infection include: haematoma, poor nutritional state, diabetes mellitus, reduced immunity, nasal carriage of *Staphylococcus aureus*.

Symptoms and signs

Painful red incision with discharge. General malaise. Examination reveals pyrexia, red, hot, tender wound. A purulent discharge may be apparent.

Treatment
1. If pus is present, it should be evacuated.
2. Culture and sensitivity of pus.
3. Appropriate antibiotic if cellulitis present or compromised patient, e.g. diabetic, steroids.
4. If cavity present, pack with alginate dressings, e.g. Sorbsan. A larger cavity may require a period of vacuum assisted closure, e.g. VAC.

Wound breakdown
Factors which delay wound healing include: old age, obesity, malnutrition, poor vascularity, sepsis, carcinoma, jaundice, uraemia, steroids, haematomas, raised intra-abdominal pressure.

Burst abdomen
This is a sudden bursting of the wound revealing bowel. This is often preceded by discharge of a salmon pink fluid (Pink sign). Usual cause is inadequate suturing of abdominal wall. Coughing, straining at stool, may be contributory. Cover the abdominal contents with sterile saline-soaked packs. Return the patient to theatre and repair with large bites of whole thickness of the abdominal wall using deep tension sutures. This complication has a mortality around 20%.

Incisional hernia
The overall incidence is about 10%. In addition to factors delaying wound healing, causes include poor suture technique, raised intra-abdominal pressure (e.g. paralytic ileus), coughing, straining (e.g. constipation), prostatism. Rarely a broken suture is responsible. These herniae often have a wide neck and strangulation is rare.

Treatment
If the patient is unfit, a surgical belt may be worn. If the patient is fit, surgical repair should be carried out.

Anastomotic breakdown
This is a major cause of postoperative morbidity and mortality after bowel surgery.

Causes
These include:

- Poor surgical technique
- Ischaemia at the anastomosis
- Perioperative sepsis
- Distal obstruction
- Residual inflammatory disease, e.g. Crohn's or malignant disease
- General condition, e.g. uraemia, jaundice, malnutrition, steroids.

Anastomotic breakdown may result in generalized peritonitis, paracolic abscess, abscesses between loops of bowel or fistula formation. However, presentation can be surprisingly subtle with mild pyrexia, persistent tachycardia and general failure to progress as the only signs of anastomotic leak (→ Chs 6 and 14).

Haematoma

This is a localized collection of blood beneath the wound. May be an obvious tender mass with surrounding bruising. Treatment is by aspiration percutaneously or may require opening of the wound and clot evacuation.

Seroma

This is a localized collection of serous fluid. Often where skin flaps have been raised, e.g. chest wall in mastectomy, or where lymphatics have been divided, e.g. groin or axilla. Examination reveals a non-tender fluctuant mass. Small areas may be left and may absorb spontaneously or they may be needled percutaneously. Large ones may need formal drainage.

Stitch sinus

Sutures may act as nidus of infection, especially at the knot. Less common, since absorbable sutures and monofilament nylons replaced silk. Often the suture will extrude through the sinus spontaneously and the sinus will then heal. Occasionally, exploration and removal of the suture is required.

CARDIOVASCULAR PROBLEMS

Cardiac arrest following surgery is usually due to an underlying cardiac condition aggravated by a precipitating cause, e.g. hypoxia, shock, MI, anaesthetic overdose, hyperkalaemia, hypokalaemia or drug reactions. Cardiac arrest may follow respiratory arrest, e.g. following an obstructed airway (laryngeal oedema or tongue blocking airway) or inhalation of vomit. DVT may follow prolonged bed rest.

LUNG PROBLEMS

Lung complications are a common postoperative problem. They include atelectasis, aspiration, pneumonia, PE, pulmonary oedema, pneumothorax and ARDS.

Atelectasis

Mucus is retained in the bronchial tree, blocking the smaller bronchi and resulting in absorption of alveolar air with collapse of an area of lung. Infection may then occur and progress to pneumonia. Minor degrees are common. Smoking and COPD are predisposing factors. Anaesthesia may increase bronchial secretions and depress ciliary action. Postoperative abdominal pain inhibits coughing and allows secretions to accumulate.

Symptoms and signs

Minor atelectasis may be accompanied by mild pyrexia alone; greater degrees are accompanied by dyspnoea, tachypnoea, rapid pulse and elevated temperature. Major degrees may be accompanied by cyanosis and respiratory collapse. The signs include widespread rales, reduced air entry and dullness to percussion.

Diagnosis

Clinical:

- CXR
- ABG
- Sputum culture.

Treatment

Minor degrees require only chest physiotherapy. Adequate pain relief facilitates mobility and physiotherapy. Nebulized bronchodilators. More severe degrees may require bronchoscopy to remove mucus plugs. The most severe case may require intubation and ventilation.

Aspiration

Aspiration pneumonitis following inhalation of acidic gastric contents is known as Mendelson's syndrome. This tends to affect the right lung more than the left as the right bronchus is wider and more in line with the trachea. Aspiration may occur during induction, or at the termination, of anaesthesia. It may also occur in patients with bowel obstruction or paralytic ileus who vomit in the early postoperative period. Prevention includes preoperative 'nil by mouth' in elective cases, nasogastric suction in the emergency case and cricoid compression in 'crash' induction. If aspiration occurs, suction, intubation and saline lavage should be carried out. Steroids may help. Antibiotics will prevent super-added infection. Oxygen by mask.

Pneumonia

Predisposing factors include smoking, atelectasis, COPD, aspiration, debilitated patients.

Symptoms and signs

Cough, respiratory distress, sputum. Signs include fever, tachypnoea, tachycardia, cyanosis, consolidation and rales.

Diagnosis

- Sputum culture
- CXR
- ABG.

Treatment

Chest physiotherapy. Antibiotics, e.g. Amoxicillin or Septrin until results of culture are known. Oxygen by mask. If no improvement with basic measures the patient may need to be moved to a critical care facility for CPAP or intubation and ventilation.

Pulmonary oedema

Usually elderly patient with compromised cardiac function or young patient with history of cardiac or renal disease.

Symptoms and signs

Tachypnoea, tachycardia, orthopnoea, raised JVP, pink frothy sputum, widespread crepitations.

Diagnosis

- CXR
- Raised JVP
- Elevated CVP.

Treatment

Stop i.v. fluids. Sit patient upright. Oxygen by face mask. Give i.v. furosemide. Small doses of opiates. GTN/i.v. infusion of nitrates.

Pulmonary embolus (PE)

Complication of silent or overt DVT. Passage of a clot from pelvic or leg veins into the pulmonary artery. Major PE with overt DVT is usually obvious clinically. In some cases, diagnosis relies on a high index of clinical suspicion.

Symptoms and signs

Usually 4–10 days postoperatively. Sudden dyspnoea and collapse. Hypotension. Pleuritic chest pain. Haemoptysis. Pleural rub.

Diagnosis

- CXR: wedge-shaped collapse
- ECG: right heart strain, S1, Q3, T3 pattern
- ABG: hypoxia
- V/Q scan: mismatch of ventilation/perfusion areas, i.e. ventilation normal but perfusion deficient (rarely performed now)
- CT pulmonary angiogram (CTPA) – most commonly used test
- Pulmonary angiography is most accurate – used prior to surgery or thrombolysis.

Treatment

- *Patients without shock.* They may be treated by i.v. heparin sufficient to maintain the APTT at 2.5 × normal. Start warfarin after 2 days of heparin and continue for 6–9 months. With recurrent pulmonary emboli it should be continued for life.
- *Profound shock.* Inotropic support. Urgent pulmonary angiography. Thrombolytic therapy or pulmonary embolectomy.
- *Recurrent pulmonary embolus.* This should be treated by insertion of a filter, e.g. Greenfield filter percutaneously via the venous route into the IVC.

Pneumothorax

Rare complication of surgery. Rupture of subpleural bulla or complication of insertion of central line perioperatively.

Symptoms and signs

Respiratory distress. Reduced breath sounds and hyper-resonance to percussion of affected side.

Treatment

- Small: treat expectantly
- Large: chest drain.

Adult respiratory distress syndrome (ARDS; shock lung)

This is acute respiratory failure with tachypnoea, hypoxia, decreased lung compliance and diffuse pulmonary infiltrates on CXR. The exact aetiology is unknown but there is interference with the pulmonary epithelial/endothelial cell

TABLE 5.2 Causes of ARDS

Infection	Septicaemia
Inhalation	Smoke, vomit, water, high O_2 concentrations, chlorine, ammonia
Embolism	Fat, amniotic fluid, air
Cerebral	Head injury, cerebral haemorrhage
Drugs	Opiates, barbiturates
Others	Pancreatitis, DIC, blood transfusion, cardiopulmonary bypass, major trauma with shock

interface with increased interstitial oedema, vascular congestion and ultimately fibrosis (Table 5.2).

Symptoms and signs
Present a few days after diagnosis of a serious underlying condition. Breathlessness, deterioration in clinical condition.

Investigations
● CXR shows whiteout with sparing of costophrenic angles
● ABG: hypoxia resistant to oxygen administration
● May be difficult to distinguish from pulmonary oedema in early stages but latter usually shows cardiomegaly on CXR and response to diuretics.

Treatment
1. Treat the underlying disease, e.g. septicaemia.
2. Treat the pulmonary problem:
   — mechanical ventilation to maintain PaO_2. PEEP may be necessary
   — monitor fluid balance. CVP to monitor right atrial pressure. Left atrial pressure is monitored as pulmonary wedge pressure with a Swann–Ganz catheter
   — careful monitoring for development of secondary lung infection. Administration of appropriate antibiotics
   — renal failure is a common complication. Early administration of dopamine in renal doses may be appropriate.

The mortality rate for ARDS is 70–90%.

CEREBRAL PROBLEMS

Confusion
Confusion postoperatively is not uncommon, especially at night in the elderly. However, there may be an underlying cause, e.g. sepsis, hypoxia, alcohol withdrawal, electrolyte or glucose imbalance, cerebral bleed, postoperative pancreatitis, opiate analgesia.

Investigations
● Hb
● FBC
● U&Es

- Glucose
- Amylase
- ABGs
- Blood culture
- Urine analysis
- Sputum culture
- CXR
- Brain scan.

Treatment

- Correct electrolyte or glucose disturbance.
- Correct hypoxia – 35% oxygen by mask or nasal cannula.
- Investigate and treat any sepsis.
- Tranquillizers may be required, e.g. chlorpromazine or haloperidol.
- For acute alcohol withdrawal, i.v. clomethiazole and parenteral vitamin B may be used, although 60 mL of medicinal brandy may be more appropriate.

Stroke

May occur in the elderly postoperatively. Avoid intraoperative hypotension in patients with TIAs or carotid bruits.

URINARY TRACT PROBLEMS

Acute retention

Common postoperatively, especially in elderly males.

Symptoms and signs

Usually suprapubic discomfort, although this may not be apparent because the patient has been given analgesia postoperatively. Usually nurse reports that patient has not passed urine for several hours postoperatively. Examination reveals a palpable bladder dull to percussion. If the patient has no desire to micturate and the bladder is not palpable, oliguria must be considered and corrected.

Treatment

Conservative. Ensure adequate analgesics. Stand patient up. If no benefit, and the patient is fit enough, take to bathroom and leave tap running to encourage micturition. If conservative measures fail, pass a urinary catheter.

Urinary tract infection (UTI)

This is common, especially in females. Catheterization may predispose.

Symptoms and signs

Dysuria/frequency/dribbling/smelly urine. May be found on investigation of undiagnosed pyrexia postoperatively.

Investigations

MSSU.

Treatment
Appropriate antibiotic.

Acute renal failure (ARF)
Oliguria is passage of <30 mL of urine per hour. Anuria is failure to pass any urine.

Causes
Prerenal. Reduced cardiac output, shock, e.g. hypovolaemic, cardiogenic, septic.

Renal. Pre-existing renal disease, e.g. diabetes, glomerulonephritis. Nephrotoxic drugs, e.g. gentamicin. Myoglobinuria in crush syndrome. Haemoglobinuria with haemolysis.

Postrenal. Obstruction, e.g. damage to ureters, benign prostatic hypertrophy.

Treatment of anuria/oliguria
1. Check that the catheter is patent. If patient not catheterized, then pass catheter.
2. Check BP to exclude hypotension.
3. Fluid challenge, e.g. 1 L normal saline over 1 h. Give sufficient fluid to restore CVP. If elderly patient, a fluid challenge is best done with CVP monitoring.
4. If no improvement in urine output after adequate fluid administration and the BP is low then the patient may require transfer to a critical care/high dependency facility for inotropic support.
5. Check ABG (for acidosis), K^+ and HCO_3^-. Serum urea and creatinine. ECG (signs of hyperkalaemia).
6. Stop any nephrotoxic drugs.
7. Contact renal physician and manage jointly. In the presence of hyperkalaemia and metabolic acidosis, dialysis will be required until a diuresis ensues. Fluid overload may be treated with CVVH.
8. Furosemide is generally not used to increase a patient's urine output unless they are in CCF.

GASTROINTESTINAL PROBLEMS

Paralytic ileus
This is the cessation of GI motility. Aetiological factors include fractures of the spine and pelvis, retroperitoneal haemorrhage, peritonitis, hypokalaemia, drugs, e.g. ganglion blockers and anticholinergic agents, abdominal surgery, immobilization. Atony of the bowel may be expected for 24–48 h postoperatively. Paralytic ileus continuing after 48 h may have an underlying cause.

Symptoms and signs
Abdominal distension, vomiting, constipation. Tense tympanitic abdomen. Absent bowel sounds (Table 5.3).

Investigations
AXR: gaseous distension with fluid levels throughout the large and small bowel.

TABLE 5.3 Factors distinguishing paralytic ileus and mechanical obstruction

	Ileus	Obstruction
Time	Usually settles in 3–4 days	May persist longer
Bowel sounds	Absent	High-pitched and tinkling
Pain	Painless	Colicky abdominal pain
AXR	General gaseous dilatation of small and large bowel	Localized small bowel distension with absent gas in colon and rectum

Treatment
1. Pass NG tube and aspirate hourly.
2. Ensure adequate hydration.
3. Correct any potassium imbalance.
4. Paralytic ileus rarely lasts for more than 4 days.
5. If symptoms persist, look for continuing cause and exclude mechanical obstruction with an abdominal CT.

Mechanical obstruction

Early (within 2 weeks of surgery)
May be due to *fibrinous* adhesions. Obstruction may settle with i.v. fluids and nasogastric suction or it may progress and require laparotomy.

Late (after 2 weeks)
May be due to obstruction by adhesions – fibrous bands arising as part of peritoneal healing. Symptoms may settle with i.v. fluids and nasogastric suction. If they do not or signs of strangulation appear, laparotomy will be necessary.

Gastric dilatation
Acute gastric dilatation may occur in the early postoperative period and may be associated with shock. Vomiting with aspiration may occur.

Treatment
NG suction, which may aspirate several litres of brownish/black fluid with altered blood. Fluid and electrolyte losses must be replaced.

Constipation
Uncomfortable for patient. Precipitating factors include starvation, dehydration, inactivity, opiates.

Treatment
1. Check daily if patient has had bowels open. Do not delay treatment.
2. Lactulose should be given as soon as the patient is eating.
3. Glycerine suppositories. PR to exclude faecal impaction.
4. Enemas may be required. With faecal impaction, oil enemas may be necessary.
5. Attention to diet. High-fibre diet or bulking agent.

POSTOPERATIVE PAIN RELIEF

> Pain must be expected from most surgical procedures but it usually subsides gradually over the first few days. Patients respond differently to pain. However, excess pain in the postoperative period may be a symptom of a developing complication.

METHODS OF POSTOPERATIVE PAIN CONTROL

Full explanation of the operation and postoperative course and an attempt to relieve preoperative anxiety may reduce the severity of postoperative pain.

Oral analgesia

First-line analgesia for patients that are tolerating diet usually used for mild to moderate pain, e.g. groin hernia repair or varicose vein surgery. Suitable agents include paracetamol, NSAIDs, nefopam, weak opioids such as codeine and oral morphine (Oramorph).

Parenteral analgesia

Intermittent intramuscular opiates. Commonly used. Usually given p.r.n., 4-hourly. Many patients still complain of pain.

Intravenous opiates. Given for acute pain. Dose titrated to gain adequate pain relief. Beware respiratory depression in the elderly and patients with renal failure.

PCA pump. This device allows patients to self-administer a preset dose of analgesic drug by pressing a button connected to a pump. This in turn is connected to an i.v. cannula. There is a preset interval before the infusion will deliver another dose, i.e. the 'lock-out' time. This is a very effective method of pain control but is expensive.

PCEA pump. This is similar to the above but is administered as an epidural.

Spinal. LA is placed in the intrathecal space. This allows a period of regional anaesthesia for several hours or may be 'topped' up if a catheter is left *in situ*. Not used for pain relief in the postoperative period.

Epidural. A catheter is placed in the epidural space and LA or opioids may be infused. This can be as a continuous infusion or as a patient controlled pump.

Intercostal nerve blocks

These are useful for upper abdominal surgery or in thoracic injuries, e.g. fractured ribs

Direct infiltration

Bupivacaine, a long-acting local anaesthetic, can be injected directly into the wound, e.g. for repair of an inguinal hernia. It may be also injected around the nerve supplying the area of the wound, e.g. the ilioinguinal nerve in hernia repair. Infiltration of local anaesthesia may be continuous with catheters placed in between the muscles of the abdominal wall in which the sensory nerves run.

BLOOD TRANSFUSION

Blood transfusion is not without risk. Decision to transfuse blood should have a clear indication and alternative therapy, e.g. plasma substitutes for hypovolaemia and iron therapy for anaemia should be considered first. Screening programmes for HIV, hepatitis B and C have made transfusions safer. Unless a patient has severe cardiorespiratory disease (generally need Hb >10 g/dL in these patients) there is no change in cardiac output until Hb falls below 7 g/dL. In chronic anaemia, even lower levels may be tolerated.

There are numerous different blood types but the two most common systems are the ABO system and the Rhesus status. ABO is divided into type O (46%), A (42%), B (9%) and AB (3%). Rhesus is divided into positive (85%) and negative (15%). Therefore O Rh positive is the most common and AB Rh negative is the rarest.

BLOOD PRODUCTS AND ALTERNATIVES TO TRANSFUSION

Blood products used in clinical practice include:

- *Whole blood.* Rarely used.
- *Packed cells.* Used in major haemorrhage or treatment of anaemia. Can be stored at 5°C for approximately 30 days. Increases Hb by 1 g/dL per unit transfused.
- *Human albumin* (5 or 20%). Main use is in hypoproteinaemic state, e.g. nephrotic syndrome, ascites in chronic liver disease. Also used as a plasma substitute, e.g. in burns.
- *FFP.* Contains all the clotting factors in plasma. Dose is 10–15 mL/kg. Main indications for use include reversal of warfarin, DIC, massive transfusion and liver disease.
- *Cryoprecipitate.* Contains FVIII, FXIII, fibrinogen and von Willebrand's factor. It is pooled from 10–20 adult donors. Used in hypofibrinogenaemia (<1 g/dL), massive transfusion, DIC and haemophilia.
- *Platelet concentrates.* Stored at room temperature for 5–7 days. Main indications are for massive transfusions, DIC and thrombocytopaenia with active bleeding or in a thrombocytopaenic patient requiring surgery.

Alternatives to the use of stored blood include:

- *Autologous transfusion.* This includes preoperative autologous donation (blood is donated by the patient prior to surgery for that same patient), acute normovolaemic haemodilution (blood is removed immediately preoperatively; this is replaced with crystalloid) and perioperative red cell salvage (includes blood from drains being re-transfused, e.g. after knee replacements and cell salvage intraoperatively).
- *Pharmacological methods.* These include aprotinin (a serine protease inhibitor that inhibits fibrinolysis and has been shown to reduce blood loss in cardiac surgery), tranexamic acid (inhibits fibrinolysis), desmopressin (increases factor VIII – used in mild haemophilia and von Willebrand's disease) and erythropoietin (can be used to stimulate red blood cell production preoperatively).

- *Blood substitutes*. Largely in the research stage. However, some oxygen carrying fluids such as fluorinated organic compounds, have been tested.
- *Plasma substitutes*. Include gelatin solutions (Gelofusine, Haemaccel). They are used to restore circulating volume until blood becomes available.

CLINICAL ASPECTS OF BLOOD TRANSFUSION

1. The patient's ABO and Rh groups are established.
2. Each unit of group compatible blood is then cross-matched against the recipient's serum.
3. Minor incompatibilities may occur and require further cross-matching.
4. If blood is required urgently, O negative (universal donor) may be given in an emergency with comparative safety.
5. 'Group and save'. In some operations, transfusion is unlikely but occasionally possible. Blood is taken preoperatively and grouping assessed. The serum is retained in the laboratory and blood is cross-matched as required.
6. For some operations, blood should be immediately available. Blood is grouped, cross-matched and available on the day of surgery.
7. Mistakes with mismatched transfusions often have serious and occasionally fatal consequences. To avoid mistakes, blood specimens sent to the laboratory must be carefully labelled with the name, date of birth and hospital unit number of the patient.
8. Each unit of blood subsequently transfused must be carefully matched to make sure that the label of the bag of blood corresponds with the name, blood group and hospital number of the patient.

COMPLICATIONS OF BLOOD TRANSFUSION

Acute

Haemolytic transfusion reaction. This is secondary to ABO incompatibility and is usually due to human error. Patient may have a temperature, shortness of breath, rigors, loin pain, hypotension and oliguria. Jaundice and haemoglobinuria may occur. If the patient is unconscious, a pyrexia and a drop of BP >10 mmHg should cause concern. Initial management includes ABC, stopping the transfusion, checking the identity of the patient, checking blood group of patient and donor blood group, taking blood for haemolytic screen and clotting. Management involves maintaining a diuresis with fluids and mannitol. ARF may occur and should be treated appropriately. Reaction to other red blood cell antibodies is not as dramatic.

Allergic reaction. Itching, skin rashes and urticaria may occur. Slow down or discontinue transfusion and administer antihistamine. Rarely anaphylaxis may occur.

Transfusion related acute lung injury (TRALI). Similar to ARDS. Due to agglutination of WBCs due to HLA antibodies in the donor plasma (usually occurs in multiparous women).

Non-haemolytic febrile transfusion reaction (NHFTR). Fever or rigor. Due to prior sensitization to WBC antigens, e.g. after pregnancy or previous transfusions (possible to get leukocyte depleted blood). Managed by slowing transfusion and giving paracetamol.

Bacterial sepsis. Uncommon.

Circulatory overload. Blood should be given slowly in the elderly or those in heart failure. Each unit of blood may be given with a small dose of furosemide.

Hypothermia.

Hyperkalaemia.

Delayed

Delayed haemolytic transfusion reaction (DHTR). Occurs when a patient has been exposed to red blood cell antigens, e.g. previous transfusion. After 5–10 days an immune response develops and the transfused cells are destroyed. It presents with fever, anaemia, jaundice and haemoglobinuria.

Iron overload.

Graft versus host disease. Rare. Donor lymphocytes engraft into the recipient's marrow. They then recognize the recipient as foreign and cause an immunologic reaction.

Immune modulation. Increased risk of infection and increased risk of tumour recurrence.

Infections. Rare. All blood is checked for HBV, HCV, HIV and syphilis. Bacterial contamination of blood products can occur.

Post-transfusion purpura. Rare. Occurs 5–10 days and is due to HLA antibodies in the recipient. Presents with low platelets and bleeding. May be treated with i.v. steroids and immunoglobulins.

Massive blood transfusion

This is defined as a transfusion equal to or greater than the whole blood volume in <24 h. Specific complications include thrombocytopaenia, decreased coagulation factors, hypothermia, hypocalcaemia due to citrate-binding, hyperkalaemia and acidosis. In major trauma, it has been shown that transfusion of blood, FFP and platelets in a 1:1:1 ratio is associated with improved survival.

FLUID AND ELECTROLYTE BALANCE

> The basic principle of fluid and electrolyte balance is that which is lost must be replaced.

Water loss in a normal individual is approximately 2500 mL/day (urine = 1–1.5 L, faeces = 100 mL, sweating = 600 mL and water vapour via breathing = 400 mL). In the uncomplicated patient, 2.5–3 L of fluid replacement is adequate. In the postoperative patient these losses may be much greater. Sources include sweating (10% increase in insensible losses for every 1°C rise in temperature) and GI losses from vomiting, diarrhoea and fistulae. In addition to water replacement, it is important to consider electrolyte replacement, mainly Na^+ and K^+. The loss of Na^+ is around 100 mmol/day (mainly from the urine) but 40 mmol/day is lost in sweat (therefore it is more in the febrile patient). Some 80 mmol/day of K^+ is lost in the urine and a small amount in the faeces (more if diarrhoea). Generally GI losses can be replaced with normal saline. The amount of 'fluid' a patient needs should be based on their size. This can be calculated either from the 4/2/1 (4 mL/h for the first 10 kg; 2 mL/h for the second 10 kg and 1 mL/h for every kg thereafter = hourly rate of fluid); or 100/50/20 rule (100 mL/kg for first 10 kg; 50 mL/kg for next 10 kg and 20 mL/kg thereafter = 24 h fluid requirement). In a 70 kg man this is around 2.5 L/day or 110 mL/h. It is also important to replace electrolyte losses. These can be calculated as 1–2 mmol/kg per day for Na^+ and 0.5–1 mmol/kg per day for K^+.

Before understanding the effects that different fluids have on a patient's circulation, it is necessary to understand a few important physiological points:

- In a 70 kg man, the total body water (TBW) is 42 L
- $2/3$ or 28 L is intracellular fluid (ICF)
- $1/3$ or 14 L is extracellular fluid (ECF) – $2/3$ of this or 10 L is interstitial and $1/3$ or 4 L is plasma
- A small amount of fluid is termed transcellular and is not exchangeable, e.g. CSF, aqueous humour.

CRYSTALLOID AND COLLOID

Intravenous fluids can be divided into crystalloids and colloids.

Normal saline. 0.9% saline solution with 154 mmol of sodium and chloride. pH 5.5. This fluid is isotonic and therefore stays in the ECF (i.e. is distributed over 14 L). Therefore, as the intravascular part is only 3.5 L, only 25–30% of a litre of fluid remains in the intravascular compartment.

5% dextrose. The added glucose is metabolized (giving 837 kJ/L of energy). This means the fluid is no longer isotonic but hypotonic and thus distributes over the TBW. As plasma only contributes 7–8% of the TBW, only 7–8% of a litre of 5% dextrose remains intravascular.

Dextrose saline. Contains 1/5 the amount of sodium of normal saline, i.e. 30 mmol/L and 4% dextrose.

Hartmann's solution. This has a chemical composition closer to plasma. Contains 131 mmol Na^+, 112 mmol Cl^-, 5 mmol K^+, 2 mmol Ca^{2+} and 28 mmol HCO_3^-.

With this in mind, a suitable regime of postoperative fluids may include:

- 1 L normal saline and 2 L of 5% dextrose with 20 mmol KCl in each of the bags. Each bag is given over 8 h and provides 3 L of fluid, 154 mmol Na^+ and 60 mmol K^+.
- 3 L dextrose saline with 20 mmol KCl in each bag. Each bag is given over 8 h and provides 3 L of fluid, 90 mmol Na^+, 60 mmol K^+. This regime is better in the

first 24 h postoperatively as the adrenal response to surgery/trauma tends to conserve sodium.

- 1 L Hartmann's fluid (no K^+ added) with 2 L of 5% dextrose each with 20 mmol KCl. Each bag is given over 8 h and provides 3 L of fluid, 131 mmol Na^+ and 45 mmol K^+. This is a good regime after surgery due to lower sodium and lower potassium (K^+ is released with tissue damage during surgery, thus requirements are lower).

Fluid and electrolyte depletion

Surgical patients may suffer large losses of fluid and electrolytes as part of the disease process, operation or postoperative complications. In addition to obvious losses, e.g. vomiting and diarrhoea, fluid may be lost into 'new' spaces resulting from the disease process, e.g. the intestine during paralytic ileus, the peritoneum in peritonitis, the retroperitoneum in acute pancreatitis or intracellular shifts in shock. These losses are called 'third space' losses and must be promptly replaced, as the problems they cause are just as important as external losses. These fluids are eventually reabsorbed and care must be taken that circulatory overload does not occur.

Management of Na^+ and K^+ imbalance

Hyponatraemia (i.e. low Na^+). In a surgical patient, this is usually due to water overload and results from administration of inappropriate amounts of 5% dextrose. If the hyponatraemia associated with fluid overload is mild, it is best treated by restricted fluid intake, avoiding the administration of saline, and giving furosemide i.v. to force a diuresis. Electrolytes should be checked twice daily. Hyponatraemia is associated with symptoms, e.g. confusion, convulsions, coma, if the Na^+ falls below 120 mmol/L. In hyponatraemia with hypovolaemia, saline should be given.

Hypernatraemia (i.e. high Na^+). This is uncommon in the surgical patient. It may occur during dehydration and in the postoperative period if too much saline is given at a time when aldosterone secretion is high and sodium is being conserved. Rarely it may be caused by Conn's syndrome ($\rightarrow$ Ch. 11). If the cause is dehydration (i.e. clinically dry with low CVP and oliguria), the patient will need water replacement, whereas in the postoperative period with normovolaemia, sodium restriction is required.

Hypokalaemia (i.e. low K^+). Preoperatively, this may be due to diuretic therapy, diarrhoea, fistula or excessive mucus loss from a villous adenoma of the rectum. Postoperatively it is usually due to inadequate K^+ replacement. It may occur with pyloric stenosis (with an associated metabolic alkalosis). Symptoms include muscle weakness, cardiac arrhythmias (T wave flattening on ECG) and paralytic ileus. Treatment is by K^+ replacement but this should not exceed 15 mmol/h as cardiac arrhythmias may arise with high infusion rates.

Hyperkalaemia (i.e. high K^+). Preoperatively, this may be due to CRF, crush injuries or absorption from massive haematomas. Massive transfusions of stored blood may also cause hyperkalaemia. Postoperatively, it is usually due to excessive administration and is usually asymptomatic. A K^+ above 7 mmol/L is an emergency.

Intravenous insulin and glucose should be given and the K^+ checked. ECG changes include elevated T waves. If ECG changes are marked, calcium gluconate should be given i.v. Other methods of reducing the serum K^+ include calcium resonium orally or rectally, and, if renal function is compromised, dialysis.

Acid–base balance

Abnormalities of acid–base balance usually occur in seriously ill patients and include:

Metabolic acidosis. Severe tissue hypoxia, e.g. septicaemia, hypovolaemia or cardiogenic shock; renal failure; diabetic ketoacidosis; and after aortic surgery when the clamp is removed. The patient compensates by rapid deep respiration to 'blow off' CO_2. Excretes acid urine. ABGs show pH ↓, HCO_3 ↓, PCO_2 ↓. Management involves treatment of the underlying condition. Bicarbonate infusion may be necessary in severe cases.

Metabolic alkalosis. This occurs with prolonged vomiting or nasogastric aspiration. Pyloric stenosis. In order to compensate, the kidney conserves hydrogen ions at the expense of K^+ excretion. ABGs show pH ↑, PCO_2 ↑. Low K^+. Treatment is by rehydration with normal saline with potassium supplements and treatment of the underlying condition.

Respiratory acidosis. This results from CO_2 retention. After surgery, this is usually due to severe chest complications, e.g. atelectasis from sputum retention or respiratory depression due to narcotics. Respiratory acidosis is compensated for by H^+ being excreted by the renal tubules and HCO_3^- being reabsorbed. ABGs show pH ↓, PCO_2 ↑. Treatment is of the underlying cause.

Respiratory alkalosis. Hyperventilation due to anxiety. Excessive mechanical ventilation. Compensation occurs by renal excretion of HCO_3^-. ABGs show pH ↑, PCO_2 ↓. Treatment is of the underlying condition.

NUTRITIONAL SUPPORT

Poor nutrition results in increased postoperative morbidity and mortality. Poor wound healing occurs and there is a reduced resistance to infection. General examination of the patient will show evidence of weight loss, e.g. general appearance, loose skin folds. The patient will often be aware of how much weight has been lost and over what time period.

CAUSES OF MALNUTRITION

- Increased catabolism, e.g. sepsis, major surgery with complications
- Increased losses, e.g. chronic liver disease with loss of albumin, protein-losing enteropathy
- Decreased intake, e.g. dysphagia, vomiting, general debility
- Decreased absorption, e.g. intestinal fistulae, short bowel syndrome
- Other causes, e.g. major trauma, chemotherapy, radiotherapy.

INDICATIONS FOR NUTRITIONAL SUPPORT

Most patients requiring surgery are well nourished and will stand a few days starvation. They will recover from surgery sufficiently to resume eating before they become malnourished. Some patients will be clearly malnourished prior to surgery, while others may develop complications that delay resumption of normal diet and require parenteral nutrition. Others may have conditions, e.g. short bowel syndrome, which require long-term or permanent nutritional support.

Other indications for nutritional support include:

● Preoperatively in malnourished patients
● Postoperatively in malnourished patients and those who develop malnutrition because of complications
● Patients with sepsis or major postoperative complications
● Patients with fistulae
● Patients with chronic liver disease
● Patients undergoing chemotherapy or radiotherapy for certain tumours
● Patients with short bowel syndrome or malabsorption syndrome.

EVALUATION OF NUTRITIONAL STATUS

1. History: duration of illness, weight loss, change in appetite, dietary habits
2. Physical examination, general appearance, loose skin folds, loss of skin contours over bony prominences, muscle wasting, peripheral oedema
3. Weight: in relation to height
4. Anthropometric measurements, e.g. triceps skin fold thickness
5. Laboratory tests, e.g. Hb, serum albumin, serum iron.

ADMINISTRATION OF NUTRITIONAL SUPPORT

Oral nutrition

This is the most efficient, least expensive, most pleasant and safest route for the patient. If the GI tract is available and the patient able to take oral nutrition, then this method is the most appropriate. Liquidized food, Clinifeed or supplements may be given this way.

Enteral nutrition

This is used for patients with a functioning small bowel unable to take nutrients by mouth, e.g. those who are seriously ill, unable to swallow or have a mouth lesion, e.g. herpes.

Fine-bore NG tubes. Liquidized food, Clinifeed or supplements are given via a tube passed via the nose into the stomach.

Surgically created gastrostomy or jejunostomy. These are appropriate for long-term enteric feeding.

In both the above methods the feed is dripped slowly into the GI tract. Bolus feeding should be avoided as it gives marked diarrhoea and if given via a nasogastric tube in large volumes, may result in regurgitation and aspiration pneumonia.

Complications. Complications of enteral feeding depend on the route of administration and the enteral feed itself. They include:

NG feeding. Removal, blockage, aspiration, reflux, vomiting, diarrhoea, hyperglycaemia.

Gastrostomy/jejunostomy. Pain, bleeding, peritonitis, infection, blockage, diarrhoea, hyperglycaemia.

Parenteral nutrition

This is used where GI function is inadequate and nutrition is administered via the venous system.

Peripheral line. Short-term feeding (up to 5 days) may be given via drip in a peripheral vein. Solutions used with this method must be of a special type, which causes little thrombophlebitis. This method may be used preoperatively for patients with malnutrition of moderate degree for which oral nutrition is unsatisfactory, e.g. malignant strictures of the oesophagus.

Central line. This is the most appropriate route and is used for total parenteral nutrition (TPN). For short-term use, a percutaneous internal jugular line may be used. For longer-term and permanent nutrition, a tunnelled subcutaneous line (Hickman or Broviac) should be used. Hypertonic solutions are infused via the catheter into a large-bore vein with good flow to prevent thrombophlebitis.

TOTAL PARENTERAL NUTRITION (TPN)

This is usually provided in 3-litre bags either prepared in the hospital pharmacy or bought commercially. This provides all the nutrients required for a 24-hour period. Controlled rates of administration are essential and this is achieved either by a special counting device attached to the drip line or via an infusion pump. Any additional fluid and electrolyte to restore losses, or administration of drugs, should be via a separate peripheral line.

Components of TPN

- Calories: these are supplied as a combination of carbohydrate and fat. Most patients require approximately 2000 kcal/day – or more if they have sepsis or burns
- Protein: this is supplied as amino acids. Nitrogen requirements are about 15 g/day but may be as high as 30 g/day in hypercatabolic states
- Water
- Vitamins
- Electrolytes, e.g. Na^+, K^+, calcium, phosphate, magnesium
- Trace elements, e.g. zinc, copper, manganese.

Monitoring TPN

Blood sugar, U&Es should be checked daily. Until fluid and nitrogen balance is obtained the blood sugar should be monitored 6-hourly by BM stix. LFTs, calcium, phosphate, and FBC should be checked twice weekly. If the patient becomes pyrexial, blood cultures should be obtained. The site of catheter insertion should be dressed twice weekly under aseptic conditions. If the patient develops a pyrexia and no other cause is found, it may be necessary to remove the catheter and send the tip for culture. The catheter should be used for feeding only. Any other substances, e.g. additional electrolytes or drugs, should be given via a separate peripheral line.

Complications of TPN

Catheter related. Pneumothorax or arterial puncture may occur during insertion. If the catheter is not correctly positioned in a large vein but is in a chamber of the heart, arrhythmias may occur. Rarely the catheter may erode through a vessel wall and give rise to haemopericardium. Air embolus may occur when manipulating the line and this should be avoided by keeping the patient supine. Thrombosis of a central vein may occur. Prophylactic heparin 1000 units/L of the infusion is useful prophylaxis.

Metabolic. Too much or too little of components of i.v. feeding may be given. Careful monitoring for the following is required:

- Fluid overload
- Hyperglycaemia
- Hypoglycaemia (may occur if infusion of hypertonic glucose is suddenly stopped)
- Electrolyte abnormalities
- Hepatic cholestasis.

Home TPN

Long-term TPN in ambulatory patients is practicable providing it is properly monitored. Patients with short-bowel syndrome are the most appropriate. The patient or a partner is taught the technique and back-up is provided by a specially trained team able to provide regular biochemical monitoring. A Broviac or Hickman tunnelled central line is used. The feeding solution may be administered overnight and the catheter disconnected to allow activity during the day. Alternatively it may need to be administered throughout 24 h, depending on the patient's requirements.

Infection and surgery

The surgical patient is exposed to potentially harmful microorganisms prior to admission, during admission and after discharge. The outside surfaces of the body, including the aerodigestive tract, are normally colonized with bacteria – a defence mechanism that is disrupted by stress and antibiotic therapy. With the prevalence of hospital acquired infections, such as *clostridium difficile* and methicillin-resistant *staphylococcus aureus* (MRSA), and the potential for blood-borne virus transmission, the practicing surgeon needs to be aware of safe antimicrobial techniques and treatments, to protect both the patient and healthcare staff. Effective communication needs therefore to be present between surgeon and microbiologist.

PRINCIPLES OF WOUND MANAGEMENT

Healing by primary intention
When appropriate, the wound edges are approximated as soon after the injury as possible, e.g. clean traumatic wounds or surgical incisions. This is known as primary closure and the wound heals by first intention.

Healing by secondary intention
The wound edges are not apposed and the wound is left to heal by second intention. Granulation tissue grows up from the base of the wound and the skin grows over in a centripetal manner. This type of healing is appropriate for large, grossly contaminated wounds.

Delayed primary closure
The wound is left open and observed for several days. If the wound then appears healthy, it may be closed as for a primary closure. This type of closure is suitable for wounds that have low-grade infection or for surgical incisions where infection may be expected, e.g. abdominal incisions following operations for gross faecal peritonitis.

Factors affecting wound healing
Age. Younger patients heal better than older patients.
Nutritional state. Malnutrition impedes wound healing. Patients who are poorly nourished should be given appropriate feeding, e.g. TPN prior to surgery.

Drugs. Steroids delay wound healing.

Tissue oxygenation and vascularity. Hypoxaemia and ischaemia delay wound healing. Highly vascular areas, e.g. face, heal quicker than poorly vascularized areas, e.g. shin.

Radiotherapy. Causes endarteritis obliterans of small vessels resulting in local ischaemia and poor healing.

Local sepsis. This is probably the commonest cause of delayed healing.

Factors predisposing to infection in surgery

Age. Increasing age is a significant independent predictor of risk.

Underlying illness. Those with an American Society of Anesthesiologists (ASA) score of 3 or more have been found to have a significantly higher risk of surgical site infection.

Obesity and smoking. Are both associated with an increased risk of surgical site infection.

Wound classification. See below.

Classification of surgical wounds

Clean. An incision in which no inflammation is encountered in a surgical procedure, without a break in sterile technique, and during which the respiratory tract, alimentary or genitourinary tracts are not entered, e.g. varicose vein surgery, hernia repair. The risk of postoperative wound infection is about 5%.

Clean contaminated. An incision through which the respiratory, alimentary, or genitourinary tract is entered under controlled conditions but with no contamination encountered, e.g. cholecystectomy, partial gastrectomy. The risk of postoperative wound infection is about 10%.

Contaminated. An incision undertaken during an operation, in which there is a major break in sterile technique or gross spillage from the gastrointestinal tract, or an incision in which acute, non-purulent inflammation is encountered. Open traumatic wounds >12–24 h old. The risk of postoperative wound infection is >50%.

Dirty. An incision undertaken during an operation in which the viscera are perforated or when acute inflammation with pus is encountered (e.g. faecal peritonitis), and for traumatic wounds where treatment is delayed, there is faecal contamination, or devitalized tissue is present.

PREVENTION OF SURGICAL SITE INFECTION (Incorporating NICE guidelines 2008)

Preoperative precautions

- Adjust patient lifestyle. Improve diet and body mass index. Advise to stop smoking
- MRSA screening and subsequent decolonization if positive (see below)
- Consideration of delay of elective surgery if concurrent infection detected

- Advise patients to take a bath or shower using soap within 24 h prior to surgery
- If hair removal desired, use electric clippers on the day of surgery.

Perioperative precautions
- Staff to wear specific non-sterile theatre wear in operating suite, sterile gowns in the theatre
- Keep staff movements in and out of theatre to a minimum
- Operating team to remove hand jewellery, nail polish and artificial nails
- Scrub hands with nail cleaning with a brush or pick prior to the first operation
- Scrub hands prior to subsequent operations and if hands soiled
- Patient skin preparation with povidone-iodine or chlorhexidine prior to incision
- Maintain adequate patient temperature, oxygenation and perfusion throughout
- Cover surgical wounds with an appropriate dressing at the end.

Postoperative precautions
- Use an aseptic technique to change dressings
- Use sterile saline to cleanse wound up to 48 h after surgery
- Patients may shower 48 h after surgery
- Use an appropriate dressing for wounds healing by secondary intention.

ANTIBIOTICS IN SURGERY

> Antibiotics are never a substitute for sound surgical technique. Pus, dead tissue and slough need removing. Antibiotics should be used carefully and only with positive indications. Prolonged or inappropriate use of antibiotics may encourage resistant strains of organisms to emerge. Except in straightforward cases, advice of a microbiologist should be sought.

PRINCIPLES OF ANTIBIOTIC THERAPY

Selection of antibiotic
The decision to prescribe antibiotics is usually clinical and is based initially on a 'best-guess' policy, i.e. based on experience of that particular condition, what the organism is likely to be, and to what it is most likely to be sensitive. The following sequence of events usually occurs:

1. A decision is made on clinical grounds that an infection exists.
2. Based on signs, symptoms and clinical experience, a guess is made at the likely infecting organism.
3. The appropriate specimens are taken for microbiological examination, i.e. culture and sensitivity testing.
4. The most effective drug against the suspected organism is given in line with individual hospital guidelines. If doubt exists this is discussed with a microbiologist.
5. The clinical response to treatment is monitored.
6. The antibiotic treatment is altered, if necessary, in response to laboratory reports of culture and sensitivities.

Occasionally the response of the infection to an apparently appropriate antibiotic is poor. Possible causes for this include:

- Failure to drain pus, excise necrotic tissue or remove foreign bodies
- Failure of the drug to reach the tissues in therapeutic concentrations, e.g. ischaemic limbs
- Organism isolated is not the one responsible for the infection
- After prolonged antibiotic therapy, new organisms develop due to selection pressure
- Inadequate dosage or inappropriate route of administration.

Route of administration

Antibiotics should be given i.v. in severe infections in seriously ill patients. Some antibiotics, e.g. gentamicin, can only be given by the parenteral route. When the patient improves and the GI tract is functioning satisfactorily, drugs may be given orally.

 It is best to avoid the intramuscular route if possible as it is uncomfortable for the patient and in shocked patients absorption would be inadequate.

Duration of therapy

This depends on the individual's response, laboratory tests and the underlying cause of infection. For most infections that show an appropriate response to treatment after 48 h, a suitable 'course' should be for 5–7 days. Infections such as osteomyelitis require prolonged courses of antibiotics administered long after symptoms and signs of infection have resolved.

Dosage

The dosage may need to be modified in renal and liver disease.

Complications of antibiotic therapy

- Adverse reactions
  - Side-effects, e.g. nephrotoxicity, ototoxicity
  - Hypersensitivity
  - Anaphylaxis
- Development of resistance
- Iatrogenic infection, e.g. *Clostridium difficile* with the use of cephalosporins, clindamycin.

PROPHYLACTIC ANTIBIOTICS

Despite aseptic techniques, some operations carry a high risk of postoperative wound infection, bacteraemia or septicaemia. Administration of antibiotics in the perioperative period will reduce the risks.

Indications for prophylactic antibiotics

These include:

- Implantation of foreign bodies, e.g. cardiac prosthetic valves, artificial joints, prosthetic vascular grafts
- Patients with pre-existing cardiac disease who are undergoing surgical procedures including dental procedures, e.g. patients with mitral valve disease as prophylaxis against infective endocarditis
- Organ transplantation
- Immunosuppressed patients
- Diabetics
- Amputations, especially for ischaemia or crush injuries, where there is dead muscle; risk of gas gangrene is high especially in contaminated wounds; penicillin is the antibiotic of choice
- Compound fractures and penetrating wounds
- Surgical incisions, where there is a high risk of bacterial contamination, e.g.
  (1) clean/contaminated wounds – prophylactic antibiotics are indicated;
  (2) contaminated – antibiotics are given as therapy not prophylaxis;
  (3) dirty – antibiotics are given as therapy not prophylaxis.

Most prophylactic antibiotics are given to prevent wound infection. In some cases, they are given prior to instrumental procedures in potentially infected sites, e.g. when performing cystoscopy, when they are given to prevent septicaemia. In most cases, one dose is given preoperatively either orally if under LA (1 h preoperatively) or i.v. if under GA. The aim is to achieve therapeutic levels at the time of surgery. Individual hospital policy should be followed with regard to the use of specific agents and their duration as prophylaxis.

SPECIFIC ANTIBIOTICS (→ Table 6.1)

SURGICAL INFECTIONS

SEPSIS

Sepsis is generally related to the body's response to infection. However, sepsis is probably better defined as a group of conditions that include:

- Systemic inflammatory response syndrome (SIRS) which is defined as any two from:
  — pyrexia – $>38°C$ or $<36°C$
  — tachycardia – >90 beats/min
  — tachypnoea – >20 breaths/min
  — WCC – >12 or <4
- Sepsis – SIRS plus a documented infection
- Sepsis syndrome – sepsis plus organ dysfunction and hypoperfusion
- Septic shock – refractory hypotension plus documented infection.

SIRS is seen in many surgical patients and does not always result from an infective process. It is commonly seen in pancreatitis, trauma and burns. SIRS is a

TABLE 6.1 Some commonly used antibiotics

Class	Antibiotic	Route	Activity	Uses	Side-effects	Cautions
Penicillin	Benzylpenicillin; Phenoxymethylpenicillin	Oral, i.v.	Streptococcus Pneumococcus Clostridia Neisseria	Soft tissue and wound infection	Hypersensitivity Urticarial rash Anaphylaxis Cross-sensitivity Convulsions at high doses	Allergy to penicillins Renal failure Cardiac failure (i.v. forms contain K^+ and Na^+ salts)
	Flucloxacillin	Oral, i.m., i.v.	Staphylococcus	Soft tissue and wound infection		
	Amoxicillin; Ampicillin	Oral, i.m., i.v.	Strep. faecalis H. influenzae	UTI Chest Infection		
	Co-amoxiclav	Oral, i.v.	Coliforms Staphylococcus Bacteroides	Soft tissue infection Prophylaxis for GU, HPB and bowel surgery		
	Meropenem; imipenem	i.v.	Broad spectrum Anaerobes, aerobes	Life-threatening sepsis		
	Piperacillin	i.m., i.v.	Bacteroides Coliforms Klebsiella Pseudomonas	Used with tazobactam for severe sepsis chest, soft tissue and skin infection		
Cephalosporin	Cephradine	Oral, i.m., i.v.	Broad spectrum Including E. coli, Klebsiella, Proteus Staphylococcus	Second-line in UTI, chest infection, soft tissue infection	10% cross-sensitivity with penicillin allergy Rashes Pyrexia Transient elevation in LFTs Pseudo-membranous colitis (C. diff)	Dose reduction in renal failure
	Cefuroxime	Oral, i.m., i.v.	Broad spectrum	Prophylaxis with metronidazole in colorectal and hepatobiliary surgery		
	Cefotaxime/ Ceftazidime	i.m., i.v.	Broad spectrum Also Pseudomonas	Sepsis due to Gram −ve bacilli		

Continued

TABLE 6.1 Some commonly used antibiotics—cont'd

Class	Antibiotic	Route	Activity	Uses	Side-effects	Cautions
Sulphonamide and trimethoprim	Co-trimoxazole (Sulfamethoxazole and trimethoprim)	Oral, i.m., i.v.	Broad spectrum	UTI Chest infection	Nausea Vomiting Rash Mouth ulcers	Avoid in pregnancy Potentiates action of warfarin and ciclosporin
	Trimethoprim	Oral, i.v.	Broad spectrum	UTI Chest infection	Marrow suppression	
Macrolide	Erythromycin	Oral, i.v.	Broad spectrum Streptococcus Clostridia Staphylococcus Campylobacter	Used as second-line agent in patients sensitive to penicillins Skin and soft tissue infection Chest infection Legionnaire's disease Campylobacter enteritis	Diarrhoea (oral administration) Phlebitis (i.v.)	Potentiates action of warfarin and ciclosporin
Aminoglycoside	Gentamicin	i.m., i.v.	Gram −ve Coliforms Pseudomonas Staphylococcus	Prophylaxis against UTI during catheterization Therapeutic effects dependent on renal function	Ototoxicity (vertigo, deafness) Nephrotoxicity	Monitor serum levels Caution in impaired renal function
Quinolone	Ciprofloxacin	Oral, i.v.	Broad spectrum Pseudomonas Staphylococcus	UTI Skin and soft tissue infection Chest infection	Nausea Diarrhoea Vomiting Anxiety Insomnia Nervousness Convulsions Pseudo-membranous colitis (C. diff)	Potentiates action of warfarin

	Drug	Route	Organisms	Uses	Side effects	Notes
Glycopeptide	Vancomycin	Oral (does not cross gut lining) i.v.	Staphylococcus MRSA Streptococcus Clostridia	Severe infections Oral for pseudomembranous colitis	Phlebitis (i.v.) Ototoxicity Nephrotoxicity	Monitor serum levels to control dosage Renal failure Hepatic failure
	Teicoplanin	i.v., i.m.	Staphylococcus Streptococcus Enterococcus Listeria Anaerobes	Longer duration of action than vancomycin		
Other	Metronidazole	Oral, i.v., topical, p.r.	Anaerobic bacteria Protozoa	Prophylaxis in colorectal surgery Intraperitoneal sepsis Gynaecological sepsis Giardiasis Amoebiasis Amoebic liver abscess	Anorexia Sore tongue Metallic taste Disulfiram-like reaction if taken with alcohol	Potentiates action of warfarin
	Clindamycin	Oral, i.v.	Staphylococcus Streptococcus Bacteroides	Inhibits toxin synthesis therefore used in necrotizing fasciitis, skin and soft tissue infections	Pseudo-membranous colitis (C. diff) Diarrhoea Nausea Vomiting	Not to be used with macrolides
	Fusidic acid	Oral, i.v.	Staphylococcus Corynebacterium	Osteomyelitis	Jaundice	Pregnancy

normal response to injury and in the early stages, is protective. A number of stages in the evolution of SIRS may occur:

- In the region of injury there is local production of inflammatory mediators and cytokines. These lead to vasodilatation, increased vascular permeability and the recruitment of cells that fight infection.
- In more severe injury the cytokine release has a systemic effect; this includes the production of acute phase proteins, pyrexia and an increase in peripheral leukocytes. This response is regulated by a group of counter-regulatory cytokines.
- In patients with SIRS there is an exaggerated response and the production of cytokines exceeds the counter-regulatory mechanisms. Cytokines such as IL-1 and TNF-α produce vasodilatation leading to hypotension, increased vascular permeability leading to oedema and third space fluid loss. There is also widespread activation of leukocytes that can cause damage in organs distant from the site of injury, e.g. lungs.

Management of SIRS
- Resuscitation
- Identify source of sepsis. Likely possible sources include: the wound; intravascular access (arterial, central venous, cannulas); urinary catheters/urinary tract infection; prosthetic implants; chest infection
- Administration of appropriate antibiotics – empirically initially and then changed after antibiotic sensitivities are known
- Definitive management of the course of sepsis, i.e. surgical or radiological guided drainage of abscess.

CELLULITIS

A spreading inflammation of connective tissue. It is usually subcutaneous and caused by β-haemolytic *Streptococci* or *Staphylococcus aureus*.

Symptoms and signs
Redness, oedema, and localized tenderness. A scratch, insect bite, ulcer or surgical wound may be apparent. There is usually fever and malaise. Lymphangitis or lymphadenitis may be present. Lymphangitis produces red tender streaks in the line of lymphatics extending from the area of cellulitis towards the regional lymph nodes. Lymphadenitis is represented by enlarged tender regional lymph nodes. Occasionally the overlying skin is red and the glands may be fluctuant.

Investigations
- WBC
- Blood cultures
- CRP
- Blood glucose.

Drawing a line around the erythema with permanent marker pen enables observation of progression/regression of the leading edge, and can be used to gauge response to treatment.

Treatment

Streptococcus and Staphylococcus are usually sensitive to flucloxacillin. Elevation of a limb may be required. Occasionally an abscess with thin watery pus forms and requires drainage.

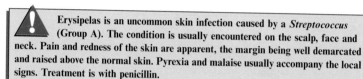

Erysipelas is an uncommon skin infection caused by a *Streptococcus* (Group A). The condition is usually encountered on the scalp, face and neck. Pain and redness of the skin are apparent, the margin being well demarcated and raised above the normal skin. Pyrexia and malaise usually accompany the local signs. Treatment is with penicillin.

NECROTIZING FASCIITIS

This is a rapidly progressive and potentially fatal bacterial infection that spreads along fascial planes and causes vascular thrombosis resulting in necrosis of the tissues involved. If present in a limb distal to the elbow or knee, organisms often involved include β-haemolytic streptococci and staphylococci. Coliforms and Gram-negative anaerobes may be synergistically involved elsewhere such as the scrotum (Fournier's gangrene). Necrotizing fasciitis may result from a small puncture wound, surgical incision or penetrating trauma of a hollow viscus.

Symptoms and signs

Pain and tenderness at the leading edge of the infection can be agonizing. Redness, oedema, necrotic insensate skin patches, haemorrhagic bullae, crepitus and discharge. The patient is febrile and exhibiting signs of systemic sepsis. A test incision either at the bedside or in an operating theatre producing a grey/brown 'dishwater' exudate aids diagnosis, as does a 'sweep test' where a finger placed into the test incision and turned into the soft tissues easily separates the tissue planes digested by bacterial enzymes.

Investigations

- WBC
- Blood culture
- Swabs – culture and sensitivity
- Radiograph may show gas in tissues.

Treatment

Patients should be resuscitated and transferred urgently to the operating theatre for surgical debridement of all infected and dead tissue. A critical care bed should be requested for postoperative recovery. The tissue is usually oedematous, grey and smells. The subcutaneous fat and fascia are involved. Muscle is often viable. The microbiologist should be informed if a diagnosis of necrotizing fasciitis is suspected. Fresh specimens of tissue should be sent for urgent Gram stain and microscopy. Antimicrobial treatment is usually with clindamycin (which inhibits the production of streptococcal toxins) and benzylpenicillin intravenously. Meropenem may be used instead of benzylpenicillin in cases requiring anaerobic cover. Antibiotics are changed according to culture and sensitivities. The patient's systemic state is observed carefully postoperatively and the wound is inspected regularly, often with a planned second look under general anaesthetic at 24 or 48 h, and any further necrotic tissue excised. When the infection has been controlled, large skin defects can be reconstructed with skin grafts. Mortality rate is about 25% in extensive cases.

GAS GANGRENE

Myositis and cellulitis caused by *Clostridium perfringens*, an anaerobic, spore-forming and gas-producing organism. The organism is found in soil and faeces. It is an infection associated with deep, penetrating, contaminated wounds usually involving an extremity, and rarely is seen as a complication of amputation of an ischaemic limb. Intravenous drug users may inadvertently inject *Clostridia* (*perfringens* or *tetani*) into the soft tissues. It may involve the abdominal wall following penetrating trauma of, or surgery to, the GI tract.

Symptoms and signs
Acute onset 6 h to 3 days after injury. Severe pain at site of injury. The tissues are swollen; brownish, serous, malodorous fluid may drain from the wound. Patchy necrosis and crepitus occur. The patient is toxic and may be confused or delirious. The temperature is not always elevated.

Investigations
- WBC
- Bilirubin raised because of haemolysis
- Gram-stain of discharge shows Gram-positive bacilli
- Radiograph shows gas in tissues.

Treatment
Prophylactic. Adequate debridement of wound at time of initial injury. All contused and dead tissue should be removed and the wound thoroughly irrigated and left open. Prophylactic penicillin should be given to all patients with contaminated wounds and to patients with ischaemic limbs undergoing amputations.

Therapeutic. Radical debridement of all necrotic tissue is mandatory. If the muscle of a limb is involved, amputation will be necessary. This should be done at a level where the muscle bleeds and contracts when cut. Large doses of penicillin should be given intravenously. Anti-gas gangrene serum either prophylactically or therapeutically is of unproven value.

TETANUS

This is a rare condition in the UK owing to widespread immunization. It is caused by *Clostridium tetani*, an anaerobic Gram-positive bacillus that produces a neurotoxin. It is found in soil and faeces. The neurotoxin enters peripheral nerves and travels to the spinal cord where it blocks inhibitory activity of spinal reflexes resulting in the characteristic features of the disease. The disease follows the implantation of spores into deep, devitalized tissues.

Symptoms and signs

History of injury. This may be as minor as the prick of rose thorn. The incubation period is 1–30 days. Muscle spasm usually occurs first at the site of inoculation and is followed by trismus resulting in the typical risus sardonicus (lock-jaw). Stiffness in the neck, back and abdomen follow together with generalized spasms, which may cause asphyxia. The muscles remain in spasm between convulsions. Opisthotonos (arching of the back and neck due to spasm) may occur. This stage is followed by convulsions which are extremely painful and during which the patient is conscious. Death may occur from asphyxia due to involvement of respiratory muscles or from inhalation of vomit with aspiration pneumonia.

Differential diagnosis
- Strychnine poisoning: the muscles are flaccid between convulsions
- Tetany: usually carpopedal spasm and does not affect the trunk
- Epilepsy
- Meningitis: there is usually only neck stiffness but convulsions may occur
- Hysteria.

Treatment

Prophylactic
- Active immunization with tetanus toxoid. All children should be immunized and this is repeated at 6 weeks and 6 months after the initial dose. Booster doses should be given at 5-yearly intervals. All patients attending an A&E department with new trauma, however mild, should have a booster, unless one has been given within the previous 5 years.
- Contaminated and penetrating wounds should be debrided and prophylactic penicillin administered. A tetanus toxoid booster dose should be given to the previously immunized patient. Those not previously immunized should be given human antitetanus immunoglobulin.

Therapeutic
1. Involve the critical care team. Discuss with microbiology.
2. Isolate the patient in a quiet darkened room. Give diazepam or chlorpromazine. In severe cases, the patient will need to be paralysed and ventilated. Feeding should be given via a fine-bore nasogastric tube. Ventilation may need to be continued for up to 4 weeks. A trial period of weaning off relaxants without recurrence of spasm will indicate when ventilation is no longer required. Tracheostomy may be required.
3. Administer penicillin, tetanus toxoid, and human antitetanus immunoglobulin.
4. Excise and drain any contaminated wound.
5. Regular physiotherapy will be required during the recovery period.

Prognosis
The mortality rate is inversely proportional to the length of the incubation period. If spasm occurs within 5 days of the time of injury, the prognosis is poor. The mortality rate is also directly proportional to the severity of the symptoms.

METHICILLIN-RESISTANT *STAPHYLOCOCCUS AUREUS* (MRSA)

MRSA is a major nosocomial pathogen. It may cause severe morbidity and mortality. Up to 40% of nosocomial *Staph. aureus* infections may be methicillin resistant. They are also resistant to flucloxacillin, amoxicillin, co-amoxiclav, cephalosporins and Tazocin. Many inpatients are colonized or infected and up to 25% of hospital personnel may be carriers. The organism may be carried in the anterior nares, inguinal, perineal and axillary areas. Spread often occurs by the hands, usually of nursing or medical staff.

Risk factors for colonization. These include advanced age, previous hospitalization, length of hospitalization, stay in ITU, chronic illness, prior and prolonged antibiotic therapy, presence of a wound, exposure to colonized or infected patients, presence of invasive indwelling devices, nursing home residency.

Clinical presentation. These principally include line sepsis, surgical site infection and pneumonia.

Infection control. This includes screening of patients and staff. If MRSA is suspected, swabs should be taken from the hairline, nose, axilla, groin, perineum. Important factors in infection control include hand washing, use of gowns and gloves, isolation of infected or colonized patients (barrier nursing) and environmental cleaning.

Management
Carriers. Carriers may be treated by application of antiseptics, e.g. mupirocin to nose; use of antiseptic soaps and shampoos for five days. Check swabs should be taken at 2, 9 and 16 days after use of antiseptics.

Patients with MRSA infection. These patients should be nursed using special precautions. Vancomycin is the antibiotic of choice. Linezolid and daptomycin are alternative treatments.

INFECTION AND THE SURGEON

The surgeon – as indeed are any medical, nursing, or paramedical personnel – is at risk from three main viral infections: HIV, hepatitis B, hepatitis C.

HIV

Infection with HIV is permanent and it is likely that all carriers will eventually develop AIDS. Surgical personnel are at high risk. Infection with HIV results from the passage of infected body fluid (usually blood) from one person to another. Needlestick injuries and scalpel injuries are possible sources of infection. In the general population, HIV may be transmitted by unprotected anal, vaginal, and oral intercourse, sharing needles in drug abuse, and infected blood products (e.g. as has happened in the past with haemophiliacs).

Risk categories

The following are at risk of becoming HIV-positive: homosexual or bisexual males; prostitutes (male and female); intravenous drug abusers; haemophiliacs who were treated before routine testing became available, i.e. October 1995; sexual partners of the above and children of infected mothers.

Prevention of HIV

Care at operation needs to be exercised with patients who are known to have AIDS or be HIV-positive. Patients with anorectal disease related to homosexuality, haemophiliacs and sexual partners and children of the above should be treated with appropriate caution.

Counselling is required and consent must be obtained for HIV testing. If a patient refuses and is suspected of being HIV-positive, then precautions must be taken with nursing care and any invasive procedures from simple venepuncture to major surgery.

The chance of seroconversion from a needlestick injury is approximately 0.3%.

HEPATITIS B

Infection is largely blood-borne. It may be transmitted by blood transfusion; inoculation via sharp injuries from blood or blood products; droplet transmission; syringe and needle sharing in drug addicts; sexual intercourse with an infected partner; homosexual practices; tattooing or ear piercing, etc. with unsterile equipment. Antigen carriage is a risk for hospital staff, especially those in 'high-risk' areas, e.g. theatre staff. Dialysis units are often quoted as being a 'high-risk' area, but following outbreaks many years ago, all staff and patients are tested for HBsAg.

Hepatitis B vaccine is offered to all high-risk staff. These categories include: surgeons; theatre nurses; other operating department personnel; pathology department staff; A&E unit staff; liver transplant unit staff; gastrointestinal unit staff; workers in residential units for the mentally handicapped; staff of infectious and communicable diseases units.

The chance of seroconversion from a needlestick injury in unvaccinated individuals is approximately 30%.

HEPATITIS C

Hepatitis C (HCV) is present in blood and spreads in the same way as HBV, by blood transfusion; syringe and needle sharing in drug addicts; mother-to-baby transmission; sharps injuries; tattooing, ear piercing, etc. with unsterile equipment; sharing toothbrushes and razors. Sexual transmission occurs but is uncommon. The incubation period is 6 weeks to 2 months. About 0.7% of the population are chronically infected with HCV.

The disease is often asymptomatic, only about 25% becoming symptomatic and jaundiced. Around 20% of those infected will clear the virus in the acute stage. Of those that do not, some will never develop liver damage; many will develop only moderate liver damage, with or without symptoms; 20% will progress to cirrhosis during 20 years or so and of that 20%, some will progress to liver failure and some will develop hepatocellular carcinoma. Carriers are a source of infection and include drug addicts; recipients of blood and blood products before September 1991; children of infected mothers; and healthcare workers from occupational injuries.

The chance of seroconversion from a needlestick injury is approximately 3%.

PRECAUTIONS FOR THE CARE OF KNOWN AND SUSPECTED HIV, HBV AND HCV CARRIERS

Sources of infection are:

● Contact – blood, urine, faeces, saliva, tears, CSF
● Air-borne – use of power tools
● Inoculation – sharps injuries, e.g. needlestick, scalpels.

Universal precautions
This refers to those precautions taken to protect theatre staff from infection in all cases. They include:

● gowns
● masks
● surgical gloves
● 'no touch' technique.

Special precautions
These are used for all high-risk patients, e.g. hepatitis, HIV or patients suspected of having these conditions:

● All personnel involved in patient care should be aware of the risk.
● Any patient considered as a risk should be indicated as belonging to a high-risk category on the operating list (*under no circumstances should the actual disease causing the risk be placed on the operating list for reasons of patient confidentiality*).
● Arrangements should be made for contaminated fluid, dressings, etc. to be handled and disposed of correctly.
● Appropriate theatre techniques should be adopted:
  — minimize theatre staff; only essential personnel – no spectators
  — remove all but essential equipment
  — disposable drapes and gowns
  — double-gloving and use of 'indicator' glove systems
  — visors to prevent splashing in eyes
  — blunt suture needles
  — stapling devices rather than needles where possible
  — pass instruments in kidney dish
  — 'no touch' technique
  — all disposable equipment should be removed in specifically marked containers
  — the theatre should be thoroughly cleansed with dilute bleach solution at the end of the procedure
  — recovery staff must also be aware of the risk.

MANAGEMENT OF SHARPS INJURIES

- Let the site of injury bleed.
- Wash area with soap and water.
- Immediately report the incident to supervisor/senior officer/occupational health.
- Visit the Occupational Health Department or nearest emergency department as soon as possible.

Procedure at Occupational Health or Emergency Department

- Take detailed information – details of injury; how long ago it occurred; was the skin penetrated; did it bleed; was the sharp visibly contaminated with blood; was the source patient known to be infected and with what; any first aid measures used.
- Explain transmission risk is small.
- Offer blood test but only after appropriate counselling.
- If the source patient is known (i.e. the original user of the needle in needlestick injuries) they should be asked to consent for testing for HIV, HBV or HCV. They should be counselled before the tests are done.
- The person sustaining the sharps injury should be advised about the risks of transmission until such time as test results are received. They should practice safe sex and not donate blood.

Post-exposure prophylaxis

Hepatitis B

- If the source patient tests positive for HBV, the healthcare worker should have been vaccinated and serum antibody positive.
- If antibody levels are low, a dose of hyperimmune anti-hepatitis B IgG plus one dose of vaccine should be given.
- In the unvaccinated, one dose of hyperimmune anti-hepatitis B IgG should be given and a course of vaccination commenced.
- Similar procedures should be followed when the source patient cannot be identified or refuses to be treated.

Hepatitis C

- After 6 weeks and 12 weeks, serum analysis with polymerase chain reaction. If positive, then can give interferon and ribavirin.

HIV

- Carry out tests after counselling at 3 months and 6 months.
- No vaccine available.
- Post-exposure prophylaxis should be given within 1 hour of exposure in cases involving high-risk or known HIV carriers.

Triple agent prophylaxis may include zidovudine, lamivudine and nelfinavir.

Management of malignant disease

Patients with malignant disease form a major part of the workload of a surgical unit. They are assessed and decisions on management are made as part of a multidisciplinary team of surgeons, oncologists, specialist radiologists and pathologists, nurses, dieticians, etc. The total number of patients with malignant disease is rising owing to increased life expectancy. Where possible, the aims should be to prevent malignancy, e.g. cessation of smoking in the prevention of lung cancer, and the avoidance of excessive ultraviolet light in the prevention of skin cancer. Screening programmes should be instituted to make earlier diagnoses of the common forms of cancer and hopefully maximize the cure rate.

SCREENING

This is the examination of an asymptomatic population at risk of a particular condition, with a view to early diagnosis and consequent increase in cure rate. The basis for screening a normal population is to diagnose cancer at an asymptomatic stage, treatment at which point results in greater survival than cancers diagnosed at a symptomatic stage. For a screening programme to be successful it must adhere to certain principles:

- The cancer being detected must be common enough to represent an important health problem.
- The natural history of the cancer should be established, i.e. its development from a latent phase to symptomatic disease.
- A test should be available to detect the latent stage; the test should be sensitive and specific to the cancer and be acceptable and safe to the patient.
- Early detection of the cancer should lead to a benefit in terms of cost of treatment and survival of the patient.

Examples of screening programmes being carried out at present are:

- Cervical smears for cervical carcinoma
- Mammography for carcinoma of the breast
- Faecal occult bloods for carcinoma of the colon.

PREMALIGNANT CONDITIONS

It is important that these conditions are recognized and appropriate action taken.

Examples of premalignant conditions include:

- *Skin*: actinic keratoses, Bowen's disease, erythroplasia of Queyrat (penis).
- *GI tract*: leukoplakia (mouth and tongue), Plummer–Vinson syndrome, Barrett's oesophagus, villous adenoma, familial polyposis coli, ulcerative colitis, Crohn's disease, Ménétrièr's syndrome.
- *GU tract*: leukoplakia of the bladder, bilharzia.

GENERAL SYMPTOMS AND SIGNS OF MALIGNANT DISEASE

These may relate to the primary tumour, metastases, or generalized systemic manifestations.

They may be broadly classified as follows:

Primary tumour

Palpable swelling. This is usually painless unless invading other structures. Common examples include the palpable masses of the primary tumour in carcinoma of the breast, carcinoma of the thyroid, carcinoma of the caecum.

Obstruction. Examples include dysphagia in carcinoma of the oesophagus, obstructive jaundice in carcinoma of head of pancreas, large bowel obstruction in carcinoma of the colon, vomiting in gastric outlet obstruction from carcinoma of the gastric antrum.

Bleeding

- Overt: haemoptysis, haematemesis, haematuria, rectal bleeding
- Occult: carcinoma of the stomach or carcinoma of the caecum. Anaemia occurs.

Symptoms due to compression or invasion of local structures. SVC obstruction with bronchial carcinoma; back pain with retroperitoneal invasion with pancreatic cancer; invasion of nerves, e.g. facial paralysis with carcinoma of the parotid gland, recurrent laryngeal nerve palsy with anaplastic carcinoma of the thyroid.

Metastases

- Enlarged lymph nodes: may be discrete or hard, irregular and matted
- Hepatomegaly: primary in stomach, colon, bronchus, or breast
- Jaundice: from nodes in the porta hepatis, with primary in the stomach, pancreas, or colon
- Ascites: ovarian or any GI malignancy

- Abdominal mass due to omental secondaries – often in association with ascites
- Pathological fractures from bony metastases, e.g. breast, bronchus, thyroid, prostate, kidney
- Pleural effusion, e.g. from breast cancer
- Fits, confusion, personality change from cerebral metastases, e.g. breast, bronchus, malignant melanoma.

Generalized manifestations. Examples include cachexia, PUO (lymphoma, hypernephroma), hypertrophic pulmonary osteoarthropathy (carcinoma of the bronchus), thrombophlebitis migrans (carcinoma of the pancreas), neuropathies and myopathies (carcinoma of the bronchus), endocrine manifestations, e.g. ADH or ACTH production in bronchial carcinoma.

Asymptomatic incidental findings. Axillary lymphadenopathy on routine examination, e.g. with small impalpable carcinoma of the breast. Silent pulmonary primary or metastases on routine CXR.

DIAGNOSTIC PROCEDURES

Biopsy. This is mandatory, and may be carried out in a variety of ways:

- Fine-needle aspiration using a 22G needle: smear produced on slide; read by experienced cytologist
- Core biopsy, e.g. Tru-Cut: core of tissue removed for histological examination
- Incisional biopsy: removes a small accessible piece of the lesion for histological examination
- Excisional biopsy: the complete removal of a discrete lesion without a wide margin and without it being considered curative of the malignancy
- Evaluation under anaesthetic: to assess presence or extent of disease, e.g. staging laparotomy (largely superseded by CT scanning), panendoscopy, mediastinoscopy, bronchoscopy with biopsy of suspicious or high-risk areas.

Imaging (e.g. ultrasound, CT or MRI). This is used for confirming a suspected diagnosis and assessing spread. A negative study does not exclude microscopic disease.

Positron emission tomography (PET). This is complementary to other imaging modalities but differs from them as the scanner detects the metabolic activity of cancer cells via their increased uptake of a radioactive tracer (fluorodeoxyglucose) and subsequent emission of positrons. It can be used to detect the site of an unknown primary malignancy in the patient who presents with metastatic disease that cannot be identified by conventional clinical, radiological or histological means (e.g. SCC of the head and neck); for identification of metastases, e.g. lung cancer or non-Hodgkin's lymphoma; or for monitoring of response to therapy, and evaluation of recurrence. Further evidence is required to evaluate the roles for this relatively new modality.

STAGING AND GRADING OF CANCER

The extent of the malignancy of a tumour may be established clinically to provide an indication of the prognosis and to act as a guide for the type of treatment. It is also necessary for comparing the efficacies of different treatments in clinical trials. Three methods may be used – clinical, pathological and histological. Pathological staging is very subjective and there is a degree of observer variation. A tumour's apparent growth rate may be graded according to its histological appearance and its resemblance to mature cells of its lineage (degree of differentiation) can be commented on to indicate aggression.

CLINICAL STAGING

An example of this is the Manchester Classification of carcinoma of the breast (→ Ch. 10). This is based purely on clinical findings but is somewhat imprecise.

CLINICAL AND PATHOLOGICAL STAGING

The TNM Classification is recommended by the International Union Against Cancer. This method uses both clinical and laboratory results to grade the tumour. The clinician assesses three factors:

- Extent of the tumour (T)
- Node status (N)
- Presence of metastases (M).

(→ Ch. 10).

A method that is based on pathological staging only is Dukes' Classification for colorectal carcinoma (→ Ch. 14).

GRADING OF TUMOURS

The histological appearance of specimens are graded according to various criteria such as the proportions of cells undergoing mitosis, the degree of differentiation, the degree of nuclear pleomorphism, etc. This represents the 'aggressive' nature of the cancer. Examples include Broder's grading of squamous cell carcinoma or the Bloom-Richardson grading of breast carcinoma.

THE MULTIDISCIPLINARY TEAM (MDT) MEETING

Patients' case histories are presented at a regular MDT meeting comprising of specialists, e.g. surgeons, oncologists, radiologists, pathologists, nurses, etc. who manage those particular conditions, e.g. breast, head and neck, skin, sarcoma. The clinical findings are correlated with the radiological and pathological investigations, including staging and grading where known, and if the findings are concordant with a diagnosis, a course of action is decided. This may be, for example, surgery with curative or palliative intent, primary radiotherapy or chemotherapy, neo-adjuvant therapy or further investigation prior to treatment.

TUMOUR MARKERS

These are substances present in the body in a concentration related to the presence of a tumour. They are rarely sufficiently specific to be of diagnostic value. The tumour marker may be a substance secreted into the blood or other body fluid or expressed at the cell's surface by malignant cells in larger quantities than that of their normal counterparts. Detection is by measuring the concentration of the marker in the body fluids, usually by immunoassay, although some markers may be detected in histological sections by immunohistochemistry. The main value of tumour markers is in following the course of a malignant disease and monitoring the response to treatment and hence determining the prognosis. They may also be used for tumour localization and antibody-directed therapy. The following are examples of tumour markers in common use.

α-fetoprotein (AFP). Normally synthesized in the fetal yolk sac and liver. It is increased in hepatocellular cancer and germ cell tumours, i.e. testicular teratoma. It can be useful in monitoring the presence of metastases and response to treatment. Non-neoplastic causes of a raised AFP include cirrhosis, hepatitis and pregnancy.

Carcinoembryonic antigen (CEA). Normally produced by the fetal gut, liver and pancreas. It is raised in tumours of the colon, pancreas and stomach. In colonic malignancy, CEA is raised in 3% of Dukes A, 25% of Dukes B, 45% of Dukes C and 65% of metastatic cancer. It can be useful in assessing response to treatment and diagnosing recurrence before clinical detection. Non-neoplastic causes of raised CEA include ulcerative colitis, Crohn's and cirrhosis.

Human chorionic gonadotrophin (hCG). This was one of the first tumour markers to be recognized. It is raised in choriocarcinoma and hydatidiform moles. β-hCG is a valuable tumour marker for testicular cancers.

Prostate-specific antigen (PSA). PSA is a serine protease. Its normal function is to liquefy gel around spermatozoa. It is a very useful marker in prostatic cancer – it is organ-specific and is elevated in a higher proportion of patients than prostatic acid phosphatase (PAP). In patients with a PSA of 4–10 ng/mL, 20–30% will have prostate cancer. With a PSA <20 ng/mL, bony metastases are rare. Non-neoplastic causes of a raised PSA include benign prostatic hypertrophy and prostatitis.

CA 19-9. A tumour antigen elevated in gastrointestinal malignancy. It is not diagnostic but has been used commonly in association with pancreatic malignancy. It has a sensitivity and specificity of 80–90% for pancreatic cancer and is used to monitor the success of chemotherapy. It can also be elevated in pancreatitis, gallstones, cholecystitis and cirrhosis.

CA125. Most commonly used tumour marker in ovarian malignancy. It is associated with non-mucinous tumours. An elevated level is not diagnostic of ovarian malignancy – fewer than 50% of patients with stage I have a raised CA125. In addition, raised levels are also seen in pregnancy, endometriosis and cirrhosis. CA125 is also elevated in advanced non-ovarian malignancies.

CA15-3. This is a mucin marker used in the assessment of breast cancer. Patients with stage I disease may only show raised CA15-3 in approximately 10–20% of cases. In advanced cancer, the number of patients with increased levels is 50–100%. Benign breast disease may lead to elevated levels. However, CA15-3 has been used in assessing recurrence and has been shown to be prognostic – initially elevated levels are associated with a poorer prognosis. CA15-3 levels may also be raised in benign breast or ovarian disease or endometriosis.

TREATMENT OF CANCER

> Major treatments are surgical excision, radiotherapy, chemotherapy and hormonal manipulation.

SURGERY

Curative

The ideal operation for cancer is the one that completely eradicates the tumour. This may require wide excision of the tumour together with removal of the lymph nodes in continuity with the tumour. Sometimes, when the tumour is explored, it is found that it cannot be removed. On other occasions, the tumour is operable, i.e. the primary tumour can be removed but tumour remains behind, in which case it is incurable. Pre-malignant conditions may be treated by surgery, but other modes of management such as curettage and cautery, cryotherapy or photodynamic therapy (the ablation of pharmacologically photosensitized cells using a laser), e.g. in Bowen's disease or Barrett's oesophagus are also available.

Palliative

When operating on a tumour, it may be discovered that it is impossible to remove the primary lesion. However, a palliative operation may be carried out, e.g. bypassing an obstructing tumour in the GI tract to prevent the symptoms of intestinal obstruction.

Occasionally, operations are undertaken purely for palliative reasons when it is known that it will be impossible to remove the primary tumour, e.g. for bleeding, pain, obstruction. Occasionally, surgery is used to 'debulk' a tumour. This is often the case in extensive ovarian malignancy where removal of the greater mass of tumour will improve the efficacy of subsequent chemotherapy. Metastasis may also be excised, such as solitary lung metastases, subcutaneous metastases, etc. for local control. Other modes of therapy include radiofrequency ablation for liver metastases.

RADIOTHERAPY

Delivery of radiotherapy

Radiotherapy can be delivered to the site of a tumour in three ways:

- External beam radiation
- Implantation radiotherapy
- Systemic irradiation.

Radiation damages cells by inducing DNA damage. Cancer cells are affected more than normal cells because their DNA repair mechanisms are impaired. As a general rule, the higher the mitotic rate of a tumour, the greater the response to radiotherapy.

The absorbed dose of radiotherapy is quantified as the SI unit, the Gray (Gy) where $1 \text{ Gy} = 1 \text{ J.kg}^{-1}$. The total dose (typically around 50 Gy in solid tumours) is often divided into multiple exposures, or fractions to enable normal cells to recover, and to ensure more cancer cells are exposed during radiosensitive points in the cell cycle.

External beam radiation. This method is the most commonly used form of radiotherapy for skin and deeper tumours. The doses from beams from several angles can summate deep to the skin, thus avoiding the severe skin lesions that previously were a side effect of radiotherapy. Three-dimensional conformational mapping using a planning CT scan, and intensity modulated radiotherapy (IMRT) enables accurate dosing of radiotherapy fractions through computer-controlled X-ray accelerators for deep asymmetric tumours while minimizing collateral damage.

Implantation radiotherapy (e.g. intracavitary or intralesional). The source of irradiation may be placed within a cavity, e.g. in the vagina for irradiation of the cervix or directly into the lesion, e.g. iridium-192 (^{192}Ir) wires in carcinoma of the tongue.

Systemic irradiation. ^{131}I can be administered orally for follicular and papillary carcinoma of the thyroid gland. Experimentally, radioisotopes can be directed at cancer cells by attaching them to tumour-specific antibodies.

Use of radiotherapy

Radiotherapy can be used in four ways:

- Primary treatment (radical radiotherapy)
- Neoadjuvant prior to surgery and adjuvant after surgery
- Palliation
- Systemic treatment.

Primary treatment. Radiotherapy is used as the primary treatment with a view to a cure. Certain tumours, e.g. laryngeal, have a cure rate equal to surgery. Examples of tumours treated by radiotherapy include:

- Basal cell and squamous cell carcinoma of the skin
- Some head and neck tumours and laryngeal tumours
- Hodgkin's disease
- Lymph node metastases of a testicular seminoma following orchidectomy.

Adjuvant and neoadjuvant treatment. Neoadjuvant treatment is used preoperatively to down-stage tumours, i.e. decrease size and potentially convert an inoperable tumour into an operable one. Adjuvant radiotherapy aims to control microscopic tumour deposits that have spread beyond the resection margins or are spilt during surgery. An example is radiotherapy to the scar, axillary nodes, supraclavicular and internal mammary nodes in breast cancer.

TABLE 7.1 Complications of radiotherapy

General	Tiredness, malaise
Skin	Rashes, moist desquamation
Blood vessels	Endarteritis obliterans. Impairs blood supply. Progresses for many years after treatment. Many of the effects on other systems may have endarteritis obliterans as a precipitating cause
Healing	This is delayed, e.g. failure of skin grafts, anastomotic breakdown, intestinal fistulae
Renal tract	Frequency, cystitis
GI tract	Nausea, vomiting, anorexia. Irradiation proctitis (after irradiation of the cervix), causes rectal bleeding and tenesmus. Small bowel irradiation may give rise to intestinal fistulae and strictures
Head and neck	Xerostomia (dry mouth). Epiphora (red-watery eye) due to damage to tear duct

Palliative radiotherapy

● Bony metastases – pain relief is often dramatic
● Cerebral metastases
● Ulcerating or fungating breast cancer – controls oozing and bleeding and allows skin healing
● Lung cancer – to prevent cough and haemoptysis.

The complications of radiotherapy are shown in Table 7.1.

Systemic. Two types of systemic radiotherapy are used:

Total body irradiation. Leads to bone marrow failure and thus necessitates a bone marrow transplant; it is used in the treatment of leukaemias.

Radioactive isotopes. This form of radiotherapy uses radioisotopes that are concentrated in the tumour and lead to local irradiation of the tumour. Examples include ^{131}I in thyroid cancer and strontium-89 in prostatic metastatic disease.

CHEMOTHERAPY

Chemotherapeutic agents destroy tumour cells in a variety of different ways. Most tumours are treated by a combination of cytotoxic drugs, the combinations being chosen so that their toxic effects on any particular organ are minimized. The most appropriate combinations have usually been established by clinical trials based on initial empiricism. Drugs are usually given in short courses with a period of rest between courses to allow recovery of the normal tissues. The response of tumours to chemotherapy is very variable. Some are highly sensitive while others are insensitive.

Highly sensitive tumours in which there are prospects of a cure include Hodgkin's disease, testicular teratoma, childhood leukaemias, osteogenic sarcoma (lung secondaries).

Moderately sensitive tumours where palliation is the aim include ovarian tumours, breast cancer, and bronchial carcinoma.

TABLE 7.2 Side-effects of chemotherapy

Non-specific	Nausea, vomiting, metallic taste, general malaise
GI tract	Oral ulceration, diarrhoea
Reproductive system	Loss of libido, sterility, mutagenesis
Bone marrow	Bone marrow suppression with anaemia, thrombocytopenia, (bleeding), leukopenia (infection)
Immune system	Immunosuppression. Opportunistic infections, e.g. candidiasis, and *Pneumocystis carinii*
Skin	Rashes, ulceration, hair loss (regrows after course is stopped)
Urinary tract	Cystitis (cyclophosphamide), gout due to massive tumour destruction, leads to hyperuricaemia, which may lead to renal failure – prevented with allopurinol
Oncogenesis	20-fold increase in incidence of other malignancies

Apart from oral and intravenous administration, cytotoxic agents may be directly administered into a tumour, e.g. 5-fluorouracil for liver metastases and close intra-arterial injection in malignant melanoma; instillation into the bladder for superficial bladder tumours.

Side-effects

Chemotherapy is not only toxic to malignant cells but also to normal body cells, especially those with a high turnover rate, e.g. bone marrow and GI epithelium. Many side-effects are extremely unpleasant and should be carefully explained to, and discussed with, the patient prior to starting the course (→ Table 7.2).

HORMONAL MANIPULATION

This is applicable to carcinoma of the breast and carcinoma of the prostate. Removal of the source of hormones or blocking their effect may inhibit tumour growth.

Breast

The options available for hormonal treatment in breast cancer include:

● Inhibition of ovarian function
● Blocking the binding of oestrogen to cancer cells
● Blocking peripheral oestrogen production.

Inhibition of ovarian function. There are three methods available to decrease oestrogen production by the ovaries:

● Surgery – oophorectomy
● Pelvic irradiation – radiotherapy
● LHRH agonists, i.e. goserelin.

Inhibition of ovarian function is important in the management of breast cancer in premenopausal women. Meta-analysis of various trials of ovarian ablation in women <50 years old demonstrated a 26% reduction in annual recurrence and 25% reduction in the annual death rate.

Blocking the binding of oestrogen to cancer cells. The anti-oestrogen tamoxifen is effective in pre- and postmenopausal women with oestrogen receptor positive breast cancer. Tamoxifen is a non-steroidal drug that competes with oestrogen to bind the oestrogen receptor. Meta-analysis of trials demonstrated a 25% reduction in annual recurrence and a 17% reduction in annual death rate. Tamoxifen is also a first-line drug in metastatic disease. Long-term use may be associated with an increased risk of endometrial cancer. Fulvestrant is a new anti-oestrogen that causes downregulation of the oestrogen receptor. It can be used in tamoxifen-resistant metastatic disease.

Blocking peripheral oestrogen production. Following the menopause, the main source of oestrogen production is by the peripheral conversion of adrenal androgens in liver, muscle, breast and fat – this is mediated by the aromatase enzymes. The aromatase inhibitors, e.g. anastrozole, are useful in first-line treatment and in patients who have tamoxifen-resistant metastatic disease.

Prostate

The main aetiological factor in prostate cancer is dependence on testosterone. A number of modalities are available to reduce androgen exposure.

Surgical orchidectomy. The gold standard; has become less popular with the advent of medical alternatives.

LHRH analogues, e.g. goserelin. This results in chemical castration by the downregulation of receptors in the pituitary gland. It must be remembered that initial use will stimulate androgen production before inhibition (androgen flare). This may result in an exacerbation of symptoms and thus should always be given with an anti-androgen.

Oestrogen, e.g. diethylstilboestrol. Rarely used due to considerable side-effects. Results in castrate levels of androgens in 1–2 weeks.

Anti-androgens. These may be steroidal or non-steroidal. Steroidal anti-androgens, e.g. cyproterone acetate, inhibit LH release from the pituitary and decrease the binding of dihydrotestosterone to androgen receptors. Non-steroidal anti-androgens, e.g. flutamide, block dihydrotestosterone binding but not LH production.

Inhibition of adrenal enzyme synthesis. Used as second- or third-line treatment. Ketoconazole at 6× the normal dose causes chemical castration in 24 h.

BIOLOGICAL THERAPIES

Man made agents targeting specific cellular processes, rather than the DNA itself, have been developed and are used in certain cancers.

Examples include tyrosine kinase inhibitors (e.g. Imatinib for gastrointestinal stromal tumours) and monoclonal antibodies (MAb).

Examples of MAb agents currently in use include:

- Trastuzumab (Herceptin) in HER2 receptor positive breast cancer
- Rituximab targeting the CD20 antigen over-expressed in non-Hodgkin's lymphoma
- Bevacizumab (Avastin) targeting vascular endothelial growth factor (VEGF) to inhibit angiogenesis in bowel cancer.

TERMINAL CARE

Most patients with disseminated malignancy deteriorate until they reach a terminal phase. This phase is often accompanied by many unpleasant symptoms that are difficult to control. Support should not only be medical but should be emotional, psychological and spiritual. Initially, it may be possible to manage the patient at home with the support of family, friends, Macmillan nurse and family doctor. Death should be met with privacy and dignity. Eventually, hospitalization may be required for terminal care. Patients may be best managed in a hospice where all expertise is available to support the patients and their relatives.

PRINCIPLES OF TERMINAL CARE

1. Assess prognosis.
2. Discuss prognosis with patient and relatives.
3. Inform the family doctor of the situation and encourage regular visits. Maintain continuity out-of-hours.
4. Ensure all support that the patient may need to remain at home as long as possible, e.g. commodes, home help, district nurse, Macmillan nurse.
5. Provide support for carers.
5. Anticipate symptoms and try to prevent them, e.g. nausea, constipation, pain.
6. Regular review of medication to make sure pain relief is adequate and nausea and vomiting are well controlled.
7. Arrange appropriate hospital, or preferably hospice, accommodation when/if required.

TREATMENT OF SYMPTOMS

Pain
Regular opiates are needed to prevent 'breakthrough' pain. Suitable analgesics include MST tablets, fentanyl patches, morphine elixir, subcutaneous morphine, PCA via pump and spinal opioids; local blocks may help. In addition, steroids and chlorpromazine may be helpful. The correct dose of analgesic is that which relieves the pain. Opiate dependency and respiratory depression are irrelevant in the dying patient.

Nausea and vomiting
Anti-emetics should be given, e.g. metoclopramide, domperidone, prochlorperazine. Ondansetron is a very effective anti-emetic. If there is a mechanical reason for the nausea and vomiting, it may be difficult to control. If possible, a tube gastrostomy carried out under local anaesthetic may help. It allows the patient to swallow a suitable liquidized diet, which will then drain through the gastrostomy tube without subsequent vomiting.

Constipation
Regular laxatives and enemas may be required.

Dysphagia

A stent may be already *in situ*. Tasty liquidized food is helpful.

Mouth care

Careful attention to oral hygiene may prevent problems. 'Swish and swallow' nystatin may prevent candidiasis. If ulcers develop they may be treated with local anaesthetic gel and metronidazole gel.

Cough

This may be treated with morphine or codeine.

Insomnia

Treat with chlorpromazine or benzodiazepines.

Head, neck and otorhinolaryngology

The majority of head and neck problems seen in a surgical clinic are usually lumps. Often it is difficult for the family doctor to decide whether the lump lies in the field of the general surgeon, ENT surgeon, dental surgeon or dermatologist. The conditions described in this chapter are those that one may expect to see in a general surgery clinic or in an ENT clinic. The speciality of otorhinolaryngology (ear, nose and throat – ENT) is diverse. A multidisciplinary approach is mandatory and involves allied professionals such as audiologists, speech and language therapists, dentists, specialist nurses and prosthetists. ENT surgeons possess a detailed knowledge of the anatomy of the head and neck and its related benign and malignant pathological conditions, and have developed a variety of surgical techniques to manage these. Head and neck cancers are discussed at diagnosis in the context of a multidisciplinary team.

SCALP SWELLINGS

> These include sebaceous cysts, lipomas, papillomas, squamous cell and basal cell carcinomas and melanoma ($\rightarrow$ Ch. 19). Other swellings of the scalp include those described below.

Cephalhaematoma
This is a subperiosteal haematoma. It occurs following birth trauma or direct injury in babies. The haematoma occurs beneath the periosteum and is limited by the suture lines. It usually resolves spontaneously.

Ivory osteoma
Osteoma of the outer table of skull is a smooth hard swelling, and skin moves over it freely. It is confirmed by radiograph. It is asymptomatic and should be left or excised if it enlarges.

Cock's peculiar tumour

This is a suppurating sebaceous cyst with granulation tissue. It may be mistaken for a squamous cell carcinoma.

FACIAL SWELLINGS

> These include boils, sebaceous cysts, dermoid cysts, squamous cell carcinoma, basal cell carcinoma, malignant melanoma (→ Ch. 19).

SWELLINGS IN THE NECK

A convenient classification of these is: superficial, lymph nodes and deep swellings (→ Table 8.1).

The key to assessment and diagnosis of soft tissue neck swellings is careful history-taking, examination of the site, size and nature of the swelling (soft or firm, mobile or fixed, transilluminates, presence of a bruit). Fine needle biopsy is indicated for non-pulsatile masses. If the cytology is not definitive, then ultrasound core biopsy may be indicated if the imaging suggests it. The definitive investigation for soft tissue swellings is MRI.

In general, in patients over 45 years of age, assume a neck lump is metastatic malignant disease until proven otherwise.

TABLE 8.1 Swellings in the neck	
Superficial	Sebaceous cyst
	Lipoma
	Dermoid cyst
	Abscess
Lymph nodes	
Deep	
Anterior triangle	Move on swallowing:
	• thyroid
	• thyroglossal cyst
	• lymph node
	Do not move on swallowing:
	• salivary glands
	• branchial cyst
	• carotid body tumour
	• carotid aneurysm
	• sternomastoid 'tumour'
Posterior triangle	Cervical rib
	Subclavian artery aneurysm
	Pharyngeal pouch
	Cystic hygroma

SUPERFICIAL

Superficial lumps include sebaceous cysts, lipomas, dermoids and infective lesions, e.g. boils and abscesses. A common site for lipomas is in the midline posteriorly at the level of the collar line (→ Ch. 19).

LYMPH NODES

The majority of swellings in the neck, especially in children, are likely to be lymph nodes. The lymph nodes of the head and neck are basically arranged in two circles; an outer superficial one including submental, submandibular, preauricular, and occipital nodes; and an inner one surrounding the trachea and oesophagus and including the paratracheal and retropharyngeal nodes. Both the superficial and deep groups drain into a chain of deep cervical lymph nodes that surround the internal jugular vein. Lymph from there drains into the thoracic duct on the left and into the right lymphatic duct. The causes of cervical lymphadenopathy are shown in Table 8.2.

Investigation of cervical lymphadenopathy

Clinical examination. Look for local lesions, e.g. scalp, face, neck, mouth, tonsil. A full general examination of chest, breast, abdomen, testes and lower limb is required. Check for axillary and inguinal lymphadenopathy. Check for hepatosplenomegaly.

- Hb, FBC, ESR, Paul–Bunnell, *Toxoplasma* screen, viral antibodies, HIV
- CXR for hilar nodes or primary lung tumour
- Laryngoscopy and examination of postnasal space
- FNAC
- Ultrasound guided core biopsy of node
- Excisional biopsy of node – if lymphoma suspected

TABLE 8.2 Causes of cervical lymphadenopathy	
Infection	Local lesions on head and neck Upper respiratory tract infection Tonsillitis Glandular fever Toxoplasmosis Tuberculosis HIV Cat-scratch disease
Malignancy	Primary: • lymphoma • lymphosarcoma • leukaemia Secondary: • almost anywhere in the body, e.g. breast, lung, testis
Sarcoidosis	

- MRI or CT of the head and neck to examine nodes and look for possible primary
- Examination under anaesthetic by panendoscopy of nasopharynx, oropharynx, hypopharynx, larynx, trachea and upper bronchi, oesophagus and stomach and biopsy of suspicious areas and likely primary sites, i.e. nasopharynx, tongue base and the pyriform and tonsillar fossae.

DEEP SWELLINGS OF THE ANTERIOR TRIANGLE

Swellings that move on swallowing

Thyroid
Swellings of the thyroid gland are dealt with in Chapter 11.

Thyroglossal cyst
This is an embryological remnant of the thyroid and may present as a fluctuant swelling in the midline of the neck. It may occur anywhere along the line of thyroid descent but is most common just above the body of hyoid bone and attached to it.

Symptoms and signs. Usually a painless, cystic swelling in the midline of the neck that moves on swallowing. It also moves on protrusion of the tongue. Occasionally may become infected, with pain, tenderness, and increased swelling.

Treatment. This is by excision.

Lymph node
Occasionally a lymph node may be attached to thyroid isthmus and this will move on swallowing.

Swellings that do not move on swallowing

Salivary glands: inflammatory
The parotid gland is included here, although only a part of the gland extends into the neck under normal conditions. In pathological conditions it may present with the swelling largely in the neck. The causes of swellings of the salivary glands are shown in Table 8.3.

Acute sialadenitis. This is most common in the parotid gland and is due to epidemic viral parotitis of mumps. It is bilateral. Occasionally sialadenitis of both

TABLE 8.3 Swellings of the salivary glands	
Inflammatory and infective	Acute sialadenitis, e.g. mumps parotitis Chronic sialadenitis, e.g. calculus, duct stenosis
Neoplastic	Benign: • adenolymphoma • pleomorphic adenoma Malignant: • adenocarcinoma
Autoimmune	Mikulicz's syndrome Sjögren's syndrome

parotids and submandibular glands can be caused by poor oral hygiene, dehydration or duct obstruction by stone or stenosis. Acute bacterial sialadenitis is often unilateral.

Symptoms and signs. Sudden onset of pain and swelling over salivary glands. Made worse by eating. General malaise. Examination reveals redness, tenderness and swelling in the region of the gland.

Treatment. *Viral parotitis* – treat symptomatically with analgesics. Acute bacterial sialadenitis is treated by antibiotics, e.g. flucloxacillin. If an abscess forms, drainage is required. Recurrent parotitis should be investigated by sialography to exclude sialectasis and areas of duct stenosis.

Chronic sialadenitis. This is usually due to calculus in the duct or duct stenosis. Salivary calculi are composed of calcium or magnesium phosphate and are usually radio-opaque.

Symptoms and signs. Pain and swelling of the affected gland occur on eating and drinking. The swelling can be reproduced in clinic by putting lemon juice on the tongue. If the stone becomes impacted, the gland remains swollen. Infection and abscess formation may ensue. Inspect the duct orifice. In the case of submandibular calculi, the swelling may be seen in the duct in the floor of the mouth. Feel along the duct with a gloved finger in the floor of the mouth, palpating bimanually from the outside with the other hand. The calculus may be felt.

Investigations
● Plain radiograph
● 'Floor of mouth' view for submandibular calculi
● If no stone is seen, arrange sialogram.

Treatment
● Stone in the submandibular duct may be removed by incising directly over the stone into the duct in the floor of the mouth. The stone is extracted leaving the duct marsupialized.
● With duct stenosis, a ductoplasty (widening of the duct orifice) is carried out.
● For the stones in the gland itself, total (submandibular) or partial (parotid) removal of the gland is indicated.

Salivary glands: tumours

Salivary gland tumours are rare; 85% arise in the parotid gland, 8–15% in the submandibular gland, and 5–8% in the sublingual gland. Of these, the majority are benign and in the parotid, are usually pleomorphic adenomas. The minor salivary glands are submucosal around the oral cavity. In general, the smaller the gland, the more likely a neoplasm will be malignant.

Benign: Pleomorphic adenoma. Some 90% occur in the parotid. The old name of 'mixed parotid' tumour arose from the histological appearances of mixed element, i.e. epithelial, fibrous, myxomatous and 'pseudocartilaginous'. The latter was, in fact, mucus. They are slow growing and may enlarge over many years. The tumour sends processes into the surrounding parotid tissue, thus explaining why shelling out (enucleation) of these lesions may leave tumour behind with a high recurrence rate. After many years (10–30 years of slow growth), some pleomorphic adenomas develop into invasive malignant tumours.

Symptoms and signs. Early and middle adult life. Painless swelling on side of face. Slow growing. Examination reveals a non-tender, diffuse swelling in the angle between the mandible and mastoid process. It may extend down into the neck and forward on to the cheek overlying masseter. Test the integrity of the facial nerve. Diagnosis is made on clinical history and examination.

Differential diagnosis. Parotitis, sebaceous cyst, lipoma, preauricular lymph node, tumour of ramus of mandible.

Treatment. Superficial parotidectomy, i.e. removal of the gland superficial to the facial nerve. Enucleation is associated with a high incidence of recurrence.

Complications. Facial nerve palsy either temporary or permanent. Salivary fistula – usually dries up spontaneously. Frey's syndrome, i.e. facial flushing and sweating on eating, occurs in areas supplied by the auriculotemporal nerve.

The patient should be warned of these complications, especially the facial nerve palsy, prior to informed consent being obtained.

Benign: Adenolymphoma (Warthin's tumour). This is a cystic tumour that contains epithelial and lymphoid elements. It is benign.

Symptoms and signs. Middle and old age. More common in males. Slow-growing, painless swelling over angle of jaw. It is soft and well defined.

Treatment. Surgical excision. If patient is elderly and diagnosis is certain, these can be left alone. Recurrence is rare.

Malignant. Usually affects parotid and may arise in a longstanding pleomorphic adenoma. Mucoepidermoid tumours are primary squamous cell tumors of the parotid gland and are of variable grade.

Adenoid cystic carcinoma is associated with early perineural spread and skip lesions which normally requires adjuvant radiotherapy following removal of the gland and nerve branch. Patients may have a long latency period before haematogenous lung, liver or bone metastasis become clinically evident.

Symptoms and signs. The gland becomes hard, irregular and painful. Facial nerve palsy may develop.

Treatment. Radical parotidectomy with sacrifice of the facial nerve. Neck dissection may be required. Radiotherapy is of limited value. The prognosis is poor.

Secondary squamous cell carcinoma or melanomas of the head and upper aerodigestive tract may present with a lump in the parotid gland. These are treated with total parotidectomy and ipsilateral neck dissection.

Lymphomas may arise in the parotid gland. Surgery is confined to incisional biopsy prior to definitive oncological therapy.

Salivary glands: autoimmune

This is a slow painless enlargement of salivary glands. The glandular tissue is invaded by lymphocytes.

Mikulicz's syndrome. This causes symmetrical enlargement of the salivary glands, both parotid and submandibular. There is involvement of lacrimal glands and a dry mouth (xerostomia).

Sjögren's syndrome. This has the same symptoms as Mikulicz's disease but in addition has keratoconjunctivitis sicca (dry eyes) and seronegative arthritis.

Treatment. No treatment may be required but steroids may help. Dry eyes may be treated with hypromellose drops (artificial tears).

Branchial cyst

This is a remnant of the second branchial cleft. It may be associated with a sinus or fistula.

Symptoms and signs. It appears in early adult life, usually with soft swelling but consistency varies with tension in the cyst and some may be firm. It occurs at the level of the junction of the upper third and lower two-thirds of sternomastoid, appearing from under the anterior border of that muscle. It may be associated with the branchial sinus that opens over the anterior border of sternomastoid at the junction of the middle and lower thirds of that muscle. The sinus may extend up between the internal and external carotid arteries and open as a fistula into the side-wall of the pharynx.

Differential diagnosis of a branchial cyst. This is a lymph node. Diagnosis can be confirmed by aspirating the cyst and examining the fluid under the microscope, when cholesterol crystals will be seen.

Treatment. Surgical excision of cyst, sinus or fistula tract.

Carotid body tumour

This is a chemodectoma; a slow-growing tumour arising from the carotid body at the carotid bifurcation. It is usually benign but rarely does become malignant. Pathologically, it is described as a 'potato' tumour because of the shape and consistency when it is cut.

Symptoms and signs. Age 40–60 years. Painless, slow-growing lump with transmitted pulsation. May be associated with fainting attacks from pressure on the carotid sinus.

Investigations
● CT scan
● Angiography: shows a tumour blush at carotid bifurcation with splaying of the bifurcation (this investigation has largely been superseded by CT scanning).

Treatment. Surgical excision. Large tumours may require carotid bypass grafting.

Carotid aneurysm

A true aneurysm is extremely rare. A false aneurysm may arise following penetrating trauma of the neck. A tortuous carotid artery appearing from under the anterior border of sternomastoid may give the impression of an aneurysm. Careful examination will reveal the tortuosity and lack of an expansile area.

Sternomastoid 'tumour'

This is a swelling of the middle third of sternomastoid in neonates. It consists of oedematous and infarcted muscle.

Symptoms and signs. Neonates. Difficult birth, e.g. breech or forceps. Lump or torticollis. Pain on attempting to straighten neck. Head becomes turned to opposite side and tilted towards shoulder on side of lesion.

Treatment. Sternomastoid tenotomy.

DEEP SWELLINGS OF THE POSTERIOR TRIANGLE

Cervical rib

This may cause neurological or vascular symptoms in the arm (→ Ch. 15). It is often asymptomatic. Occasionally the rib is palpable.

Symptoms and signs. Vascular symptoms, e.g. Raynaud's phenomenon or venous thrombosis in the arm. Neurological symptoms, e.g. wasting of the small muscles of the hand (T1 myotome). Paraesthesia on the inner upper aspect of the arm in the dermatomal distribution of T1. May be a palpable lump in the supraclavicular fossa.

Diagnosis
- CXR to include thoracic inlet
- Count the ribs – if there are 13, there is a cervical rib.

Treatment. Excise the rib if causing symptoms.

Subclavian artery aneurysm

This is often just a poststenotic dilatation distal to a cervical rib. True aneurysms are rare. Treatment is by excision if symptomatic.

Pharyngeal pouch

This is a pulsion diverticulum of the pharynx occurring between the thyropharyngeus and cricopharyngeus muscles of the inferior constrictor, i.e. through Killian's dehiscence. The swelling is thought to be due to formation of a high-pressure area at Killian's dehiscence because of incoordination of the contraction of the two parts of the inferior constrictor of the pharynx.

Symptoms and signs. Middle or old age. Regurgitation of food on lying down. May develop aspiration pneumonia. Dysphagia due to pouch pressing on oesophagus. May gurgle on palpation. Halitosis.

Diagnosis. Barium swallow. *Never* endoscopy – the pouch may be perforated if the endoscope passes into it.

Treatment. Endoscopic diverticulotomy with external excision and cricopharyngeal myotomy if this is not possible.

Cystic hygroma

This is a collection of dilated lymphatic sacs that occur near the right lymphatic duct or thoracic duct in the lower part of the posterior triangle. They probably arise because of failure of the lymph channels to connect with main lymphatic drainage.

Symptoms and signs. Swelling in the lower part of the posterior triangle present at birth or occurring in the first few years of life. Soft, lobulated, fluctuant, compressible and brilliantly transilluminable.

Treatment. Surgical excision. Cyst walls are gossamer thin and rupture easily. Difficult to excise completely and therefore risk of recurrence.

ORAL DISORDERS

STOMATITIS

Stomatitis is a general term used to describe inflammation of the lining of part, or the whole, of the mouth (→ Table 8.4).

Symptoms of stomatitis
A sore dry mouth; mastication is painful. There may be painful cracking at the corners of the mouth.

Specific causes

Candida stomatitis
It is found in children and adults with debilitating disease, those on immunosuppressive drugs, and those with AIDS. It is also found in diabetics.

Symptoms and signs. Clinically small red patches appear which are then covered by a white membrane.

Investigations
● FBC
● Blood sugar
● Oral swab
● HIV test (if suspected and only after counselling).

Treatment. Nystatin mouth washes.

TABLE 8.4 Causes of stomatitis	
Local	Ill-fitting dentures Sharp teeth Smoking Local ulceration Infections, e.g. herpes simplex, candida, Vincent's angina Trauma, e.g. chemical, thermal, irradiation
General	Haematological: • leukaemia • agranulocytosis • anaemia • vitamin deficiency B and C Debilitating illness: • cancer • tuberculosis • following major surgery

Vincent's angina (acute ulcerative gingivitis)

It is caused by *Borrelia vincentii* (a spirochaete), and *Fusobacterium fusiformis*, which are Gram-negative anaerobes.

Symptoms and signs. Swollen, painful, inflamed gingiva. Ulcers develop which may spread to the tonsils and buccal mucosa. Other signs are bleeding, halitosis, cervical lymphadenopathy.

Investigations. Mouth swab.

Treatment. Penicillin, metronidazole.

Angular stomatitis (cheilosis)

Inflamed fissures at the corner of the mouth. The common cause is dribbling saliva at the corners of the mouth. It may occur in school-age children who lick the corners of the mouth. Treatment is aimed at adequate diet, improving oral hygiene, and local application of Vaseline.

General principles of management

History. Smoking, drugs, hot spicy foods, dentures, antibiotics.

Examination. Check dentures, check for sharp teeth, check general oral hygiene. Examine clinically for other signs of vitamin deficiency or haematological disease.

Investigations

- Hb
- FBC
- ESR
- Blood sugar
- CXR
- VDRL
- Mouth swab with film for fungus and culture and sensitivity for bacteria.

Treatment. Treatment is that of the underlying disease.

ULCERS

Traumatic

Caused by a sharp tooth or ill-fitting dentures. They heal rapidly when the causative agent is removed.

Aphthous

A small white deep painful ulcer, it may be solitary or multiple and heals spontaneously. Pain is relieved by local anaesthetic gel.

Herpes simplex

Multiple small painful ulcers of mouth or lips, they usually appear in debilitated patients. They may also appear as part of AIDS. Treat with topical acyclovir cream, oral or intravenous acyclovir.

Syphilitic

These are rarely seen. Chancre in primary, 'snail track' in secondary, and gumma in tertiary syphilis.

Tuberculous
These are rare, and usually found on the tongue. Painful ulcers with undermined edges, they are associated with advanced pulmonary tuberculosis.

Malignant
See below.

LEUKOPLAKIA

Leukoplakia may occur anywhere within the mouth but is common on the tongue. Areas affected by it appear thickened, white and may show cracks and fissures. Unlike *Candida* it cannot be rubbed off. It is a premalignant condition.

CYSTIC LESIONS OF THE LIPS AND MOUTH

Mucous retention cyst
These occur on the inner surface of the lips and anywhere in the mouth where there are mucus-secreting glands. Obstruction to the duct causes the cyst.

Symptoms and signs. Painless cystic lesion. Pinkish grey. Transilluminates.

Treatment. Excision or it may burst spontaneously.

Ranula
A large mucus retention cyst of the floor of the mouth, it looks like a frog's belly (*ranula* is Latin for frog). It occurs in children and young adults.

Symptoms and signs. A swelling in floor of mouth between symphysis menti and the tongue in the midline. Soft, fluctuant, transilluminates, bluish in colour.

Treatment. Complete excision or marsupialization.

Sublingual dermoid
Although congenital, these are rarely noticed before the age of 10. Usually midline, it results from inclusion of the ectoderm during fusion of mandibular processes.

Symptoms and signs. Swelling in floor of mouth. Usually painless. May present as 'double chin' if below mylohyoid. In the latter case it may be mistaken for a thyroglossal cyst.

Treatment. Excision or leave alone if diagnosis known.

TONSILLITIS
The tonsils are mucosal-associated lymphoid tissue (MALT) lying in the space bounded by the anterior faucial pillars formed by the palatoglossus and the posterior faucial pillars formed by palatopharyngeus. Infection, most commonly viral (e.g. rhinovirus, adenovirus).

Symptoms and signs. The patient complains of a sore throat, difficulty in swallowing, earache and general malaise. Patients may be pyrexial. Bacterial tonsillitis (β-haemolytic *streptococcus, staphylococcus, haemophilus influenzae*) may present with pus on the tonsils (follicular tonsillitis) which is an indication for broad spectrum antibiotic therapy.

Investigations
● Throat swab
● Paul Bunnell test for infectious mononucleosis (glandular fever).

Treatment. Broad spectrum antibiotics if considered bacterial. Amoxicillin should not be given if infectious mononucleosis is suspected as it may be complicated by a rash.

Lymphoid neoplasias such as lymphoma and leukaemia should form part of the differential diagnosis of tonsillar enlargement.

Tonsillectomy
Tonsillectomy is not generally indicated in isolated episodes of tonsillitis. Recurrent bacterial tonsillitis, multiple quinsy or respiratory obstruction may necessitate removal. This is performed under general anaesthetic. An incision is made in the mucosa of the anterior faucial pillar and the tonsil dissected from its fossa. Bleeding may be prevalent from its inferior aspect where it merges with the base of the tongue. Postoperative bleeding may occur immediately or within 48 h of surgery, and warrant re-exploration, or may occur several days postoperatively, normally due to infection.

CARCINOMA OF THE UPPER AERODIGESTIVE TRACT

THE ORAL CAVITY

Squamous cell carcinoma may present as a lump or ulcer on the lips, in the mouth, or on the tongue. It spreads via the lymphatics to glands in the neck. It is usually a disease of the elderly and more common in males.

Predisposing factors
The six 'Ss': smoking, syphilis, sharp tooth, spirits, spices, sunlight. Alcohol and smoking have a synergistic effect on predisposition. These agents may predispose to chronic superficial glossitis, which results ultimately in leukoplakia, which then results in malignant change with frank carcinoma. Exposure to sunlight may predispose to carcinoma of the lip.

Carcinoma of the lip
Symptoms and signs. An ulcer that does not heal in those aged 60 years and above. More common in men than women. Preceded by leukoplakia, it may occur in pipe smokers. A non-tender ulcerative lesion, it may be associated with lymphadenopathy.

Investigations. Excision or incisional biopsy depending on size.

Treatment. Wide excision. Block dissection of neck if nodes involved. Radiotherapy.

Carcinoma of the tongue

Although it is more common in males, the incidence has been decreasing over the past 25 years. The incidence is stable in females but the overall incidence remains higher in the male. Most frequently it appears on the lateral margins of the anterior two-thirds of the tongue as a small warty growth, ulcer, or indurated fissured area. Initially painless it becomes painful when secondary infection occurs or invasion is deep into the tongue. Pain may be referred to the ear, being referred from the lingual branch of the trigeminal nerve, which supplies the tongue to the ear via the auriculotemporal nerve. If the tumour is extensive and is on the posterior one-third of the tongue, swallowing and speaking may be difficult.

Investigations
- Biopsy, incisional or excisional depending on size of tumour
- Panendoscopy and biopsy should be performed on patients with oral cavity tumours to exclude synchronous tumours (1–6% of patients).

Treatment
- Small tumours less than 1 cm can be treated by simple excision or brachytherapy.
- Larger lesions may be treated with radiotherapy or more extensive surgery, e.g. subtotal glossectomy and block dissection of neck (40% of patients have nodal involvement at the time of presentation, 20% bilateral disease). Occasionally this may require removal of part of the mandible with major plastic reconstruction.

Carcinoma of the floor of the mouth

Often these are extensive ulcerating tumours that may invade the floor of the mouth and extend into the root of the tongue and the gums. Spread to regional lymph nodes occurs early.

Investigations
- Biopsy
- CT scan.

Treatment. Wide excision, with or without mandibulectomy, with block dissection of the neck and plastic reconstruction. Radiotherapy may be the most appropriate treatment in some cases and can be given by either external beam or implants.

Prognosis. For small cancers of the lips, 5-year survival rates of 90% have been reported. However, overall carcinoma of the lip has a 5-year survival of over 60%. Tumours of the tongue and floor of the mouth have a poorer survival, being about 30% at 5 years.

Carcinomas can occur anywhere in the oral cavity in the buccal mucosa, retromolar trigone, alveolar ridge and hard palate.

SQUAMOUS CELL CANCER OF THE PHARYNX AND LARYNX

The upper aerodigestive tract can be divided into the nasopharynx (from nasal choana anteriorly to soft palate inferiorly), oropharynx (from palatoglossus anteriorly, including posterior third of tongue and soft palate, to upper border of epiglottis), hypopharynx (from upper border of epiglottis superiorly to cricoid cartilage inferiorly, the larynx anteriorly).

Carcinoma of the nasopharynx

Rare in the Western population but a much higher prevalence in China. Predisposing factors include Epstein–Barr virus (EBV) and nitrosamine-containing foods, but less evidence of causative effects of tobacco and smoking. Local invasion can occur into sphenoid sinus, oropharynx, orbit or skull base.

Symptoms and signs. Patients often present late with enlarged nodes in the neck (often bilateral). Other symptoms include epistaxis, nasal obstruction, conductive deafness, otitis media, tinnitus, sore throat or CNIII–VI palsy.

Investigation
- MRI head and neck
- Panendoscopy and biopsy
- FNAC
- US guided core biopsy of lymph node.
- If lymphadenopathy of uncertain cause then polymerase chain reaction (PCR) of specimen can amplify and identify EBV DNA to support diagnosis of occult tumour.

Treatment. Chemoradiation is treatment of choice. Neck dissection if lymph nodes involved.

Carcinoma of the oropharynx

Most tumours are squamous in origin, however the higher density of lymphoid tissue means that higher proportions of lymphoma are found in this region. Local invasion can occur into sinuses, sphenoid,

Symptoms and signs. Patients often present late with enlarged nodes in the neck (often bilateral). Referred otalgia. CNIX or X palsy.

Investigations
- MRI head and neck
- Panendoscopy and biopsy.

Treatment. MALT lymphoma is radiosensitive. Early SCC treated with chemoradiotherapy. More advanced lesions may require surgical resection. Access can be difficult. Tumours on base of tongue may require exposure via a lip splitting, lateral pharyngotomy or mandibulotomy approach. Laryngeal wall tumours may require laryngopharyngectomy. Neck dissection is performed if involved nodes present or access required to vessels for free flap reconstruction. Tracheostomy is performed initially.

Carcinoma of the hypopharynx and cervical oesophagus

Hypopharyngeal carcinoma most frequently involves the pyriform sinuses, and when advanced, has a high rate of pulmonary metastatic spread.

Symptoms and signs. Dysphagia, CN IX referred otalgia. Palpable lymphadenopathy.

Investigations
- Barium swallow
- MRI head and neck
- Panendoscopy and biopsy.

Treatment. Chemoradiation is becoming treatment of choice. If early stage or chemoradiation has failed, then surgery is an option. Partial laryngopharyngectomy may be performed for small hypopharyngeal lesions, total laryngopharyngectomy if more extensive. Gastrointestinal continuity can be reconstructed with a gastric pull up, free radial forearm or free jejunal flaps. Pedicled pectoralis major flaps can be used for salvage cases or high anaesthetic risk. Neck dissection may be performed for microsurgical access or in presence of lymphadenopathy. Total oesophagectomy and gastric pull-up may be required for extensive oesophageal lesions.

Carcinoma of the larynx

Divided into supraglottic (above vocal cords), glottic (vocal cords – most common), subglottic (below vocal cords – rare).

Symptoms and signs. Voice change, hoarseness.

Investigations
- MRI head and neck
- Panendoscopy and biopsy.

Treatment. Dependent on site and size. Options include transoral laser ablation, chemoradiation, partial laryngectomy and closure or reconstruction with a free radial forearm flap, total laryngectomy. Elective neck dissection for supraglottic tumours, as >20% have occult metastatic spread to lymph nodes – rarely with glottic tumours.

Neck dissection

Removal of the lymph nodes draining the head and neck by block dissection of soft tissue between superficial and visceral/deep layers of deep cervical fascia.

Cervical nodal basin divided into levels I–VI (Sloan Kettering nomenclature):

I.   Submental/submandibular nodes – triangle bounded by hyoid, mandible and posterior belly of digastric
II. Upper jugular – skull base to level of hyoid bone
III. Middle jugular – hyoid bone to level of cricoid cartilage
IV. Lower jugular – cricoid cartilage to clavicle
V.   Posterior triangle – bounded by clavicle, sternomastoid, trapezius
VI. Anterior nodes.

Indications. Clinical or radiological evidence of lymph node secondaries from head and neck cancer. If no evidence of lymphadenopathy may be performed if high probability (arbitrarily >20%) of occult metastases, or if access to branches of the external carotid artery/internal jugular vein (IJV) required for microsurgical anastomosis in free flap reconstruction.

Classification. Traditionally, radical neck dissection removes levels I–V sacrificing the XI accessory nerve, internal jugular vein and sternomastoid muscle.

Modified radical neck dissection preserves one or more of these structures.

Selective neck dissection takes specific levels of drainage, e.g. supraomohyoid dissection (levels I–III), lateral (II–IV) – determined by likely levels of lymphatic spread from anatomic location of primary. Sentinel node biopsy helps to further define the locale of lymph node spread.

Extended neck dissection – Levels I–V plus other levels or non-lymphatic structures, e.g. parotid, anterior level VI.

Complications. Bleeding, pneumothorax, air embolus, carotid artery injury, cerebrovascular accident, carotid blow-out, skin flap necrosis, infection, marginal mandibular (VII), XI, XII, phrenic or lingual nerve injury, chyle leak.

DISORDERS OF THE EAR

Otitis externa

Infection of the external auditory canal to the tympanic membrane. Infective causes include β-haemolytic *streptococcus, Staphylococcus aureus, Pseudomonas aeruginosa*, anaerobes or fungi, e.g. *aspergillus*. Skin allergies, swimming in dirty water, chemical irritants (e.g. shampoo, hairspray), foreign bodies (e.g. cotton buds) and diabetes predispose. Furunculosis can occur around an infected hair follicle.

Symptoms and signs. Pain, swelling and itching of pinna, discharge from the canal, conductive hearing loss.

Treatment. Topical antibiotic (gentamicin, chloramphenicol) and steroid eardrops normally lead to resolution. Malignant otitis externa can occur in diabetics leading to skull base destruction and cranial nerve palsy, therefore requires surgical debridement and parenteral antibiotics.

Acute otitis media

Common middle ear infection in infants and young children. Acute otitis media is associated with a middle ear effusion. Causative organisms viral or bacterial (*Strep. pneumoniae, Haemophilus influenzae, Moraxella catarrhalis*). Acute otitis media is often associated with an upper respiratory tract infection due to migration along the eustachian tube.

Symptoms and signs. Peak incidence at 6–15 months. Pain, fever, malaise, vomiting, red and bulging eardrums, pus discharge from perforated eardrum. Child is unlikely to report hearing loss.

Treatment. Most cases resolve spontaneously. Indications for antibiotic therapy are controversial. In general, if the child is under 2 years of age, pyrexial, or has evidence of purulent discharge prescribe antibiotics (co-amoxiclav). Otherwise consider delaying therapy for 2–3 days. Perforated eardrums should heal within 2–3 weeks.

Complications. Chronic serous otitis media (glue ear) can persist and hearing can become impaired. Audiometry is used to assess hearing loss. A child >3 years with bilateral OME (otitis media with effusion) may develop problems with language development and therefore myringotomy and insertion of grommets may be required. These small tympanic tubes equalize the pressure between the middle and external ear. Other complications include chronic suppurative otitis media, mastoiditis, labyrinthitis, meningitis, intracranial abscess.

Chronic suppurative otitis media (CSOM)

This can arise in cases of recurrent acute otitis media due to a cycle of inflammation, ulceration, infection and granulation tissue formation in the middle ear.

In 'unsafe' CSOM there is associated cholesteatoma (squamous epithelial implantation into the middle ear causing destruction of middle ear contents).

Symptoms and signs. Cheese-like, purulent or clear otorrhoea; hearing loss; swollen auditory canal, tympanic perforation with erythematous, oedematous middle ear mucosa beyond. Unsafe CSOM may also be complicated by labyrinthitis, cerebral sinus thrombosis and embolism, facial paralysis, vertigo, meningitis, intracranial abscess. May ultimately cause conductive deafness.

Investigations
- Audiometry – conductive hearing loss
- CT scan to identify cholesteatoma.

Treatment. Regular aural toilet. Topical antibiotic therapy and steroid therapy to control granulation. Surgery for failed medical therapy includes tympanomastoidectomy to clear the middle ear of disease, with a tympanoplasty to seal the perforated eardrum. If cholesteatoma is present then a classical or modified radical mastoidectomy may be indicated. In hearing loss, cochlear implants may be considered once disease eradicated.

Benign paroxysmal positional vertigo (BPPV)

Vertigo is the hallucination of movement and BPPV is the commonest form. It is caused by dislodged vestibular calcium carbonate particles (otoconia) entering the semicircular canals (particularly posterior canal) causing abnormal stimulus of the hair cells.

Predisposing factors. Labyrinthitis or head trauma.

Symptoms and signs. The patient feels the room moving around them, for about 10–20 s after rotational head movement or looking up.

Diagnosis. Can be precipitated and diagnosed by quickly moving a patient from sitting upright face forward, then rotating the neck laterally at 45°, then moving to a lying down position with the neck hyperextended 20° (Dix–Hallpike manoeuvre). Nystagmus after a latency of 5–10 seconds is positive for BPPV. The fast phase of the nystagmus is towards the affected ear.

Treatment. May resolve spontaneously over weeks or months; may respond to manipulations of the head (e.g. Epley or Semont manoeuvre).

Ménière's disease

Inner ear condition of unknown cause. Associated with increased pressure in the endolymphatic sac; 1:100 incidence. Onset commonly at 20–50 years.

Symptoms and signs. Triad of vertigo, tinnitus and deafness. Progressive. Initial paroxysmal (minutes to hours' duration) vertigo with nausea and vomiting. Tinnitus and transient hearing loss may develop. Periods of remission become more variable until the deafness and tinnitus becomes permanent. Later, the vertigo may resolve. Balance becomes difficult.

Investigations. With pure tone audiogram, balance and other specialized tests.

Treatment
- Vertigo attacks treated with prochlorperazine or cinnarizine
- Preventive treatment with betahistine and low dose diuretic may control symptoms
- Vestibular rehabilitation exercises
- White noise generators can help to mask the tinnitus
- Hearing aids for deafness.

Refractory treatment may require local gentamicin injection into middle ear, endolymphatic sac decompression, section of the vestibular nerve or labyrinthectomy.

Labyrinthitis

Inflammation of the labyrinths housing the vestibular system. Commonly viral in origin but may be a bacterial cause.

Symptoms and signs. Patient presents with vertigo, imbalance, nausea, vomiting and sometimes tinnitus or hearing loss. Vestibular neuritis (inflammation of CNVIII) presents in similar fashion but without the hearing loss.

Ramsay Hunt syndrome = Herpes zoster reactivation in geniculate ganglion of CNVII with external vesicular rash and facial nerve weakness. CNVIII affected as in close proximity. Symptoms may improve on lying down. Treat with acyclovir and steroids (prednisolone).

Treatment. Acute labyrinthitis treated symptomatically with prochlorperazine. If bacterial, then amoxicillin. Resolves within 8 weeks as brain compensates for changes in vestibular signalling. Uncompensated labyrinthitis may cause chronic symptoms. Additional treatment includes vestibular rehabilitation therapy (VRT) using eye, head and body exercises.

Deafness and hearing aids

Hearing loss can be conductive (CHL) or sensorineural (SNHL); congenital or acquired.

CHL is impairment of the airwave signal from the external ear to the cochlea. Acquired causes include foreign body, earwax (cerumen) impaction, cholesteatoma (see above) and benign tumours, e.g. glomus jugulare or haemangioma.

Otosclerosis

Otosclerosis is the commonest cause of CHL affecting 1% of the population in the third decade. This has a genetic predisposition and is caused by osteoblasts forming dense bone around the ossicles. The stapedial footplate can become involved and fixed to the oval window causing CHL. Patients can present with associated tinnitus and vertigo. Fine-cut CT scan and pure tone audiometry may confirm the diagnosis. Amplification hearing aids may improve function. Surgery is highly successful, involving removal and replacement of the stapes with a prosthesis (stapedectomy). However, it may not cure the tinnitus and there is a risk of deafness.

SNHL is the impairment of the transmission of the hearing signal after the cochlea. This may be caused by damage to the cochlea hair cells or CN VIII, e.g. due to trauma, surgery or acoustic neuroma. Congenital causes are numerous and may be syndromic (associated with other congenital anomalies) or non-syndromic. Positive family histories and known causative genetic mutations have been identified.

Prenatal cytomegalovirus, rubella virus or exposure to teratogens predispose, as does perinatal sepsis, administration of ototoxic medication (e.g. aminoglycosides), childhood meningitis or mumps.

Investigations. Neonates in the UK are routinely screened for audio-evoked brainstem response (ABR), looking for nerve signal activity to the brain in response to an audible stimulus. This does not distinguish between SNHL and CHL. Pure tone audiometry (PTA) can be used from age 4–5 and can distinguish.

Treatment. Ongoing cause of CHL caused by otitis media should be treated with, e.g. antibiotics, myringotomy, grommets. An amplification hearing aid may help in both CHL and SNHL to provide as much audio input as possible. Speech therapy can prevent delayed language development. Hearing aids may be bone-anchored (BAHA) in the case of a congenitally absent or malformed pinna. SNHL may be treated surgically with a cochlear implant. These are surgically implanted into the cochlear and convert sound frequencies into electrical impulses that stimulate the CN VIII.

DISORDERS OF THE NOSE

The nose can be examined using a headlight or head mirror, and nasal speculum. A nasendoscope can be used to examine the nasal cavity.

Nasal obstruction

May be caused by inserted foreign bodies, inflammation secondary to allergic rhinitis or infectious rhinosinusitis, nasal polyps, tumours, granulomas (sarcoidosis, Wegener's granulomatosis, tuberculosis).

Foreign bodies are associated with a purulent discharge and swelling. May require examination and removal under general anaesthetic.

Infectious rhinosinusitis

Can be caused by viruses (rhinovirus, influenza, parainfluenza), bacteria (*Haemophilus influenzae, Streptococcus, Staphylococcus*) or fungi (*aspergillus*). Aggressive infection may spread to the orbit, skull base or intracranially, causing an intracerebral, extradural or subdural abscess. Changes in vision, conscious state, drowsiness, meningism or lateralizing neurological signs, indicate an urgent CT scan and subsequent definitive drainage.

Polyps

Polyps are pedunculated masses of oedematous mucosa that arise from the sinuses or the lateral nasal wall. They are most commonly idiopathic, but can be secondary to cystic fibrosis, asthma or aspirin sensitivity. They can be surgically removed or treated symptomatically with intranasal or systemic steroid therapy.

Tumours

Tumours of the sinuses are rare. They may present with epistaxis, and in adults are most commonly squamous cell carcinomas. These can present with recurrent epistaxis and chronic nasal obstruction. Nasopharyngeal cancer can present with nasal obstruction.

MRI and CT scans will help identify the extent of the tumour and help plan surgical resection after discussion in the MDT. Adjuvant chemotherapy and radiotherapy may be indicated.

Lesions of the maxilla may require access via a Weber–Ferguson incision – an incision extending vertically along lip philtrum, along the ipsilateral nasal-cheek margin (lateral rhinotomy) and along the eyelid-cheek margin. Partial or total maxillectomy may be required for clear margins and the orbital floor can be reconstructed with calvarial bone grafts, and the cavity including the hard palate filled with a prosthetic obturator or free microvascular muscle transfer, e.g. rectus abdominis (→ Ch. 19).

ENT EMERGENCIES

EPISTAXIS

Acquired causes of nose bleeds include local trauma, anticoagulants, massive transfusion, benign and malignant tumours, allergic rhinitis, liver and renal failure, and blood dyscrasias, such as primary and secondary thromobocytopaenia, lymphoma, leukaemia and aplastic anaemia. Congenital causes include hereditary haemorrhagic telangiectasia, haemophilia and von Willebrand's disease.

Little's area (anterior nasal septum) is the most common site of bleeding. Minor bleeds may cease with local pressure, topical application of local anaesthetic with adrenaline, or cautery with a silver nitrate stick.

Heavier bleeds can be packed with Merocel nasal tampons or a ribbon gauze layered within the nasal cavity. Posterior nasal bleeding may be controlled by passage of a Foley catheter into the nasopharynx and inflation of the balloon to apply pressure to the area. Uncontrollable bleeding may require urgent referral to the interventional radiologist for embolization or arterial ligation may be required.

In the case of heavy bleeding, the patient should be investigated for cause with full blood count and clotting studies. They may need resuscitation with fluids and blood products.

NASAL TRAUMA

A simple 'broken nose' may be reducible by manipulation if managed within 2 hours of injury, after which swelling obscures the deformity. However, manipulation can be attempted at 10 days once the swelling has resolved and before the fractures have become too sticky.

Submucosal nasal septal haematomas require urgent incision and drainage to prevent cartilage necrosis and a resultant 'saddle-nose' deformity.

Nasal trauma with broadening of the distance between the medial canthi (telecanthus) implies a nasoethmoidal fracture which may require reduction and fixation, and should therefore be investigated with a CT scan. Any nasal trauma associated with a high-energy blow and other deformity (e.g. malocclusion, trismus, diplopia) should also be investigated with a CT scan.

SWALLOWED FOREIGN BODY

Chicken or fish bones can become entrapped in the oropharynx. This may be in the palatine or lingual tonsils. The patient presents with drooling and a feeling of irritation at the back of the throat. These can be removed under local anaesthetic, using forceps.

Foreign bodies can become lodged in the hypopharynx, above the cricopharyngeal sphincter, sometimes causing dysphagia, pain and a change in the voice. Surgical emphysema around the neck would suggest perforation by a sharp body such as a bone. If suspected, an urgent barium swallow should be requested and endoscopy may be required for removal. In cases of perforation, there is a risk of mediastinitis and the patient should commence broad-spectrum i.v. antibiotics and be observed while 'nil by mouth'.

Larger foreign bodies, such as marbles or coins swallowed by children may become trapped at the upper oesophageal sphincter and in extreme cases, may present with stridor and respiratory compromise. These may be radio-opaque and therefore an X-ray investigation is indicated.

PERITONSILLAR ABSCESS (QUINSY)

The peritonsillar or quinsy abscess is an acute suppurative infection in the peritonsillar space following an episode of acute tonsillitis. Patients present with trismus and drooling with a foul smelling breath. It can cause necrotizing fasciitis, airway compromise and haemorrhage. The abscess is treated by incision and drainage under local, or occasionally general anaesthetic.

DEEP INFECTIONS OF THE NECK

Acute peritonsillar infection or oropharyngeal foreign bodies may give rise to a deep neck abscess in the lateral parapharyngeal space between the deep and superficial cervical fascia, superior to the hyoid bone and anterior to the carotid sheath. These are treated by external incision and drainage with adjunctive antibiotic therapy. Children can be affected by a suppurative infection of the retropharyngeal nodes. Similar retropharyngeal abscesses can be seen in adults following endoscopy, intubation or oropharyngeal/middle ear infections. These present with sore throat, fever, dysphagia and neck pain. Urgent incision and drainage is recommended.

ACUTE EPIGLOTTITIS

Caused by *Haemophilus influenzae* type B, acute epiglottis is a potentially fatal infection presenting in children 2–7 years of age. Symptoms include stridor and dyspnoea – worse on lying supine, dysphagia and excessive drooling. The child sits upright and is distressed. Widespread vaccination has reduced the incidence of this, and it responds to amoxicillin therapy. On presentation, humidified oxygen should be administered. Direct laryngoscopy may cause life-threatening obstruction, and should only be performed by staff with the means to secure the airway. Orotracheal intubation may be difficult, and therefore needle cricothyroidotomy may be life-saving until a definitive airway can be established.

ACUTE HEARING LOSS

Sudden deafness is most often conductive, caused by occlusion of the external ear canal by wax, foreign body or haematoma. Middle ear causes include perforation of the tympanic membrane caused by otitis media or direct trauma, and ossicle dislocation. Sensorineural hearing loss is most commonly idiopathic, probably viral or vascular in nature, but can also be secondary to acoustic trauma, barotrauma (in divers) or ototoxic drugs such as gentamicin. Associated vertigo or tinnitus would suggest a sensorineural cause. Care must be taken to exclude a retrocochlear cause such as acoustic neuroma. Inspection of the ear canal, tympanometry, pure tone audiogram and imaging with CT scan may be indicated to aid diagnosis. Treatment depends on cause.

Procedure

Open tracheostomy

This is a planned elective procedure, usually performed on a patient who is anticipated to require airway protection and ventilation for longer than 10 days. A tracheostomy reduces the dead space compared to an orotracheal tube, making gas exchange more efficient; reduces ulceration around the mouth and facilitates upper airway suction. A patient who is anticipated to need weaning from assisted ventilation over a long period will cope much better with a tracheostomy. Complications include bleeding, infection, tracheomalacia and tracheal stenosis.

- This is performed in an operating theatre with the patient under general anaesthetic, positioned supine with the neck extended and a sandbag between the shoulder blades.
- The intended tracheostomy tube is selected and the cuff checked for leaks and that the introducer fits inside the tube with ease.
- A 4 cm transverse skin incision is made one or two finger breadths above the sternal notch, below the palpable cricoid cartilage. Any anterior jugular vein is ligated and divided.
- Dissection through the superficial fascia proceeds in a longitudinal direction and the strap muscles (sternohyoid and sternothyroid) are separated from their counterparts.
- The isthmus of the thyroid gland is divided using bipolar diathermy to prevent bleeding. A self-retaining retractor is placed to visualize the trachea.
- The anterior trachea is dissected to visualize the underlying tracheal rings.
- The anaesthetist is informed that the trachea is about to be opened and they will advance the orotracheal tube caudally, moving the cuff away from the planned incision.
- The stoma is incised below the first tracheal ring, either as a longitudinal split or excised disc through the second, third and fourth rings.
- The introducer is made ready inside the tracheostomy with the cuff deflated and the anaesthetist deflates the orotracheal cuff and draws the tube in a cephalic direction until the tube is clear of the stomal opening. The introducer and tracheostomy tube are passed into the stoma and the introducer removed and the cuff inflated. This is then attached to the anaesthetic circuit.
- Breath sounds and chest expansion is checked bilaterally, and leaks excluded. If present, this may require a larger tube.
- The wound is partially closed with skin sutures around the tube, and the tube secured into place with the supplied neck tape or with sutures.

Thorax

HEART AND GREAT VESSELS

PRINCIPLES OF CARDIAC SURGERY

Surgery for heart disease has advanced to a point where safe and effective treatment can be offered for most conditions. Assessment of patients has become more refined with the development of special diagnostic techniques, e.g. echocardiography, scintigraphy, cardiac catheterization and cineangiography. Improvements in diagnostic techniques, anaesthesia, surgical techniques and postoperative management have led to better results with lower mortality rates and a reduction in complications.

Indications for surgery
- Failed medical treatment
- Where the mortality and morbidity of a surgical procedure is perceived to be less than that of the condition.

Contraindications for surgery
Correction of a defect alone may be contraindicated in the presence of the following:

- Irreparable myocardial damage
- Irreversible failure of other organs, e.g. kidneys and lungs.

However, it is now possible to correct these problems with multiple organ transplants and the above are only contraindications to repair of the defect alone.

Preoperative preparation
- Accurate diagnosis. This requires not only a full examination but a variety of investigations, including CXR, ECG, echocardiography, Doppler's, cardiac catheterization, MRI, cardiac CT, radionuclide scanning, pulmonary function tests
- Psychological preparation, especially for intensive care
- Control of cardiac failure with drugs
- Correction and/or investigation of anaemia
- Correction of electrolyte imbalance
- Correction of nutritional deficiencies
- Chest physiotherapy, bronchodilators, antibiotics, cessation of smoking.

Surgery

Most open-heart surgery is carried out via a median sternotomy incision. Closed mitral valvotomy used to be carried out via a left thoracotomy – the operation is rarely performed nowadays. A left posterolateral thoracotomy is used for ligation of a patent ductus arteriosus.

Cardiopulmonary bypass

The heart and lungs are excluded from the circulation, being replaced by a pump and membrane oxygenator. Venous blood returning to the heart is diverted, through tubes inserted into the right atrium, to an oxygenator. A roller pump is used to return oxygenated blood to the patient through a cannula placed in the ascending aorta, which is cross clamped below its point of entry. A small amount of blood returning to the LA from the bronchial arteries via the pulmonary veins is sucked out by additional suckers, defoamed and returned to the oxygenator. When the aorta is occluded, the myocardium becomes ischaemic. Two methods are available to preserve the myocardium:

- Intermittent or continuous coronary perfusion
- Depression of myocardial metabolism (cardioplegia).

The former consists of cannulation of either of the coronary ostia and infusion of blood or intermittent release of the aortic cross clamp. Reduction of myocardial metabolism is accomplished by cooling the heart with a 'cardioplegic' solution at 4°C infused into the coronary arteries, which arrests the heart in diastole. Aortic occlusion is well tolerated for 1–2 h using cold blood. After closure of the cardiac incisions, the heart is allowed to fill up with blood, air is removed from the heart, the aorta unclamped, the heart restarted and bypass discontinued.

Postoperative complications

Low cardiac output. This may result from haemorrhage, cardiac failure, tamponade, pulmonary hypertension, or cardiac arrhythmias.

Respiratory failure. This may be due to pulmonary oedema or atelectasis giving rise to hypoxia. Pain from the surgical incision reducing respiratory effort may be contributory.

Renal failure. Due to ATN, resulting from renal hypoperfusion. Haemofiltration/haemodialysis may be required.

Jaundice. Usually a result of transfusions or haemolysis, occurring as a result of cardiopulmonary bypass. Occasionally, liver failure occurs because of low cardiac output.

Cerebral damage. May be due to anoxia, air embolism, thrombus, cerebrovascular disease or fat embolism. Cerebral oedema may occur.

Postoperative treatment

Maintenance of cardiac output. Ensure adequate filling pressure of ventricles (preload). Maintain adequate CVP. Ensure myocardial contractility – inotropes. Maintain heart rate around 90/min. Use isoprenaline or pacing wires inserted at surgery. Reduce peripheral resistance (afterload) with vasodilators, e.g. GTN.

Metabolic acidosis may occur and is an indication of poor perfusion. Aortic balloon pumping may be used to reduce cardiac afterload. Haemorrhage and tamponade require urgent re-exploration. Pulmonary hypertension may respond to prostacyclin. Arrhythmias require drugs, cardioversion or pacing.

Prevention of respiratory problems. Optimize cardiac output. Use positive pressure ventilation, diuretics, pain relief, physiotherapy.

Maintenance of urine output. Optimize cardiac output, diuretics, e.g. furosemide, renal dose of dopamine.

Prevention of cerebral problems. Maintain normal BP. Reduce CO_2 by positive pressure ventilation, avoid hyperpyrexia, give dexamethasone.

CONGENITAL HEART DISEASE

> This occurs with an incidence of 8:1000 live births. Aetiological factors include maternal rubella, Down's syndrome and maternal drugs, e.g. warfarin and phenytoin.

The following lesions are most commonly encountered (in order of decreasing frequency): VSD, ASD, PDA, pulmonary stenosis, aortic stenosis, tetralogy of Fallot, coarctation of the aorta and transposition of the great vessels. Congenital heart disease may be classified as cyanotic (significant R-to-L shunt) or acyanotic (L-to-R or no shunt). The reader is referred to a textbook of medicine for the symptoms, signs and investigations of these conditions. The treatment and prognosis are indicated below.

Acyanotic

Ventricular septal defect (VSD)
Small defects may close spontaneously but surgery is indicated for large defects, cardiac failure, increased pulmonary vascular resistance and patients with pulmonary blood flow 1.5 times greater than systemic flow. The defect is closed with a prosthetic patch using cardiopulmonary bypass. Mortality and morbidity depend on the preoperative state of the patient and degree of pulmonary vascular resistance. An uncomplicated VSD has an operative mortality of less than 5%.

Atrial septal defect (ASD)
Surgery is indicated if pulmonary flow is 1.5 times systemic. The defect is closed with a patch. Ideally, the operation should be carried out before a child goes to school. Mortality is less than 1% but increases in the presence of pulmonary vascular resistance. Percutaneous device closure is increasingly used.

Patent ductus arteriosus (PDA)
At birth, the pulmonary vascular resistance decreases markedly as the lungs inflate and the ductus arteriosus closes within a few days. Failure of closure may occur in premature babies, hypoxia or maternal rubella. In premature babies a prostaglandin synthetase inhibitor, e.g. indomethacin, may promote closure.

All persistent ducts should be closed to prevent infective endocarditis. The ductus is doubly ligated via a left thoracotomy. Endovascular techniques are now in common use. Mortality is less than 0.5%.

Coarctation of the aorta

There are two types: adult and infantile. In the adult form, the aorta is narrow in the region of the ligamentum arteriosum just beyond the origin of the left subclavian artery. Proximal hypertension and LV overload occur. Most adult types can be stented. If surgical correction is required, the ideal age is 7–15 years. Operative procedures include resection with end-to-end anastomosis. If the gap is too large, a woven Dacron graft is inserted. Complications include residual hypertension, spinal cord ischaemia during surgery, recurrent laryngeal nerve palsy, and mesenteric 'arteritis' due to increased pulse pressure. Without surgery, the majority of patients are dead before the age of 40. Death occurs from aortic rupture, infective endocarditis, LV failure, cerebral haemorrhage. The operative mortality is about 5%.

The infantile form is rare and usually preductal. It may be associated with other cardiac defects in 60% of infants. Operative mortality is high, reaching 70% for surgery in the first 3 months of life.

Coarctation is commonly now treated by angioplasty in small children.

Congenital valve disease in children

Aortic stenosis or pulmonary stenosis may occur. Treatment is by balloon dilatation during cardiac catheterization or occasionally by open surgery.

Cyanotic

Congenital cyanotic heart disease is uncommon. The two common forms are the tetralogy of Fallot and transposition of the great vessels. Cyanosis may also occur where the L-to-R shunt of a VSD reverses owing to pulmonary hypertension (Eisenmenger complex).

Tetralogy of Fallot

This consists of a VSD, overriding aorta, pulmonary stenosis and RV hypertrophy. Correction involves reconstruction of the RV outflow tract and closure of the VSD. Nearly all children are corrected by a one-stop procedure – early correction in infancy is now the procedure of choice. Very rarely, an aortopulmonary shunt is used for palliative purposes in the first instance. A Blalock–Taussig shunt is the most common. The subclavian artery is divided on one side and anastomosed to the ipsilateral pulmonary artery to improve pulmonary blood flow. The shunt is closed and the defects corrected between the ages of 3 and 5 years. There should be no mortality associated with the shunt operation. However, the quality of cardiopulmonary bypass in children has now improved considerably such that one can expect to get good results with a one-stop procedure.

Transposition of the great vessels

The aorta arises from the RV and the pulmonary artery from the LV. Survival is dependent on co-existing defects, e.g. PDA, VSD, ASD, which permit mixing of the two circulations. Definitive surgical correction involves an 'arterial switch' where the aorta and PA are transected and reanastomosed, aorta to LV and PA to RV.

This operation has to be done in the first 2 weeks of life before the LV decreases in size. Alternatively interatrial repair can be undertaken at 6 months. A 'baffle' made of pericardium is created in the atrium to direct caval blood behind the baffle to the mitral valve and LV and PA, with the pulmonary venous return channelled in front of the baffle to the tricuspid valve, RV and aorta. Operative mortality is about 10%.

ACQUIRED VALVULAR HEART DISEASE

This is limited to the aortic, mitral and occasionally tricuspid valves. The pulmonary valve is rarely affected. The valve may be narrowed (stenosis) or rendered incompetent (regurgitation), or both may occur. Except for mitral stenosis and tricuspid incompetence, surgical treatment of acquired valvular disease requires valve replacement. Some types of mitral stenosis may be treated by closed mitral valvotomy while tricuspid incompetence may be treated by valvoplasty.

Types of valve
Mechanical valves
These include: *Ball valve* – The Starr–Edwards is a metal cage with a silastic ball. It is durable for long periods (up to 25 years). Not used nowadays.

Disc valve. In the past Bjork–Shiley tilting disc valves have been used but these are no longer made.

Bileaflet valve, e.g. St Jude (most commonly implanted in USA), Sulzer-CarboMedics.

All three types require(d) lifelong anticoagulation with its attendant risks. There remains a small risk of thrombosis and embolism. Failure is sudden.

Tissue valves
These are usually porcine xenografts or bovine pericardium. They are mounted on a frame with a sewing ring. The embolic rate is very low and therefore anticoagulants are not required. They lack long-term durability, with up to 75% failure rate at 15 years. They fail gradually.

Free aortic homograft is still a major choice.

Antibiotic-preserved fresh homografts may also be used.

Human cryopreserved allograft valves
Usually aortic valve inserted without a frame. Anticoagulants are not required.

Complications of artificial valves
- Thromboses with valve dysfunction or embolism
- Failure – calcification and rupture with tissue valves; mechanical breakage with prosthetic valves
- Bacterial endocarditis
- Obstruction – tissue growth onto valve ring
- Paravalvular leakage
- Haemolysis.

ISCHAEMIC HEART DISEASE

This is the commonest cause of death in the UK. Coronary artery disease is four times more common in men than in women although the incidence in women is increasing. It accounts for one-third of all male deaths and one-quarter of all female deaths.

Aetiology. Male sex, smoking, family history, hypertension, hyperlipidaemia, diabetes, obesity, myxoedema.

Symptoms and signs. Angina, MI, CCF. Sudden death. Often nothing to find on examination. Occasionally xanthelasma. Cholesterol nodules. Arcus senilis. Stigmata of diabetes. Peripheral vascular disease.

Investigations
- Hb
- FBC
- Lipid profile
- CXR – occasionally cardiomegaly
- ECG: may be normal at rest in up to 75% of patients; S-T depression with angina – exercise ECG usually confirms diagnosis
- Echocardiogram: LV hypertrophy, ejection fraction, areas of infarction
- Cardiac catheterization and coronary angiography – contrast medium is injected into each coronary artery and views recorded by cinephotography; the site and severity of disease is assessed
- LV function is assessed by ventriculography and intracardiac pressures.

Treatment. *Conservative.* Stop smoking. Dietary restrictions. Exercise, correct hyperlipidaemia, control anaemia, control diabetes. Avoid stress. Vasodilators, e.g. nitroglycerine spray; β-blockers, e.g. propranolol. Calcium antagonists, e.g. nifedipine, diltiazem. Aspirin. Graduated exercise programme.

Percutaneous transluminal coronary angioplasty (PTCA)
This is indicated with localized proximal incomplete blocks causing angina unresponsive to medical treatment. A balloon is inserted under radiographic control and the stenosis dilated. There is a 5% risk of infarction and a mortality of less than 1%. Stenting is thought to reduce restenosis rates.

Coronary artery bypass graft (CABG)
Surgery is indicated when there is intractable or unstable angina; triple vessel disease with depressed ventricular function, and left main stem stenosis. A reverse segment of saphenous vein is anastomosed between the aorta and the coronary artery distal to the obstruction. Total arterial revascularization is increasingly common. Both right and left internal mammary arteries are used, as well as the radial artery, as an arterial replacement. The gastroepiploic artery is rarely used to anastomose to the right posterior descending. The results are good when left ventricular function is normal, with a mortality of approximately 1%. At 1 year, 85% of patients have complete freedom from angina. This reduces to 50% at 10 years. About 5% of patients suffer perioperative MI.

Surgery for complications of myocardial infarction (MI)

Ventricular aneurysm

The prognosis without surgery is poor – less than 20% of patients survive 5 years. Death is due to LVF or MI. Rupture is rare but fatal. Surgery is required for excision of the aneurysm. This is carried out on cardiopulmonary bypass with CABG if appropriate.

Mitral regurgitation

Infarct involves the papillary muscles. Treatment is by valve replacement with CABG if appropriate. However, valve repair is increasingly common and has better long-term results.

Ruptured intraventricular septum

This carries a high mortality rate. Early operative repair is advisable but the perioperative mortality rate is high. The defect is repaired with a Dacron patch.

PERICARDITIS

This is inflammation of the parietal and visceral layers of the pericardium. It may occur as an isolated lesion or as part of a systemic disease. Causes include idiopathic (probably viral), tuberculosis, bacterial (*Staphylococcus*, *Streptococcus* or *Haemophilus* septicaemia), rheumatic fever, collagen diseases, uraemia, traumatic, neoplastic (direct invasion from bronchial carcinoma), post-pericardiotomy syndrome, MI.

Symptoms and signs. Sharp precordial pain. Radiates to shoulders and neck. Malaise. Fever. Pericardial friction rub. Diminished heart sounds if effusion. If tamponade – tachycardia, hypotension, raised JVP, pulsus paradoxus.

Investigations

- Hb
- FBC
- WCC elevated
- ESR raised
- U&Es: uraemia
- Blood culture
- CXR: globular heart if effusion
- ECG: S-T elevation
- Echocardiogram: exudates may show bright echoes on pericardium – pericardial effusion
- Diagnostic aspiration
- Biopsy.

Treatment. This is of the underlying cause or of complications.

Complications of pericarditis

Cardiac tamponade

A pericardial effusion as small as 100 mL may produce symptomatic tamponade if it occurs rapidly, while larger amounts may be well tolerated if it accumulates slowly. Rapid development of an effusion interferes with diastolic filling and results in reduced cardiac output. The fluid may be blood (trauma, ruptured ventricular aneurysm) or inflammatory exudate (any pericarditis).

Symptoms and signs. Tachycardia, hypotension, raised JVP with systolic descent, pulsus paradoxus, reduced heart sounds.

Treatment. Urgent when signs of peripheral circulatory failure. Tamponade is treated by pericardiocentesis with a wide-bore needle inserted under xiphoid process. Samples are sent for bacteriological and cytological examination unless the cause is clearly traumatic. Persistence or recurrence of symptoms is an indication for surgery. The pericardium is opened via a left anterior thoracotomy. A drain is inserted. If the cause is traumatic, a co-existent laceration of the heart may require suture.

Constrictive pericarditis

The rigid pericardial sac limits ventricular filling. Aetiological factors include TB, renal failure, post-cardiac surgery.

Symptoms and signs. Dyspnoea, fatigue, oedema, abdominal swelling. Raised JVP, which rises with inspiration (Kussmaul's sign), tachycardia, reduced pulse volume, ascites, hepatomegaly.

Investigations
- ECG: low voltage, T inversion
- CXR: may be calcified pericardium
- Echocardiogram: thick and calcified pericardium.

Treatment. Surgical removal of thickened pericardium.

THORACIC AORTA

Aneurysms

Aneurysms of the thoracic aorta may be true (fusiform, saccular), false or dissecting. Causes include arteriosclerosis, syphilis, previous aortic dissection, trauma and cystic medial necrosis.

Symptoms and signs

Asymptomatic. Found on routine CXR. In ascending aorta it may be associated with valvular incompetence, hoarseness may be due to pressure on the recurrent laryngeal nerve, back pain may be due to vertebral erosion, dysphagia may be due to pressure on the oesophagus and dyspnoea may be due to phrenic nerve involvement. Rarely pain is due to erosion of the sternum.

Investigations
- VDRL: syphilis
- CXR: mediastinal widening
- CT scan.

Treatment. Indications for surgery include rupture, documented enlargement, pain, aortic incompetence. Aneurysms of the ascending aorta and arch require a prosthetic graft replacement on cardiopulmonary bypass. Replacement of the aortic valves and reimplantation of the coronary arteries may be necessary.

Aneurysms of the descending aorta are repaired using left heart bypass, replacing the aorta with a prosthetic graft. The most serious complication of repair of descending thoracic aortic aneurysms is paraplegia, occurring in about 5% of patients. Combined surgical and endovascular procedures are increasingly common.

Aortic dissection

In aortic dissection, blood breaks through the intima and creates a false passage through the media. This may rupture back into the main lumen leaving an aorta with a double lumen and the patient may survive. In other cases, rupture with exsanguination may occur, or occlusion of the normal lumen may occur with obstruction to the blood flow through the major branches. As dissection advances, occlusion of side branches may occur, e.g. carotid (hemiplegia), spinal branches (paraplegia), renal arteries (anuria and renal failure), visceral arteries (ischaemic bowel). The aneurysm may rupture back into the pericardium with cardiac tamponade and death. Aetiological factors include arteriosclerosis, hypertension, Marfan's syndrome and cystic medial necrosis.

Symptoms and signs. Sudden excruciating chest pain radiating to the back. May be difficult to distinguish from MI. Shock. Signs of cardiac tamponade. Hypotension. Disparity of pulses or BP in extremities. MI may occur if disease extends proximally.

Investigations
- ECG may exclude MI
- CXR: mediastinal widening, pleural effusion if rupture
- CT
- MRI
- Thoracic aortogram will show extent of dissection with site of intimal tear.

Treatment
Medical. Control hypertension, e.g. nitrates, alpha blockers. May prevent further dissection. Obtain CT, MRI or angiogram when BP controlled.

Surgical. If the ascending aorta is involved, surgery is undertaken immediately because of the high risk of rupture and fatal cardiac tamponade. The ascending aorta is replaced with a tube graft with or without aortic valve replacement. The principle of the operation is to replace the segment of aorta up to where the blood has entered the false channel and to reapproximate the layers of aorta at the distal suture line. Blood now enters the true lumen, decompressing the false channel and restoring blood flow through the branches. If the dissection is distal to the left subclavian artery, medical or surgical treatment may be undertaken. Surgery is indicated for rupture, failure to control BP, compromise of blood flow to kidneys and other abdominal organs. Paraplegia may occur because of compromise of blood flow to the spinal cord.

Prognosis. Operative mortality is 10–20%. Some patients do not reach hospital alive. If medical therapy is undertaken, patients need regular follow-up with adequate control of BP.

THORACIC TRAUMA

Thoracic trauma accounts for 25% of deaths from trauma. Injuries may be open or closed. Open injuries are the result of penetrating trauma from knives or gunshot wounds. Closed injuries follow blunt trauma and deceleration. The commonest cause of closed injuries is road traffic accidents. Only about 25% of chest injuries require open surgical intervention.

Open injuries

There may be catastrophic bleeding from penetration of the heart or great vessels. Haemothorax, pneumothorax, cardiac tamponade and visceral damage with mediastinitis may occur.

Closed injuries

Rib fractures, pneumothorax, haemothorax, flail chest, aortic injury, myocardial contusion, ruptured diaphragm, ruptured oesophagus, pulmonary contusion and haemorrhage.

Symptoms and signs. Shock, cyanosis, dyspnoea, pain. Hypotension, peripheral vasoconstriction, cyanosis, pulsus paradoxus, diminished heart sound, tracheal deviation, tension pneumothorax. Reduced breath sounds. Altered percussion note. Tenderness over ribs.

Investigations
- FBC: cross-match
- CXR: widened mediastinum, pneumothorax, fractured ribs, fractured sternum, pleural fluid (haemothorax), mediastinal or subcutaneous emphysema, enlarged cardiac outline, ruptured diaphragm
- Aortography
- CT
- Water-soluble contrast swallow
- Peritoneal lavage
- ECG.

Treatment. This may be required before any investigations are carried out:

1. Establish airway, breathing and circulation.
2. If dyspnoea, tracheal deviation and absent breath sounds over lung fields, insert chest drain or wide-bore needle immediately.
3. Examine for other injuries as well as chest injuries.
4. Cover or close sucking chest wounds.
5. Radiographs should be carried out when the patient is stable.

Management of specific complications of thoracic trauma

Pneumothorax *(Fig. 9.1)*

Open sucking wounds. Air is sucked into the pleural cavity during inspiration. This causes a to-and-fro movement of the mediastinum during respiration and leads to respiratory embarrassment. The open wound must be sealed immediately by application of Vaseline gauze dressings. Surgical closure is carried out as soon as possible. A chest drain should be inserted meanwhile.

Figure 9.1 A pneumothorax is visible on the right side. Note the absence of lung marking at the periphery. The lung edge is visible (arrow).

Closed pneumothorax. This results from an air leak from lung, tracheobronchial tree or oesophagus. It may occur from open or closed trauma.

Simple pneumothorax. May be associated with haemothorax. If the pneumothorax is small (<10%) on CXR, it may be reassessed later by repeat CXR. If larger, a chest drain connected to an underwater seal should be inserted. It is recommended that all traumatic pneumothoraces are drained as there is a risk of tension pneumothorax. Aspiration is appropriate for small spontaneous pneumothoraces.

Tension pneumothorax. This may cause sudden death. Chest pain, dyspnoea, cyanosis occur. Hypotension results from vena cava distortion when the mediastinum is pushed over, decreasing venous return to the heart. There is tracheal deviation to the opposite side and absent ipsilateral breath sounds. Immediate life-saving treatment is by inserting a wide-bore i.v. cannula to decompress the pleural cavity if a chest drain is not immediately available. The wide-bore needle should be replaced by a chest drain connected to an underwater seal.

Flail chest
This is due to blunt chest trauma causing multiple rib fractures, anteriorly and posteriorly, which isolate a segment of the chest wall. The classical description is

that the isolated segment moves in and out with respiration in a paradoxical fashion. There is usually associated pulmonary contusion and pneumothorax. If there is no pneumothorax or haemothorax, then the intrapleural pressure remains negative and the flail segment moves inwards as the intrapleural negative pressure increases during inspiration and outwards during expiration. Although paradoxical movement is an important physical sign, it has probably in the past received undue emphasis in the management of flail chest. Often the chest does not move paradoxically because the patient does not allow it to do so because it hurts so much. Usually flail chest is treated with epidural anaesthesia, physiotherapy and oxygen. Endotracheal intubation and intermittent positive pressure ventilation is reserved for those who decompensate. Rib cage fixation has increased in use recently, especially for young patients or those on IPPV.

Simple rib fractures

These may be very painful and inhibit breathing and coughing, leading to chest infection – especially in the elderly. Pain is best relieved by intercostal nerve blocks with a long-acting local anaesthetic. Strapping of the chest wall is a method that affords some comfort but inhibits chest wall movement and may predispose to pulmonary complications. The practice has largely been abandoned.

Cardiac trauma

This may cause damage to the following:

- The myocardium with infarction
- Valves with development of symptoms of valvular incompetence
- Conducting mechanisms with heart block and arrhythmias.

Lacerations will cause cardiac tamponade. Initial treatment is conservative unless there is cardiac tamponade, in which case, needle aspiration or open thoracotomy is required.

PLEURA AND LUNGS

PLEURAL EFFUSION

This is fluid in the pleural space and may be:

- Serous effusion, either a transudate (protein concentration less than 30 g/L) or an exudate (protein concentration greater than 30 g/L)
- Pus: an empyema
- Blood: haemothorax
- Chyle: chylothorax.

(For causes → Table 9.1).

Symptoms and signs. Pleuritic chest pain, breathlessness, signs of CCF, peripheral oedema. Ipsilateral reduced expansion, dullness to percussion, absent breath sounds.

TABLE 9.1 Causes of pleural effusions

Transudate	Congestive cardiac failure Renal failure (nephrotic syndrome) Hepatic failure (hypoproteinaemia)
Exudate	Infection: • pneumonia • tuberculosis • empyema • subphrenic abscess
Malignancy	Primary (mesothelioma) Secondary
Other	Pulmonary embolus (with infarction) Pancreatitis Haemothorax Connective tissue disease

Investigations
- CXR: dense shadow over a lung field with concave upper limit (→ Fig. 9.2). If the upper border is horizontal, then a pneumothorax is also present
- Diagnostic aspiration – assess protein content
- Culture and sensitivity
- TB culture
- Cytology for malignant cells
- Pleural biopsy.

Figure 9.2 A right-sided pleural effusion. Note the dense shadow and the concave upper limit of the effusion.

Treatment. It is of the underlying cause. Large effusions need drainage. In malignant effusions, give chemical pleurodesis by instilling a substance into the pleural cavity after drainage. Talc is the most effective, with tetracycline the second most effective. Decortication of the pleura is effective in the control of effusions.

TUMOURS OF THE PLEURA

Primary tumours of the pleura are increasing in incidence. The commonest pleural neoplasm is mesothelioma. Mesothelioma occurs in people with a history of exposure to asbestos. The disease is exceptionally rare in those who have not been exposed. It is most common in males between 40 and 50. Symptoms include malaise, weakness, cough, dyspnoea, weight loss and fever. Radiograph shows pleural fluid and thickening. Diagnosis is established by cytology or pleural biopsy. Radiotherapy or chemotherapy are palliative. Some patients benefit from extrapleural pneumonectomy. Neoplasms of the pleura may also be due to secondary spread from other tumours, e.g. bronchus, breast.

PULMONARY INFECTIONS

Bronchiectasis

This is a complication of repeated pulmonary infection where the respiratory pathways are permanently damaged and dilated. It usually affects the lower lobes. The dilated bronchi harbour infected sputum, which is expectorated, often in large amounts. Common pathogens include haemophilus and pseudomonas. Causes of bronchiectasis include cystic fibrosis, Kartagener's syndrome (bronchiectasis, sinusitis, dextrocardia), whooping cough, measles, tuberculosis, inhalation of foreign bodies, pneumonia.

Symptoms and signs. Repeated chest infections, chronic cough, copious purulent sputum. Haemoptysis, malaise, clubbing. Rhonchi, coarse crepitations.

Investigations
- CXR: cystic shadows (possibly with fluid levels), areas of fibrosis, 'tram lines' due to bronchial oedema
- Sputum culture
- Lung function tests
- Sweat test (cystic fibrosis)
- Thin section CT scan
- Differential perfusion scan – to define non-functioning lung tissue.

Treatment. Physiotherapy with postural drainage. Antibiotics. Bronchodilators. Surgery for localized disease.

Complications. Recurrent chest infections, haemoptysis (massive haemoptysis may occur), metastatic cerebral abscess. Rarely, pneumothorax may occur.

Lung abscess

The causes are bronchial obstruction due to carcinoma, inhalation pneumonitis, inhaled foreign body (especially lung abscess in a child), septic embolus, infected pulmonary infarct, transdiaphragmatic extension of subphrenic abscess.

Other causes include: infected cyst; secondary to pneumonia, bronchiectasis or TB; immunosuppression; blood-borne, e.g. staphylococcal septicaemia; fungal.

Symptoms and signs. Obviously ill. Purulent sputum. Haemoptysis. Fever. Rigors. Pleuritic pain. Pyrexial. Clubbing. Reduced breath sounds, dullness to percussion, bronchial breathing, signs of pleural effusion, metastatic abscesses, e.g. cerebral.

Investigations
- FBC
- CXR: consolidation early in disease; later, cavitation and fluid level
- Bronchoscopy to exclude foreign body and carcinoma
- Sputum culture and sensitivity
- Ultrasound scan to confirm and may be aspirated under ultrasound control.

Treatment. This is of the underlying cause. Postural drainage and antibiotics. A great majority of cases resolve on medical treatment. Surgery is only required where medical treatment fails or there is a need for treatment of an underlying cause, e.g. removal of bronchial carcinoma.

Tuberculosis
The reader is referred to a textbook of medicine. Surgery is little required in this condition at the present time, since antituberculosis therapy is effective in most cases. However, the incidence of TB is increasing and new cases are being seen associated with AIDS. Surgery is required for some of the complications of TB, e.g. bronchopleural fistula, persistent open cavities with positive sputum, bronchiectasis, haemorrhage and destroyed lung. Of historical interest are the operations of thoracoplasty and phrenic nerve crush. Patients who have had these procedures are occasionally seen (usually in finals!). The procedures are designed to collapse the chest wall and the diaphragm onto the lungs, deflating and 'resting' the lungs while healing occurs.

LUNG TUMOURS

Bronchial carcinoma
This is the commonest cancer in males in the UK accounting for approximately 50 000 deaths per year. It is the second commonest in females. Of all lung cancers, 75% are related to smoking. Other aetiological factors include chronic exposure to asbestos, nickel, arsenic, petroleum products and radioactive materials. Four histological types are described:

- Adenocarcinoma (30–45%)
- Squamous cell carcinoma (25–40%)
- Small cell (oat cell) carcinoma (15–25%)
- Undifferentiated large cell carcinoma (rarest).

Symptoms and signs
Primary. The tumour may be asymptomatic and seen on routine CXR. Cough, haemoptysis, dyspnoea, chest pain, wheeze, hoarseness, recurrent chest infections, dysphagia.

Complications
- Thoracic: pleural effusion, recurrent laryngeal nerve palsy (hoarseness), SVC obstruction, Horner's syndrome (ptosis, meiosis, enophthalmos, anhidrosis) especially with Pancoast's tumour (invasive cancer of apex of lung).
- Metastatic: cachexia, malaise; brain (headaches, fits, personality change); bone (pathological fractures); liver (jaundice); adrenal (Addison's disease).
- Non-metastatic, extrapulmonary: ADH, ACTH secretion, hypercalcaemia, myasthenic neuropathy, hypertrophic pulmonary osteoarthropathy, thrombophlebitis migrans, gynaecomastia, clubbing.

Investigations
- FBC
- ESR
- LFTs
- Calcium
- CXR: PA and lateral (→ Fig. 9.3), mass, raised diaphragm with involvement of phrenic nerve, pleural effusion
- Sputum cytology for malignant cells
- Bronchoscopy and biopsy or brushings
- Bronchoscopic biopsy is best for central lesions, percutaneous biopsy for peripheral lesions – biopsy will confirm histological type
- Pleural tap if effusion present, cytological examination for malignant cells
- CT scan: local spread and invasion

Figure 9.3 A large bronchial carcinoma in the left lung.

- Brain scan and liver scan for metastases
- Mediastinoscopy
- Lymph node biopsy
- Bone scan
- PET scan.

Treatment. Surgery offers the only hope of cure. Depends on histological type. Non-small cell tumours, if small and localized (especially if occurring peripherally), may be resected. Larger ones may respond to radiotherapy. Small cell tumours are aggressive and are usually beyond surgery, having disseminated at the time of presentation. Combination chemotherapy and radiotherapy prolong survival in small cell tumours. Squamous cell carcinoma is radiosensitive. Most patients are incurable at presentation. Symptomatic relief is the aim. Radiotherapy is appropriate for a bronchial obstruction with lung collapse, SVC obstruction, bone pain and haemoptysis. Endobronchial and SVC stenting procedures may be carried out. SVC obstruction treated by stenting has a success rate of 90% with insertion of a stent via the right femoral vein. Extensive endoluminal disobliteration can be carried out using a cryoprobe/laser and endoluminal brachytherapy.

Surgical treatment involves lobectomy or pneumonectomy and is the only potential cure. Careful selection of patients is required and operability should be assessed by bronchoscopy, CT scan, radioisotope bone scan and ultrasound scan (liver). Contraindications to surgery include distant metastases, SVC obstruction, malignant pleural effusion, recurrent laryngeal nerve and phrenic nerve involvement.

Prognosis. About 35% survive 5 years after lobectomy and 25% after pneumonectomy. Since 75% are not candidates for surgery, the overall survival for 5 years is about 5–10%. Prognosis ultimately depends on the cell type and stage of the disease at the time of diagnosis. Small cell carcinoma has the worst prognosis.

Metastatic lung tumours

Metastatic tumours are common in the lung, which in some cases may be the only site of metastases. Secondaries may be from adenocarcinoma (breast, kidney, bowel), sarcoma (bone) or malignant melanoma. Rarely, single or multiple metastatic lung tumours may be removed as part of the treatment. The primary tumour must be controlled and no metastases should be present elsewhere (CT scan, ultrasound scan, bone scan, PET scan). The best results are obtained with tumours for which there is effective chemotherapy. The best example is the surgical treatment of pulmonary metastases in patients with osteogenic sarcoma. The presence of metastatic colonic tumour in the lung is an increasing indication for 'metastasectomy'. Results are improving.

Solitary pulmonary nodules (coin lesions)

These are well-circumscribed peripheral nodules seen on routine CXRs of patients who are usually asymptomatic. The lesions may be infective, granulomatous, or neoplastic. About 10% are malignant.

Symptoms and signs. Usually asymptomatic. Smokers. Cough, haemoptysis, weight loss, hypertrophic osteoarthropathy. Beware of the overlying skin lesions seen on radiograph.

Investigations.

- Picked up on CXR: concentric or heavy calcification suggests benign lesion; documented absence of growth over 1 year suggests benign lesion
- Sputum cytology and culture
- CT scan to exclude multiple lesions.

Treatment. Surgical excision if malignancy cannot be excluded or the patient chooses surgery.

MEDIASTINUM

Mediastinal masses may be found incidentally on routine CXR or may be symptomatic. A lateral CXR and CT scan may be required to localize the mass and indicate its aetiology.

Certain lesions are more likely to occur in characteristic mediastinal sites:

- Superior mediastinum: retrosternal goitre
- Anterior mediastinum: dermoid cysts, teratoma, pericardial cysts, bronchogenic cysts, diaphragmatic hernia (foramen of Morgagni), thymoma
- Posterior mediastinum: neurogenic tumours, e.g. dumbbell tumours of neurofibroma, paravertebral mass, e.g. TB abscess, phaeochromocytoma, diaphragmatic hernia, achalasia, hiatus hernia.

In addition to the above, aneurysms and lymph nodes may be apparent in any site. Causes of lymph node enlargement include secondary deposits, sarcoid, lymphoma and TB.

Symptoms and signs. Asymptomatic, cervical lymphadenopathy, SVC obstruction, hoarseness (left recurrent laryngeal nerve palsy), Horner's syndrome.

Investigations
- FBC (blood dyscrasias)
- ESR
- Sputum culture
- Serum angiotensin converting enzyme (sarcoid)
- Thyroid scan
- CT scan
- PET scan
- Bronchoscopy
- Oesophagoscopy
- Barium swallow
- Needle biopsy under CT control
- Angiography (vascular lesions)
- Mediastinoscopy.

Treatment. Surgery may be required. Median sternotomy may be required to confirm the diagnosis and for appropriate treatment.

Breast

Whatever the presenting symptoms, the patient fears she may have cancer. A rapid, efficient and sympathetic approach, paying attention to psychological and emotional problems, is required in dealing with breast disease. The treatment of breast cancer is multidisciplinary involving surgeons, oncologists, breast care nurses, breast clinicians, specialist radiologists and pathologists.

SYMPTOMS OF BREAST DISEASE

Patients with breast disease present with either a lump, discharge from the nipple, pain in the breast, abnormality of the nipple, or a change in size of the breast (→ Table 10.1).

History. Take note of the following: the duration of symptoms, parity, age at menopause, age at menarche, breast-feeding, contraceptive pill and HRT, previous breast surgery, family history of breast cancer.

Examination
- Observe with patient sitting inclined at 45°, e.g. symmetry, masses, peau d'orange, skin dimpling, nipple retraction.
- Observe with hands raised above head, e.g. obvious skin tethering/dimpling/asymmetry.
- Examination of the nipples, e.g. nipple retraction, Paget's disease, expression of blood from a duct.
- Palpate each quadrant and the axillary tail with the flat of the hand. With the patient in the akimbo position pressing hand on hip, test for deep fixation.
- Palpate axilla. Mobile or fixed nodes.
- Palpate supraclavicular fossa. Mobile or fixed nodes.
- General examination for distant metastases, e.g. chest – pleural effusion; hepatomegaly – liver metastases. Ascites. Spinous osseous tenderness.

Investigations
- Fine needle aspiration cytology (FNAC): a negative result does not exclude carcinoma
- Mammography: 90% accurate – unreliable under the age of 35 years because of the density of breast
- Breast USS
- Core biopsy.

TABLE 10.1 Presentation of breast disease

Breast lump	Carcinoma, cyst, localized area of fibroadenosis, fibroadenoma, breast abscess, fat necrosis, duct ectasia, lipoma, galactocele, phyllodes tumour, cyst of Montgomery's glands, sebaceous cyst
Pain in the breast	Cyclical and non-cyclical breast pain Carcinoma (85% are painless) Duct ectasia (pain behind the nipple) Infection: • puerperal mastitis • breast abscess Fat necrosis Costochondritis (Tietze's disease) Mondor's disease (superficial thrombophlebitis of veins of the chest wall)
Nipple discharge	Bloodstained (intraduct carcinoma, intraduct papilloma, Paget's disease) Serous (early pregnancy) Yellowish, brown or dark green (benign nodularity) Thick and creamy (duct ectasia) Purulent (rarely in association with breast abscess) Milky (late pregnancy, post-lactation, prolactinoma)
Nipple abnormalities	Retraction (congenital, duct ectasia, carcinoma) Inflammation (eczema, Paget's disease) Destruction (Paget's disease) Mamillary fistula
Breast enlargement	Benign hyperplasia, pregnancy, cancer, giant fibroadenoma, phyllodes tumour, mammary lymphoedema

Triple assessment is the minimum standard of care for a mass or asymmetric density/thickening of the breast. Triple assessment includes examination, imaging and pathology. Imaging includes mammography + ultrasound. Pathology includes FNAC, core biopsy, vacuum assisted mammotome biopsy. As a core or mammotome biopsy offers the pathologist a sample of histological tissue with its surrounding architecture, it is more accurate for diagnosis than cells in suspension as in FNAC, and is therefore preferable.

Cases are discussed with the pathological and radiological findings at a multidisciplinary team meeting. The radiological size of a tumour and lymph node status, its histological type (e.g. ductal, lobular, mucinous) and hormonal receptor status (oestrogen receptor, progesterone receptor and HER2 protein receptor positivity) are reviewed with patients clinical and social history and a plan for both surgery and adjuvant therapy is made. The Nottingham Prognostic Index combines data of both stage and grade to offer a prognostic score, which enables the benefits of adjuvant therapies to be weighed against the risks (Table 10.2).

BENIGN BREAST DISEASE

This presents as breast nodularity; fibroadenoma; duct ectasia; fat necrosis; intraduct papilloma; breast abscess; related conditions such as Tietze's disease or Mondor's disease.

TABLE 10.2 Nottingham Prognostic Index*

Score	Prognostic group	Predicted 10-year survival (%)	
		No adjuvant chemo.	Tamoxifen if ER +ve
<2.4	Excellent	95	–
2.41–3.4	Good	85	89
3.41–4.4	Moderate I	70	78
4.41–5.4	Moderate II	50	63
>5.4	Poor	20	41

*0.2 x diameter (cm) + LN status (0 = 0, 1–4 = 2, >4 = 3) + grade (1 = 1, 2 = 2, 3 = 3)

Benign nodularity/breast pain

This occurs between 20 and 45 years and settles after the menopause. It probably results from an abnormal response of the breast to changes in the hormonal environment. The terms fibroadenosis and cystic hyperplasia describe the pathological condition well. There is exaggeration of the fibrotic element (i.e. fibrosis), the epithelial element undergoes hyperplasia (i.e. adenosis), and there is a tendency to cyst formation. The condition may be extremely painful, especially premenstrually, hence the terms cyclical mastitis or cyclical mastalgia.

Symptoms and signs. Cyclical breast pain worse before period. Intermittent breast masses or areas of thickening with no discrete mass. Discrete mass, i.e. cysts, may be noticed by patient. Examination reveals nodular breasts with multiple thickened areas (usually upper and outer quadrant) that are usually tender. Lesions change in number and size during the menstrual cycle. If condition is suspected, examination should be repeated at different stages of the menstrual cycle. If there is a dominant mass, 'triple' assessment should be carried out.

Investigations
- Mammography to exclude carcinoma
- USS – fibroadenoma, cyst – ultrasound-guided or freehand core biopsy or FNAC. Aspiration may be diagnostic and therapeutic for a cyst.

Treatment. This condition may be exceptionally painful and cause severe distress to the patient. Keeping a breast pain diary to document severity and symptoms in relation to menstrual cycle helps distinguish between cyclical and non-cyclical breast pain and the efficacy of treatment. An explanation of the condition and treatment options should be clearly and sympathetically made; 90% of patients require no further treatment.

- Firm supporting bra to 'rest' the breast. This should be worn day and night when the patient is symptomatic.
- Evening primrose oil.
- Danazol is given for severe symptoms. Androgenic side-effects need to be explained to the patient. About 50% of patients cannot tolerate danazol.

- Anti-oestrogen therapy prescribed and monitored by a specialist (tamoxifen and goserelin are excellent treatment agents but are not licensed for use with breast pain). Short-course therapy only should be given.
- Rarely, some patients are so severely troubled they become suicidal. Subcutaneous mastectomy with or without reconstruction has been used in extreme cases.
- The condition occasionally responds to hypnotherapy and acupuncture.

Fibroadenoma

This occurs at age 15–35 years.

Symptoms and signs. Very mobile breast lump noted by patient. Non-tender. On examination there is a mobile, discrete, smooth, firm and rubbery swelling in the breast. It slips under the examining fingers, hence its name breast 'mouse'. As with any discrete mass, triple assessment should be carried out to exclude carcinoma.

Treatment. Excisional biopsy if there is any doubt about the diagnosis. In young women in their teens, it is reasonable to observe. However, if observation is carried out FNAC or core biopsy should be undertaken.

Duct ectasia (periductal mastitis)

This occurs chiefly in the fifth decade. The aetiology is obscure but is associated with dilatation of the ducts behind the nipple and a periductal inflammatory reaction rich in plasma cells. The condition is sometimes called plasma cell mastitis.

Symptoms and signs. Pain and periareolar erythema. Nipple discharge may be either thick and creamy or greenish brown. There may be a periareolar tender mass. The nipple may become retracted when healing occurs by fibrosis. Occasionally infection occurs with periareolar abscess formation.

Differential diagnosis. Carcinoma of the breast with nipple retraction.

Investigations
- Mammogram: opaque mass of dilated ducts and skin indentation may be apparent.

Treatment
- If infection is present aspiration should be carried out and antibiotics given.
- If an abscess is present surgical drainage may be required.
- A mammillary fistula may occur as a complication. If it does it should be laid open.
- With severe discharge or recurrent sepsis total duct excision should be carried out (mammadochectomy). The ducts are excised through a circumareolar incision, preserving the nipple.

Fat necrosis

This is due to trauma with rupture of fat cells and a consequent inflammatory reaction, which may become calcified.

Symptoms and signs. There may be a history of trauma, often minor. The partner's teeth may be an aetiological factor and patients may be embarrassed to explain this possible cause. The lump may have decreased in size before the patient is seen in clinic. In the early phases, the lump is tender. In the later phases it is hard and irregular and tethered to the skin.

Investigations. Triple assessment to exclude carcinoma.

Treatment. Excision biopsy may be necessary ultimately to distinguish the condition from cancer of the breast. Ultimately, fat necrosis may evolve into an oil-filled cyst which can be aspirated.

Intraduct papilloma

The papilloma is usually in a solitary duct near the nipple in a young woman.

Symptoms and signs. Blood-stained discharge from a single duct on to the nipple. Occasionally a small mass may be palpable. Usually, however, no mass is palpable. Pressure over a certain spot, or the palpable mass will cause bleeding from a single duct orifice.

Investigations. Mammography may be required to exclude carcinoma.

Treatment. If the duct orifice from which the bleeding is coming can be identified, microdochectomy is carried out. If not, excision of the major nipple ducts is necessary. Histological confirmation is required to exclude *in situ* or invasive cancer.

Breast abscess

This most commonly occurs following suppuration of acute mastitis in the lactating breast. The infecting organism is usually *Staphylococcus aureus*. The early phase of acute mastitis may settle with appropriate antistaphylococcal antibiotics.

Symptoms and signs. Lactating breast. Patient generally unwell with painful, tender, red and warm swelling of breast. The swelling may become fluctuant and eventually the abscess points and discharges.

Treatment. The majority can be treated by aspiration and antibiotics. Aspiration may need to be repeated. Ultrasound guided drainage may be necessary. Loculation does not seem to be a major concern except for large abscesses. In the case of large abscesses, incision and drainage with breakdown of loculi may be required. Occasionally abscesses occur in the glands of Montgomery and appear as a boil-like lesion and should be treated as for a boil. Periareolar abscesses may occur with duct ectasia.

Related conditions

Patients may occasionally present with apparent pain in the breast, where the condition responsible for the pain is not within the breast.

Tietze's disease. This is costochondritis and usually involves the second, third and fourth costal cartilages. The cause is unknown and radiographs are unhelpful. The condition is self-limiting, although NSAIDs and infiltration with local anaesthetic and steroids may be helpful if the pain is severe.

Mondor's disease. (Superficial thrombophlebitis of the subcutaneous veins of the chest wall.) The cause is unknown and the condition self-limiting. The veins of the chest wall are felt as red, tender cords often extending on to the anterior axillary fold. The breast should be carefully palpated for underlying masses. Mammography is advised to exclude an underlying carcinoma. NSAIDs may help relieve symptoms.

CARCINOMA OF THE FEMALE BREAST

This is the most common malignancy in the female. About 42 000 women and 300 men are diagnosed annually in the UK with carcinoma of the breast. Of the women diagnosed with breast cancer, 72% live for more than 10 years. The incidence of the disease appears to be rising. The cause remains unknown. Survival rate has improved significantly over the last 10–15 years. This probably reflects screening, awareness and earlier diagnosis, use of tamoxifen and better chemotherapeutic agents.

Risk factors
- Family history – first-degree relatives with early-onset disease
- Previous breast carcinoma (recurrence versus metachronous disease)
- Atypical hyperplasia on previous biopsy
- Nulliparous women
- Early menarche
- Age (the older the more likely).

Symptoms and signs. Symptoms include: painless lump in the breast; nipple retraction or discharge; skin dimpling; breast asymmetry; erythema over skin or nipple; symptoms of metastases, e.g. bone pain, headache, breathlessness, jaundice. Examination may reveal: hard irregular mass, fixed to skin or fixed deeply; erythema; Paget's disease of nipple; peau d'orange; axillary glands mobile, fixed or matted; supraclavicular nodes palpable; signs of metastases – liver (jaundice, hepatomegaly, ascites), lung or pleural metastases (pleural effusion, consolidation), bone secondaries (bone tenderness or pathological fractures), brain secondaries (headache, fits, personality change, papilloedema).

Investigations
- Triple assessment (examination + imaging + pathology)
- Metastases screen – either (A) CXR, liver ultrasound, bone scan, LFTs and calcium, FBC or (B) CT thorax/abdomen, bone scan, LFTs and calcium, FBC. Frozen section is rarely performed nowadays as it is 35% inaccurate.
- CT scan of brain if symptoms, but not routinely performed. A mammogram of a patient with breast cancer is shown in Figure 10.1.

Clinical staging. Two forms are in wide use (Tables 10.3, 10.4).

Treatment. Surgery to the breast ranges from wide local excision (WLE) to mastectomy + oncoplastic or reconstructive options.

Important studies starting in the 1970s demonstrated that WLE with adjuvant radiotherapy produced comparable local recurrence and disease-free survival rates to mastectomy alone. WLE therefore became an option for women with smaller tumours in relatively larger breasts, i.e. where clearance is possible while still conserving the breast. Larger tumours in smaller breasts may necessitate mastectomy to achieve local control.

Adjuvant therapies include chemotherapy, anti-oestrogens (hormone) therapy and targeted therapies, e.g. trastuzumab (Herceptin) – a monoclonal antibody targeted against HER2 protein, bisphosphonates. Treatment options should be discussed

Figure 10.1 A mammogram showing a carcinoma of the breast. There is a dense mass with microcalcification. Malignant microcalcification requires careful examination of the film with magnification: it does not reproduce well in photographs.

TABLE 10.3 Manchester Classification (modified)

Stage I	Lump <5 cm; not fixed deeply
Stage II	As for stage I but mobile, ipsilateral axillary nodes
Stage III	Lump >5 cm fixed to skin with fixed ipsilateral axillary nodes, or supraclavicular nodes, or peau d'orange, or arm oedema
Stage IV	Distant metastases

with the patient. Preoperative counselling by the surgeon and a specially trained breast care nurse should explain the treatment options and prepare the patient for treatment. Recent trends are to more conservative management of breast cancer.

Alternative treatment modalities include neo-adjuvant chemotherapy (prior to surgery) which may 'downstage' a tumour to enable breast conservation in a patient with locally advanced disease that would otherwise require a mastectomy.

TABLE 10.4 TNM Classification

Primary (T)	Tis – carcinoma *in situ* T0 – no primary tumour located T1 – tumour <2 cm T2 – tumour 2–5 cm T3 – tumour >5 cm T4 – extension to chest wall
Nodes (N)	N0 – no nodal involvement N1 – mobile ipsilateral axillary nodes N2 – fixed ipsilateral axillary nodes N3 – ipsilateral supraclavicular nodes
Metastases (M)	M0 – no metastases M1 – distant metastases

Also, primary endocrine therapy for oestrogen receptor positive cancers can be offered as an alternative to surgery in patients who are at high risk of an anaesthetic, refuse surgery, or are assessed to be at a higher risk of mortality from another cause.

Surgery for ductal carcinoma in situ, *Tis (DCIS).* Forming 25–30% of screening-detected tumours, ductal carcinoma *in situ* represents an area of dysplasia reaching, but not invading the basement membrane. It can be low, intermediate or high nuclear grade and has a variety of histological subtypes. It represents a point in the evolution between atypia and malignancy. Microcalcification may be present on mammography and it may occupy a small area of the breast or be widespread. Core biopsies positive for DCIS, may not be a true reflection of the mass which may contain areas of invasion. Surgery with clear histological margins is the primary aim which, in widespread DCIS may require mastectomy. If histology confirms invasion then the axilla will require staging (see below), and adjuvant therapy is offered accordingly.

Surgery for early breast cancer (T1, T2)
- Wide local excision: removal of the lump with a margin of normal breast tissue. If the lesion is impalpable such as those detected by screening, a wire is passed to the tumour localized under ultrasound or mammographic guidance, offering the surgeon a guide to locate the tumour. Specimens are oriented with marker sutures and clips and an X-ray taken to assess clearance of margins. Surgery is now routinely performed with a view to preserving the volume and contour of the breast (oncoplastic technique).
  - Neighbouring breast tissue can be mobilized to fill the resulting defect (tissue displacement), whereas larger defects can be replaced with nearby tissue, e.g. latissimus dorsi muscle (tissue replacement) sometimes after a delay to confirm complete excision.
  - Fat injection harvested by liposuction from the abdomen or thighs is becoming increasingly popular in addressing partial defects.
  - In larger breasts, the wide local excision can be performed as part of a bilateral breast reduction (therapeutic mammaplasty).

- Simple mastectomy either with immediate or delayed reconstruction. Most common mastectomy operation is modified Patey procedure, i.e. pectoralis minor is preserved (Auchincloss mastectomy).
- Whichever excision technique is used, the nodal status of the axilla should be staged formally, either by sentinel node biopsy, axillary node sampling or axillary clearance according to local protocol. Patients with positive nodes on sampling would normally proceed to formal clearance of all the axillary lymph nodes or radiotherapy. Devices enabling the intraoperative assessment of sentinel nodes/ node samples for evidence of cancer spread are currently being introduced.

Patients with early breast cancer should be considered for systemic adjuvant treatment, i.e. chemotherapy and/or anti-oestrogen therapy. Anti-oestrogen therapy should only be used in those who are oestrogen receptor +ve. Oestrogen blockade (tamoxifen) or oestrogen deprivation therapy with aromatase inhibitors (anastrozole, letrozole, exemestane) may be used according to local protocol. Ovarian oestrogen production can be stopped with oophorectomy, radiotherapy or goserelin injections. Primary tamoxifen therapy without surgery may be used in elderly/unfit patients.

Surgery for advanced breast cancer (T3, T4)
- Locally advanced disease (no systemic disease) – neoadjuvant therapy – chemotherapy/radiotherapy/surgery
- Salvage mastectomy

Palliation (stage IV)
- Local palliation (e.g. radiotherapy for fungating lesions)
- Radiotherapy to localized bony metastases
- Aspiration of pleural effusions and instillation of cytotoxic agents
- Hormonal manipulation, e.g. tamoxifen
- Chemotherapy.

Extensive surgery may be required for chest wall defects requiring grafting with myocutaneous flaps, e.g. latissimus dorsi flaps.

Recurrent disease. Local recurrent disease may be treated by radiotherapy if this has not been given to the area before. Systemic disease may be treated by hormonal manipulation or chemotherapy.

Follow-up
- Routine self-examination of operation site and other breast
- Follow-up is in accordance with local protocols but should be continued for 5 years – patients who are disease free then should be discharged
- Mammography to contralateral breast every other year and to ipsilateral breast, if conserved, every year.

Prognosis
- Stage I: 80% 5-year survival
- Stage II: 50% 5-year survival
- Stage III: 15% 5-year survival
- Stage IV: 5% 5-year survival.

Complications of mastectomy. Wound seromas, stiffness of the shoulder. Lymphoedema of the arm is a complication of axillary node clearance. The main problems are psychological and should be managed both preoperatively and postoperatively by expert counselling and support.

Breast reconstruction. Following mastectomy, many patients are well rehabilitated with an external prosthesis that fits in a bra. Others, however, wish breast reconstruction. This may be performed immediately at the time of the initial surgery or at a later date. Reconstruction after mastectomy can be achieved using implant-based or autologous tissue according to patient choice, size of breast, fitness for surgery. Autologous transfer imports healthy tissue via pedicled or microsurgical free tissue transfer which makes it a superior choice if the chest wall has been irradiated.

Tissue can be recruited from:
- The back – pedicled latissimus dorsi muscle with overlying skin and fat based on the subscapular vessels.
- The abdomen – skin and fat with the underlying rectus abdominis muscle based on the superior epigastric vessels can be rotated into the mastectomy defect about this vascular pedicle (pedicled transverse rectus abdominis musculocutaneous flap – TRAM). The free microsurgical TRAM is based on the deep inferior epigastric vessels and a variant of this, the deep inferior epigastric perforator flap (DIEP) spares the rectus abdominis muscle.
- The buttocks – skin and fat can be harvested based on perforators from the superior or inferior gluteal vessels (SGAP or IGAP)
- The inner thigh – The free transverse upper gracilis (TUG) flap. A paddle of skin and fat is elevated with the underlying gracilis muscle based on the medial circumflex femoral vessels.

BREAST SCREENING

This is based on the premise that early detection of breast cancer improves the prognosis. Current screening in the UK invites women in the 50–70 age group to have two-view mammography every 3 years. By 2012, this age group will be extended to 47–73. Of the screened women, 5% are recalled for further investigation. Suspicious lesions on mammography are biopsied by image-guided core biopsy or mammotome biopsy – >90% preoperative diagnosis is expected by this technique. If screening biopsy does not produce a result concordant with the imaging findings, then open biopsy is required: in impalpable lesions this may be performed using a wire-localization technique (see above). If malignant, appropriate treatment is undertaken.

OTHER CONDITIONS OF THE BREAST

Paget's disease of the nipple

Associated with an intraduct carcinoma of the breast, the tumour cells spreading within the epithelium on to the nipple.

Symptoms and signs. Red, eczematous-like lesion of the nipple, which eventually erodes the nipple. There may be an associated palpable mass in the breast.

Differential diagnosis. Eczema of the nipple. However, the latter is usually bilateral, itchy, and does not destroy the nipple.

Investigations
- Mammography
- Biopsy confirms diagnosis.

Treatment. Simple mastectomy. In the absence of a palpable mass in the breast, the prognosis is excellent.

Inflammatory carcinoma (mastitis carcinomatosa)
May occur in pregnancy or lactation and is the most aggressive of breast carcinomas.

Symptoms and signs. Oedema, erythema, peau d'orange, generalized breast enlargement. Metastasizes widely and rapidly.

Diagnosis. Core biopsy.

Treatment. Palliative. Radiotherapy, tamoxifen, chemotherapy.

Prognosis. Less than 5% of patients survive 5 years.

Phyllodes tumour
This is a rapidly growing highly cellular variant of a fibroadenoma. It rarely metastasizes, but it recurs locally after an inadequate incision. It should not be shelled out like a fibroadenoma but should be excised with a rim of normal breast tissue.

Pseudolipoma
This is a soft lobulated swelling of the breast that resembles a lipoma. It is caused by an underlying carcinoma causing retraction of the suspensory ligaments of the breast resulting in bunching of the fat between the skin, septae of the breast, and the carcinoma. Beware the diagnosis of lipoma of the breast, especially in the older patient. Mammography is advised.

CONDITIONS OF THE MALE BREAST

Gynaecomastia
Gynaecomastia is benign hypertrophy of duct and connective tissue elements of the male breast. It may occur in the following instances:

- At birth (maternal oestrogens crossing placenta)
- At puberty, where it may be unilateral or bilateral (embarrassing to the patient; it may resolve or may need surgery)
- Because of drugs (cimetidine, spironolactone, digoxin, methyldopa, oestrogens)
- Because of liver failure
- Association with testicular tumours.

Carcinoma

This is rare and usually occurs over the age of 50 years. It presents with a unilateral, hard, painless mass.

Treatment. This is by mastectomy with or without axillary node clearance. Tamoxifen is given if oestrogen receptor +ve (most male breast carcinoma is oestrogen receptor +ve). The prognosis of male breast cancer is now thought to be identical to that of the female type when compared stage for stage, but the male tends to present with skin infiltration more often than the female and therefore is seen at a later stage.

Endocrine surgery

THYROID

CONGENITAL

> The embryological line of descent of the thyroid gland is from the foramen caecum of the tongue to its normal position in the neck. Occasionally, it may descend lower and even to the superior mediastinum.

Lingual thyroid

This occurs at the foramen caecum of the tongue. It may be asymptomatic or interfere with speech or swallowing. A radio-iodine scan should be performed to confirm the presence of thyroid tissue. Treatment is by suppression of TSH with thyroxine, but surgical excision should be considered if hormonal therapy is ineffective or the patient has obstructive symptoms.

Thyroglossal fistula

This is not congenital but follows rupture, or inadequate excision of a thyroglossal cyst. Recurrent inflammation occurs and the fistula intermittently discharges mucus. Treatment is by excision of the fistula and may require dissection as far as the foramen caecum of the tongue.

Thyroglossal cyst ($\rightarrow$ Ch. 8)

EXAMINATION OF THE THYROID GLAND

Inspection should be carried out initially from the front. Confirm that there is a mass in the neck in the area of the thyroid gland and that it moves up on swallowing. Place a finger in the suprasternal notch and check that the trachea is central. Examine the thyroid from behind. Place the thumbs on the vertebra prominens and the fingers on the anterior part of the neck on either side. Allow the head to tilt forwards slightly to relax the neck muscles. Feel up and down in the area of the thyroid. Applying gentle pressure to one side of the neck over the thyroid facilitates examination of the contralateral lobe. Decide whether there is a single nodule, many nodules or whether there is diffuse enlargement of the thyroid gland.

Give the patient a glass of water to swallow and check again that the gland moves up on swallowing. Palpate up and down the deep cervical chain of lymph nodes to check for lymphadenopathy. Try to get below the lower limit of the thyroid swelling to exclude retrosternal extension. Percussion over the sternum to check for retrosternal extension is inaccurate and outdated. In patients with Graves' disease auscultate over the gland. Very vascular toxic glands may have a systolic bruit.

SYMPTOMS OF THYROID DISEASE

Lump in the neck
- Smooth non-toxic enlargement of the gland. This is characteristic of a physiological goitre, which may occur at puberty or in pregnancy
- A smooth toxic enlargement of the gland associated with Graves' disease
- A smooth *firm* enlargement of the gland (occasionally asymmetrical), usually in middle-aged females and often associated with hypothyroidism, e.g. Hashimoto's disease
- A nodular non-toxic enlargement of the gland. This is characteristic of multinodular goitre
- A solitary nodule in a lobe of the thyroid gland. This may be due to a palpable dominant nodule in a multinodular goitre, a cyst, an adenoma or a carcinoma
- A rapid increase in the size of nodule associated with haemorrhage into a cyst, a rapidly growing carcinoma or thyroiditis, which may be painful
- A hard irregular goitre with infiltration of muscles and lymphadenopathy in the older patient, e.g. anaplastic carcinoma.

Hoarse voice. This is due to pressure on and/or malignant infiltration of one or both recurrent laryngeal nerves.

Dysphagia. This may occur with very large goitres.

Dyspnoea. It is due to tracheal deviation or compression. Stridor may be apparent.

Pain. This may occur with haemorrhage into a nodule, infiltration by carcinoma, subacute thyroiditis or, occasionally, Hashimoto's disease.

Eye symptoms. Staring or protruding eyes (exophthalmos) in patients with Graves' disease, double vision, dry 'gritty' eyes, difficulty closing eyes. The latter may lead to pain due to corneal ulceration.

Thyrotoxicosis. Palpitations, dyspnoea, nervousness, irritability, tremor of hands, sweating. Increased appetite with weight loss, diarrhoea. Preference for cold weather. Amenorrhoea. Pretibial myxoedema may be found in Graves' disease.

Myxoedema (hypothyroidism). Slowness of thought, speech and movement. Weight gain. Cold intolerance, tiredness, lethargy, constipation. Loss of hair. Change of voice (hoarseness). Carpal tunnel syndrome.

INVESTIGATION OF THYROID DYSFUNCTION/SWELLINGS

Patients can be euthyroid, hyperthyroid or hypothyroid. Measure TSH, free T4, free T3, thyroid antibodies. TSH is elevated in hypothyroidism. TSH is suppressed in thyrotoxicosis. Thyroid autoantibodies suggest immune aetiology of disease.

Fine needle aspiration. This will distinguish between a solid lesion and a cyst. If the lesion is solid, cells are sent for cytological examination. This is a safe technique. Usually it is possible to discriminate benign from malignant disease, although some difficulties may be encountered. In particular, cytology cannot distinguish between benign and malignant follicular lesions. Fine needle biopsy should be performed in the investigation of all thyroid nodules. Its reliability can be improved by carrying out the biopsy under ultrasound guidance.

Plain radiograph of chest thoracic inlet. May show tracheal displacement or compression. Retrosternal extension.

Ultrasound scan. It establishes the size and shape of the gland and indicates if nodules are single or multiple and their size. It will also distinguish between cystic and solid lesions.

Radioisotope scans. These are only helpful in some patients with thyrotoxicosis. In Graves' disease the uptake is increased and diffuse. In toxic nodular goitre the uptake is patchy and multiple or unifocal depending on the pathology.

GOITRE

A goitre is an enlargement of the thyroid gland (for Classification → Table 11.1).

TABLE 11.1 Classification of goitres

Simple (non-toxic goitre)	Simple hyperplastic goitre Multinodular goitre
Toxic goitre	Diffuse (Graves' disease) Toxic nodule (adenoma) Toxic multinodular goitre
Neoplastic goitre	Benign: • adenoma Malignant: • papillary • follicular • anaplastic • medullary • lymphoma
Inflammatory	De Quervain's thyroiditis Riedel's thyroiditis
Autoimmune	Hashimoto's thyroiditis

Simple hyperplastic goitre

Iodine deficiency is the commonest pathological cause. Physiological causes include puberty and pregnancy. Endemic goitres occur in childhood and are common in areas where the drinking water has a low iodine content. They are rare in the UK where iodide is added to table salt.

Symptoms and signs. The patient is usually euthyroid. Usually a smooth goitre. Iodine deficiency types of goitre may become very large.

Investigations
- Free T4 usually normal
- TSH may be raised
- CXR to exclude tracheal compression or deviation.
- CT scan (→ Fig. 11.1) – retrosternal goitre, tracheal deviation/compression.

Treatment. Addition of iodized salt to diet in areas where iodine deficiency occurs. Thyroxine orally daily to suppress TSH. Partial thyroidectomy is indicated only if the gland is very large and causing pressure effects.

Multinodular goitre

This is the commonest cause of goitre in the UK. The gland is enlarged and irregular. The condition develops spontaneously and also in simple colloid goitres. There are areas of hypoplasia and hyperplasia within the gland. The condition is more common in women. With large glands, tracheal deviation and compression

Figure 11.1 A CT scan of the neck showing a goitre (large mass in the left lobe of the thyroid gland). The trachea (arrow) is slightly deviated to the right.

may occur. Toxic change may occasionally occur with the symptoms of hyperthyroidism.

Symptoms and signs. In endemic areas, nodular goitre appears at 15–30 years, while sporadic ones occur later at 25–40 years. Occasionally only a solitary nodule is palpable. Dyspnoea, dysphagia may occur if the gland is very large. Pain may occur due to haemorrhage into a cyst.

Investigations
- TSH, free T4
- If thyroid function is normal, isotope scan is not indicated
- CXR/CT if retrosternal extension is suspected.

Treatment. If the patient is clinically euthyroid and the goitre is small, no treatment is required. If the gland is large and unsightly and causes symptoms of compression, or thyrotoxicosis occurs, thyroidectomy is indicated.

Toxic goitre
This may be a diffuse goitre (Graves' disease), toxic multinodular goitre or solitary toxic adenoma. In Graves' disease, TSH receptor antibodies are present. In toxic multinodular goitre, several nodules in a non-toxic goitre begin to function independently of TSH. A solitary toxic nodule functions autonomously. Toxic goitre is six times more common in females.

Symptoms and signs. Hyperthyroidism, tachycardia, palpitations, AF, tremor, increased tendon reflexes. In Graves' disease – exophthalmos, lid lag, pretibial myxoedema. Occasionally bruit over gland.

Investigations
- Low TSH; free T4 (↑); free T3 (↑)
- Isotope scan may show 'hot' nodules.

Treatment
Antithyroid drugs. For the patient with Graves' disease, carbimazole 40 mg daily as 'blocking' dose until euthyroid and then 5 mg t.d.s. for 12–18 months or continue 'block' and 'replace' with thyroxine. About 50% of patients with Graves' disease remain euthyroid when the drug is discontinued. Severely toxic patients may require β-blockers until euthyroid. Relapses, if they happen, usually occur within 2 years of stopping treatment. Hypothyroidism may develop. Side-effects of carbimazole include rashes and neutropenia – patients must be warned to report any sore throat or mouth ulcers occurring, especially in the initial stages of carbimazole treatment. Patients with thyrotoxicosis due to toxic multinodular goitre/toxic adenoma, can be rendered euthyroid with antithyroid drugs but require definitive treatment with radio-iodine or surgery.

Radio-iodine. ^{131}I is administered orally. It usually takes 8–12 weeks before the patient becomes euthyroid. After the ^{131}I is given, antithyroid drugs need to be taken until the symptoms settle. It is appropriate treatment for most patients with thyrotoxicosis, recurrent hyperthyroidism, and poor-risk patients. It should not be used in children and pregnant women because of potential radiation hazards. There is a high incidence of late myxoedema.

Surgery. This is the treatment of choice for younger patients, children and patients with large goitres. The patient should be rendered euthyroid prior to surgery with antithyroid drugs. Blocking therapy with carbimazole, and replacing endogenous hormone production with thyroxine administration is optimum preparation for surgery. Propranolol may be needed if control is difficult to achieve or when urgent surgery may be indicated. Total thyroidectomy is the preferred procedure. Thyroid lobectomy is the appropriate treatment for a solitary toxic nodule.

Prognosis. Hypothyroidism may occur after radioactive iodine and will occur after surgery. If subtotal resection is performed, about 4% remain toxic and around 8–10% will become toxic again at a later time. ^{131}I treatment is then appropriate. About 4% become hypothyroid immediately and up to 60% may ultimately become hypothyroid. This depends on the dose of radioactive iodine. At the low dose, 10% become hypothyroid at 1 year then cumulatively 3% per year become hypothyroid. With bigger doses (ablative), up to 60% become hypothyroid at 1 year. Lifelong monitoring of thyroid function is required.

Neoplastic goitre

Benign

Adenomas. True follicular adenomas are encapsulated and are usually >2 cm on presentation. They are solid on ultrasound and 'cold' on isotope scans. FNAC will not distinguish them from follicular carcinoma. They must be excised. Lobectomy is adequate treatment.

Malignant

The large majority are primary tumours. Aetiological factors include exposure to ionizing radiation in childhood; endemic goitre (iodine deficiency) may be associated with follicular carcinoma but the risk is small. There is also a rare association with adenomatous colonic polyps. Papillary cancer may be associated with an autosomal dominant family history. Family history may be present in patients with medullary carcinoma associated with MEN Type II. Metastatic carcinoma to the thyroid is rare but may spread via the bloodstream from breast, lung, kidney and prostate. The main types of thyroid cancer are as follows.

Differentiated (papillary and follicular)
Papillary (60%). Papillary occurs at any age with a peak incidence in the third and fourth decades. Usually a slow-growing nodule, which may metastasize early to regional lymph nodes. They are often multicentric within the thyroid gland. The tumour is TSH dependent. The condition of 'lateral aberrant thyroid' more correctly represents secondary deposit of papillary carcinoma in lymph nodes.

Follicular carcinoma (20%). Follicular carcinoma has a peak incidence in the 40–60 age group. It spreads via the blood stream. Distant metastasis is normally to lung and bone. Occasionally, the disease presents with bony secondaries.

Anaplastic carcinoma (5–8%). Occurs in old age. Usually rapidly growing and locally invasive, with early spread via the lymphatics and bloodstream to lungs, bone and brain. Stridor, dysphagia, recurrent laryngeal nerve palsy may occur.

Medullary carcinoma (5%). May present at any age. Arises from parafollicular C cells. Secretes calcitonin. Presents with solitary nodule or mass and may spread to cervical nodes. It may be familial (25%) and associated with MEN Type II. Even in the absence of a family history, screening for mutations of the ret-proto-oncogene on chromosome 10 is necessary. When present, family screening is indicated. Prophylactic thyroidectomy may be offered in gene-positive individuals.

Lymphoma (5%). May be diagnosed on FNAC or core biopsy. There is an increased incidence of lymphoma originating in the thyroid in Hashimoto's thyroiditis.

Symptoms and signs of malignant goitres. Patients are usually euthyroid. Rarely is the patient toxic. Differentiated thyroid cancer (i.e. papillary and follicular) usually presents with a thyroid nodule. Cervical nodes may be enlarged and there may be local discomfort in the neck. Bone pain may represent secondary disease and may be the presenting symptom. Cough may be due to lung metastases. Medullary carcinoma may be familial and associated with MEN. Anaplastic carcinoma occurs in the elderly. There will be a hard craggy mass, which may be locally invasive with lymph node involvement. Stridor, dysphagia, pain, and hoarseness may occur.

Investigations
- FNAC is the mainstay of preoperative investigation
- CXR: lung metastases
- Bone scan if bone pain
- Ultrasound scan for lymphadenopathy
- Calcitonin levels if medullary carcinoma suspected
- When medullary cancer is present, phaeochromocytoma must be excluded and the serum calcium checked.

Treatment
- *Well-differentiated (papillary/follicular)* Total thyroidectomy and excision of all involved nodes. ^{123}I diagnostic scanning for secondary disease and ^{131}I ablation treatment. Life-long thyroxine treatment is required as (1) replacement therapy and (2) to achieve TSH suppression. Thyroglobulin estimations should be carried out 6-monthly as a marker of recurrent disease. Subsequent ^{131}I therapy may be used for secondary disease – although bony secondaries are best treated with external beam irradiation.
- *Anaplastic* Surgery is rarely indicated. Response to radiotherapy is poor. Chemotherapy is usually ineffective. Surgical debulking to relieve pressure on the trachea and oesophagus may allow palliation.
- *Medullary* Total thyroidectomy with removal of all affected lymph nodes. Follow-up includes regular calcitonin levels. Detectable calcitonin levels suggest residual or recurrent tumour which should be sought and removed surgically. Recurrence of high calcitonin levels suggests tumour recurrence. These should be sought and removed surgically. Inoperable tumours should be irradiated.
- *Lymphoma* Treatment depends upon the type and is a matter for a specialist in lymphoma treatment.

Prognosis
- *Differentiated (papillary/follicular)*. Prognosis can be excellent. Around 9% of patients will die of the disease and 30% will need treatment for nodal/secondary disease. Adverse prognostic factors include increasing age (especially over 40) at first presentation, male gender, extrathyroidal and metastatic spread.
- *Anaplastic*. Poor prognosis – 1-year survival is <10%.
- *Medullary*. The prognosis is variable. With nodal metastases the 10-year survival is <50%.

INFLAMMATORY CONDITIONS OF THE THYROID
These are rare.

Subacute thyroiditis (de Quervain's)
This is a self-limiting condition associated with giant cells and granulomata. Symptoms include pain, swelling, enlarged tender thyroid, malaise, myalgia. The ESR is raised. Aspirin and steroids give symptomatic relief. The acute symptoms last 10–14 days.

Riedel's thyroiditis
This is a woody hard goitre that infiltrates into the adjacent muscle. It may compress the trachea and may be associated with retroperitoneal fibrosis. It must be differentiated from anaplastic carcinoma. Surgery is necessary occasionally to confirm the diagnosis and to relieve pressure on the oesophagus and trachea. Tamoxifen treatment is associated with reduction in the size of the goitre.

Hashimoto's disease
An autoimmune disease, it causes diffuse lymphocytic infiltration of the thyroid gland with destruction of the functioning thyroid tissue. Eventually the patient becomes hypothyroid.

Symptoms and signs. Occurs almost exclusively in females. Diffusely enlarged non-tender goitre. Any symptoms and signs of hypothyroidism depend on stage of disease.

Investigations
- TSH (↑)
- May be low free T4
- Many patients are euthyroid
- Antimicrosomal antibody titres and antithyroglobulin titres raised
- Diagnosis confirmed by FNAC
- Beware confusing this condition with lymphoma.

Treatment. Thyroxine to treat hypothyroidism. Surgery is only rarely required for goitres causing severe pressure symptoms. Isthmusectomy may be appropriate.

THYROIDECTOMY
Indications
These are suspected or proven malignancy, thyrotoxicosis, tracheal/oesophageal compression, cosmetic for unsightly goitre.

Preoperative preparation

Thyrotoxic patients should be rendered euthyroid preoperatively. The vocal cords should be checked preoperatively. A very few patients may show an unsuspected vocal cord paralysis preoperatively. This is an important consideration in view of possible intraoperative recurrent laryngeal nerve damage. The patient should be warned of possible nerve damage. Permanent injury occurs in 1–2% of thyroidectomies but possibly as often as 10% in re-exploration procedures.

A warning should be given regarding hypocalcaemia, which is usually a transient problem. It will be seen in about 30% of cases of total thyroidectomy with about 2% of patients still requiring replacement therapy at 3 months postoperatively.

Operations

The following operations are appropriate: solitary benign nodule requires lobectomy; cancer requires total thyroidectomy; thyrotoxicosis or large multinodular goitre requires subtotal or total thyroidectomy. Total thyroidectomy is increasingly the operation of choice.

Procedure

Principles of thyroidectomy

- General anaesthesia with endotracheal intubation
- Sandbag under shoulders and head positioned on a ring. Neck extended. Table foot down
- Skin crease incision about two fingers breadth above the sternal notch. The incision should reach the sternocleidomastoid on each side
- Raised skin flaps (including subcutaneous fat and platysma) to the thyroid notch superiorly and the sternal notch inferiorly. Flaps may then be held by a self-retaining retractor (Joll's retractor)
- Make a vertical incision through the deep fascia between the strap muscles and retract the strap muscle. If the goitre is large, the strap muscles are divided at their upper extremity because their nerve supply enters the lower part of the muscles
- Divide the middle thyroid veins
- Draw down the upper pole and identify the superior thyroid vessels
- Ligate the superior thyroid vessels close to the upper pole of the thyroid to avoid the external branch of the superior laryngeal nerve
- Draw the lobe of the thyroid gland medially and dissect the lateral connective tissue and identify the inferior thyroid artery
- Identify the recurrent laryngeal nerve
- Ligate the inferior thyroid artery in continuity lateral to the recurrent laryngeal nerve
- Ligate the inferior thyroid veins
- The lobe is now free and may be removed by dividing the isthmus, disconnecting it off the trachea and oversewing the isthmus with catgut
- If only carrying out a lobectomy, oversew the thyroid remnant to the trachea
- Meticulous haemostasis
- Suture the deep fascia between the strap muscles
- Close the wound in layers with suction drainage.

Complications

Haemorrhage

This may cause airway obstruction. Treatment is by opening the wound, evacuating the haematoma and securing haemostasis. This may need to be done on the ward.

Instruments to remove clips or stitches must be within ready reach in the postoperative period.

Laryngeal oedema

It may occur with or without compression from a haematoma. Stridor and respiratory distress occur. Intubation is required. The condition usually settles spontaneously.

Nerve damage

Recurrent laryngeal nerve. Damage to this may be unilateral, bilateral, temporary, or permanent. Unilateral injury usually causes hoarseness. If this is due to neuropraxia, the voice usually returns to normal within 3 months. If damage is bilateral, airway obstruction occurs after extubation – repeat intubation or emergency tracheostomy is required. If injury is permanent, tracheostomy will be permanent. Laser arytenoidectomy to lateralize the vocal cords is an alternative.

Superior laryngeal nerve. This may result in variable degrees of huskiness or weakness of the voice with change in volume and pitch. Singers, actors and others who rely on their voice professionally should be warned of this possible complication.

Thyroid storm (thyrotoxic crisis)

Seen rarely nowadays, because of better preoperative preparation. Hypercatabolic state due to uncontrolled thyrotoxicosis – usually in an inadequately prepared patient who is undergoing surgery for thyrotoxicosis. Symptoms include hyperpyrexia, confusion, restlessness, sweating, arrhythmias. Treatment includes propranolol, hydrocortisone and potassium iodide.

Hypocalcaemia

Tetany may occur because of ischaemia, or removal, of the parathyroids. Usually occurs within 2–5 days postoperatively. Symptoms include circumoral paraesthesia with tingling of the extremities. Chvostek's sign (tap the facial nerve in front of the external auditory meatus – with hypocalcaemia the side of the face will twitch). In severe hypocalcaemia, painful carpopedal spasms and spasm of respiratory muscles may occur. Treatment is by slow infusion of 10 mL 10% calcium gluconate followed by oral calcium administration. Usually, calcium therapy is needed for a limited period of time – up to 3 months – but long-term management will require 1α-vitamin D. This is also sometimes needed in the short term if hypocalcaemia is profound. Occasionally, parathyroid recovery can be very slow – taking up to 2 years. Calcium levels must be monitored to avoid hypercalcaemia developing.

Wound infection

This is rare.

Recurrent thyrotoxicosis

Hypothyroidism

Keloid scar

PARATHYROIDS

Hyperparathyroidism is the most common clinical disorder of the parathyroid glands. Ischaemia to the parathyroid glands may occur during thyroid surgery and result in hypoparathyroidism.

HYPERPARATHYROIDISM

Three types occur: primary, secondary and tertiary.

Primary hyperparathyroidism

This may result from a parathyroid adenoma (85%), diffuse parathyroid hyperplasia (15%) and, rarely, from carcinoma of the parathyroid. Hyperparathyroidism is the commonest component of MEN I syndrome.

Symptoms and signs. These are classically 'stones, bones, abdominal groans and moans'.

Stones. Renal calculi occur in 5% of patients with hyperparathyroidism. All patients with renal calculi should have their serum calcium and phosphate checked.

Bones. Osteitis fibrosa cystica. Bone pain and fractures may occur.

Abdominal groans. Dyspepsia, constipation and peptic ulceration may occur; pancreatitis is a complication of hyperparathyroidism.

Moans. Psychiatric manifestations may occur, e.g. confusion, depression, psychosis. However, many patients have non-specific symptoms, e.g. weakness, fatigue, lethargy, arthralgia, anorexia. Some patients are asymptomatic, hypercalcaemia being detected on routine screening performed for other reasons.

Investigations
- Ca ↑ (no tourniquet and correct for albumin concentration)
- Phosphate usually ↓
- PTH ↑
- Increased urinary excretion of calcium (calcium-restricted diet)
- Radiographs: skull may show characteristic 'ground glass' appearance
- Abnormal sella turcica if MEN associated with pituitary tumour
- Hands: subperiosteal resorption of bone (best seen on radial aspect of middle phalanges and tufts of terminal phalanges)
- Abdomen: nephrocalcinosis.

Differential diagnosis. Need to exclude other causes of hypercalcaemia, e.g. malignancy, myeloma, sarcoidosis, milk-alkali syndrome. PTH is normal or low in these conditions.

Treatment. Surgery is the treatment of choice. Some surgeons consider preoperative localization of the glands, concordant ultrasound and MIBI scans allowing a focused neck exploration to identify and remove only abnormal parathyroid tissue. If localization studies are not performed or are negative, all four glands should be identified at operation. Occasionally, there are three, five or even six glands. A parathyroid adenoma is removed. If there is hyperplasia of all glands, 3½-gland parathyroidectomy is performed. The residual gland should be marked with a surgical clip. When abnormal parathyroid tissue cannot be found in the neck, or in the superior mediastinum explored through the neck, the need for mediastinal exploration through a sternotomy should be considered. This should only be done after the missing gland has been identified by venous sampling, isotope studies, or CT/MRI scanning. The missing gland may not be in the chest – it may be intrathyroidal. Parathyroidectomy is an operation for the experienced surgeon doing this type of surgery on a regular basis. Even so, an additional parathyroid gland may be overlooked and further surgery required. Hypoparathyroidism may occur postoperatively.

Secondary hyperparathyroidism

This usually occurs in patients with chronic renal failure, although it may be seen in any situation that results in low serum calcium. Hypocalcaemia results in stimulation of the parathyroids with resulting hyperplasia. Patients in CRF are unable to synthesize vitamin D and develop hypocalcaemia, hypophosphataemia, and impaired calcium absorption.

Symptoms and signs. These are of CRF. Bone pain, pruritus, metastatic extravascular calcification. Serum calcium is normal.

Treatment. Correct the underlying cause. In CRF, patients require aluminium hydroxide to reduce phosphate, vitamin D, calcium supplements and high-calcium dialysate. Surgery is required in patients refractory to medical treatment with bone pain, pruritus and metastatic calcification.

Tertiary hyperparathyroidism

Hyperparathyroidism that persists in patients who have had successful renal transplants. Serum calcium is high. The parathyroid hyperplasia of long-term renal disease becomes autonomous despite the return of calcium levels to normal. The symptoms are those of secondary hyperparathyroidism. Treatment is by subtotal parathyroidectomy.

ADRENAL GLAND

The adrenal gland consists of an outer cortex and an inner medulla. The adrenal cortex may overfunction because of hyperplasia or tumour. This may result in an overproduction of glucocorticoids (Cushing's syndrome) or mineralocorticoids (Conn's syndrome). The most common tumour of the adrenal medulla is a phaeochromocytoma, which secretes adrenaline and noradrenaline. Adrenal insufficiency (Addison's disease) may be primary or due to tuberculosis, metastatic disease, adrenal haemorrhage or withdrawal after long-term steroid therapy.

ADRENAL CORTEX

Cushing's syndrome

This is the result of increased secretion of cortisol. Cushing's disease results from overproduction of ACTH by the pituitary resulting in bilateral adrenocortical hyperplasia. Cushing's syndrome refers to increased secretion of cortisol of any origin and includes adrenal adenoma, adrenal carcinoma, administration of exogenous corticosteroids, as well as ectopic ACTH secretion, e.g. oat cell bronchial carcinoma.

Symptoms and signs. The presentation is variable. Any or all of the following may occur: truncal obesity, buffalo hump, moon face, proximal myopathy of the limbs, skin striae, acne, hirsutism, capillary fragility with bruising, oedema, hypertension, osteoporosis, psychiatric disturbances, diabetes, peptic ulceration, pancreatitis, cataracts, skin pigmentation, avascular necrosis of bone.

Investigations
- U&Es: hypokalaemia
- Blood sugar ↑
- CXR may show bronchial carcinoma
- Plasma cortisol at midnight and morning: the diurnal variation is lost
- Overnight low dose dexamethasone suppression test – failure to suppress cortisol levels below 50 nmol/L suggests Cushing's
- Urinary free cortisol is elevated in Cushing's – beware false positives
- ACTH levels: high in pituitary-dependent cases, low or undetectable with adrenal tumour, may be very high with ectopic ACTH secretion
- CT scan or MRI scan of adrenals and pituitary fossa.

Treatment. If the symptoms are due to adenoma or carcinoma, the affected adrenal gland is removed. For bilateral hyperplasia, with ACTH suppression, bilateral adrenalectomy is indicated with permanent replacement steroid therapy. For pituitary tumours, pituitary surgery is required. This may be done by transphenoidal resection or an yttrium implant. For ectopic ACTH secretion, the source should be excised if possible, e.g. pneumonectomy for oat cell carcinoma of the lung. In inoperable cases, radiotherapy may be useful. Bilateral adrenalectomy may be required to control the symptoms. Metyrapone, which inhibits cortisol production, may also be beneficial in cases not amenable to surgery.

Primary hyperaldosteronism

There is excessive secretion of aldosterone with suppression of plasma renin. It is more common in females. The condition is usually due to unilateral adenoma (Conn's syndrome) or bilateral hyperplasia. Rarely bilateral adenomas or carcinoma. The primary type must be distinguished from secondary hyperaldosteronism where there is an increased plasma renin due to increased activity of the renin–angiotensin mechanism. This may occur in renal artery stenosis, cirrhosis, CCF or nephrotic syndrome.

Symptoms and signs. May be asymptomatic. Hypertension, lethargy, fatigue, muscle weakness (due to hypokalaemia), polyuria, polydipsia.

Investigations
- U&Es (hypokalaemia, alkalosis)
- Plasma aldosterone raised (no diuretics)
- Plasma renin levels low
- CT scan will identify adenoma.

Treatment. Unilateral adrenalectomy to remove adenoma. Preoperative preparation includes spironolactone. Bilateral adrenal hyperplasia responds to long-term spironolactone.

ADRENAL MEDULLA

Phaeochromocytoma

This is a catecholamine-producing tumour that arises from the chromaffin cells of the adrenal medulla or other sympathetic nervous tissue, e.g. aortic paraganglia. Some 10% are malignant and may be associated with other genetically determined conditions, e.g. MEN Type II, neurofibromatosis Type I, von Hippel–Lindau disease and the paraganglioma syndromes (SDH). Patients less than 40 years of age should be genetically screened.

Symptoms and signs. Paroxysmal hypertension. Headaches, palpitations, sweating, pallor, dyspnoea, anxiety, chest pain, weakness.

Investigations
- Blood sugar
- 24-hour urine for catecholamines and metanephrines
- CT scanning will locate 90% (→ Fig. 11.2)
- ^{131}I-metaiodobenzylguanidine scanning (MIBG).

Treatment. Surgical excision. Preoperative stabilization required. α-Adrenergic blockade with phenoxybenzamine. Treatment should be given prior to surgery

Figure 11.2 An abdominal CT scan showing a large phaeochromocytoma (arrow) in the left adrenal gland.

until nasal stuffiness and postural hypotension occur. High dosage may need to be gradually introduced to block the adrenergic effects of the tumour. If required, β-blockade with propranolol should be used only when α-blockade is complete. Any diabetogenic effect of the tumour should be controlled – often with insulin. Occasionally phaeochromocytomas can present acutely with cardiac arrhythmias, hypotensive episodes, encephalopathy and coma. Haemorrhagic rupture of the tumour may occur with shock. In these cases, α-adrenergic blockade with i.v. phentolamine followed by emergency surgery.

ADRENAL INSUFFICIENCY

> This may be primary (Addison's disease) when adrenal destruction may be autoimmune, or due to sarcoidosis, tuberculosis, amyloidosis, secondary deposits, adrenal haemorrhage (anticoagulant therapy) or meningococcal septicaemia (Waterhouse–Friderichsen syndrome); or secondary due to pituitary disease or withdrawal of long-term steroid therapy. Bilateral adrenalectomy is an iatrogenic cause.

Symptoms and signs
Acute adrenal insufficiency. Shock, nausea, vomiting, hyperpyrexia, rigors, abdominal pain, coma.

Chronic adrenal insufficiency. Anorexia, lethargy, malaise, hypotension, weight loss, constipation, amenorrhoea, hyperpigmentation of skin.

Investigations
- If the patient is already on steroid therapy, check that the dose is adequate
- Check BP
- U&Es: $K^+ \uparrow Na^+ \downarrow$, blood sugar $\downarrow$, serum cortisol levels reduced with inadequate response to synacthen test
- ACTH levels high in Addison's disease and low in secondary causes
- Adrenal antibody screen
- CXR: may show TB
- AXR: adrenal gland calcification in TB.

Treatment.
The acute case requires resuscitation with i.v. saline and hydrocortisone 100 mg i.v. 6-hourly. Clinical improvement is often dramatic. Chronic adrenal insufficiency is treated with oral hydrocortisone t.d.s. at a weight-related dose. Fludrocortisone as mineralocorticoid replacement (0.5–1.0 mg daily) is indicated in most patients. Fatigue, hypotension, and hyperkalaemia are signs of undertreatment. Hypertension, oedema, and hypokalaemia are signs of overtreatment. Patients on replacement therapy should be warned that increased doses are required at times of stress, e.g. surgery or an acute illness. Care should be taken in reducing steroids and discontinuing them in patients who have been on long-term therapy, e.g. for asthma or rheumatoid arthritis. In these patients, gradual withdrawal over weeks will allow endogenous steroid production to resume but in others, signs of insufficiency will appear.

ADRENAL INCIDENTALOMA

An incidentaloma is a mass lesion found unexpectedly in an adrenal gland by an imaging procedure performed for reasons other than suspected adrenal pathology. The vast majority are non-secretory benign lesions. Once discovered, the question is, are they benign or malignant and are they hypersecretory?

Symptoms and signs. Often none, as the name implies. Closer questioning may reveal signs and symptoms of a hypersecretory state, e.g. Cushing's syndrome, Conn's syndrome, phaeochromocytoma.

Investigations
- To exclude functioning tumour, e.g. Cushing's, Conn's, phaeochromocytoma (see above)
- CT scan for size and attenuation.

Treatment. None if no features of hypersecretion or malignancy. Excision if: (1) a functioning tumour; (2) >4 cm, especially if features of malignancy on CT imaging; small non-functioning tumours are best, followed by an interval scan at 6 months to exclude increase in size.

CARCINOMA OF THE ADRENAL GLAND

Adrenocortical carcinoma is rare but aggressive. It is potentially curable in the early stages but only 30% are confined to the adrenal gland at the time of diagnosis; 10% of phaeochromocytomas are malignant and occur within the adrenal medulla. Secondary deposits are more common than primary tumours, the adrenal glands being the fourth most common site of metastases after lungs, liver and bone. The most common primary sites are lung, breast, skin (melanoma), kidney, thyroid and colon.

Symptoms and signs. Signs of excess hormone production, e.g. Cushing's, androgen excess. Abdominal pain. Flank pain. Signs of spread to distant organs, e.g. abdominal cavity, lungs, liver, bone. Symptoms and signs of original primary in cases of adrenal metastases.

Investigations
- U&Es
- Circulating hormone levels
- CT
- MRI.

Treatment. Surgery, chemotherapy, radiotherapy, depending on degree of spread.

MULTIPLE ENDOCRINE NEOPLASIA (MEN)

MEN syndromes are patterns of endocrine disease inherited as autosomal dominant traits. A family history should be taken in all patients presenting with hyperparathyroidism, medullary thyroid cancer, phaeochromocytoma and pancreatic endocrine tumours.

MEN I

Manifestations are hyperparathyroidism (>90%), pancreatic tumours (>30%) with malignant potential (insulinomas, gastrinomas) and pituitary tumours (prolactinoma).

Symptoms and signs. Hyperparathyroidism may be asymptomatic and detected incidentally on checking Ca^{2+} levels. Patients can present with symptoms related to peptic ulceration (gastrinoma) or to the pituitary tumour.

Treatment. Directed at the tumours.

MEN IIa

Manifestations are medullary carcinoma of the thyroid (100%), phaeochromocytoma (30–50%) and parathyroid hyperplasia (rare).

Symptoms and signs. All patients with medullary carcinoma of the thyroid should undergo ret-mutation analysis. If a mutation is detected, family screening is necessary. If positive in the family, e.g. parents, children, brothers, sisters (and their progeny) – prophylactic thyroidectomy must be considered. Search should be made for all tumours in the syndrome prior to treatment.

Treatment. If phaeochromocytoma is located, treat this first. Then deal with thyroid and parathyroid at the same operation.

MEN IIb

Manifestations are medullary carcinoma of the thyroid, phaeochromocytoma, multiple mucosal neuromas and marfanoid habitus.

Symptoms and signs. Early appearance of marfanoid habitus and mucosal neuromas suggests diagnosis. Medullary thyroid cancer arises in the first year of life. Other symptoms are as for Type IIa. It occurs in first and second decades. Other symptoms are as for Type IIa.

Treatment. MEN IIb presents more aggressively than Type IIa and therefore prompt diagnosis and treatment are required.

Abdominal wall and hernia

HERNIAE

A hernia is an abnormal protrusion of a viscus or part of a viscus through an opening in the cavity in which it is normally contained. About 75% of all herniae occur at the groin.

Reducible hernia

This is one in which the contents of the sac reduce spontaneously or can be pushed back manually.

Irreducible hernia

The contents cannot be returned to the peritoneal cavity either because there are adhesions between the sac and contents or because of the narrow neck of the sac. Irreducible herniae may be as described below:

Incarcerated

There are adhesions between the sac and the contents, but there is no obstruction or interference with blood supply. The hernia simply will not reduce.

Obstructed

A hollow viscus is trapped within the sac and obstruction occurs. The blood supply remains intact. This is a common cause of small bowel obstruction.

Strangulated

The arterial blood supply to the contents of the sac is compromised such that unless surgical relief is undertaken the contents of the sac will become gangrenous.

GENERAL DESCRIPTION OF A HERNIA (→ Fig. 12.1)

Defect

This is in the abdominal wall (e.g. at the deep inguinal ring or femoral ring) or a defect in a surgical incision (incisional hernia).

Sac

This has a neck (which may be very narrow), a body and a fundus.

Contents of the sac. May be omentum, bowel, ovary, etc.

Figure 12.1 (A) General description of a hernia. (B) Principles of repair.

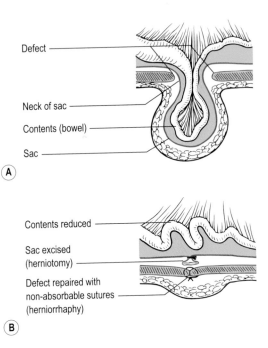

CLASSIFICATION OF HERNIA

Congenital

A congenital hernia develops in a peritoneal sac, which gives rise to a hernia in infancy, or provides a potential channel for one to form in later life, e.g. patent processus vaginalis in indirect inguinal hernia, or failure of closure of the umbilicus orifice in umbilical hernia. These sacs represent persistent embryological channels.

Acquired

Aetiological factors
- Loss of tissue strength and elasticity, e.g. direct inguinal hernia in the older patient
- Surgical trauma, e.g. incisional hernia
- Enlargement of a foramen, e.g. enlarged oesophageal hiatus allowing development of a hiatus hernia
- Nerve damage with consequent weakening of muscles, e.g. development of inguinal hernia after appendicectomy owing to damage to the ilioinguinal nerve.

If a potential weakness is present, then the following factors may predispose to hernia formation by increasing intra-abdominal pressure. These include:

- Heavy lifting or carrying
- Coughing, e.g. asthma, COPD
- Constipation
- Benign prostatic hypertrophy
- Pregnancy
- Obesity
- Ascites
- CAPD – may unmask persistent processus vaginalis with CAPD fluid filling a potential hernial sac and presenting as scrotal oedema.

TYPES OF HERNIA

Inguinal hernia

This is the most common form of hernia. There are two types: indirect and direct.

Indirect

A peritoneal sac protrudes through the deep inguinal ring, passes down the inguinal canal, and may extend as far as the upper pole of the testis. The defect is congenital and is due to a persistent processus vaginalis. It is more common in males. It may appear in infancy or early adult life. In infants, there is often an associated hydrocele and undescended testis.

Direct

This is acquired. The defect occurs in the abdominal wall, in Hesselbach's triangle (bounded by the inguinal ligament inferiorly, the inferior epigastric artery laterally and the lateral border of rectus muscle medially). It is due to a weakness of the transversalis fascia in the posterior wall of the inguinal canal. It is often bilateral and occurs in the older patient and may be associated with obesity, cough, constipation, prostatism.

Both types may occur and straddle the inferior epigastric artery, the so-called 'pantaloon' hernia.

Symptoms and signs. Often none. Occasionally aching or dragging sensation in the groin. Some patients relate the development of the hernia to an episode of straining or lifting. Some patients can push the hernia back. A painful, tense, tender lump that will not reduce indicates incipient strangulation until proved otherwise. Examine the patient standing. A hernia that descends into the scrotum is likely to be indirect. A diffuse bulge medially over the canal is likely to be direct. Locate the pubic tubercle. If the hernia is above and medial to this it is an inguinal hernia, if it is below and lateral, it is a femoral hernia. Test for a cough impulse. Lay the patient down and reduce the hernia. Apply pressure over the deep inguinal ring, i.e. 1 cm above the midpoint of the inguinal ligament. Ask the patient to cough. If the hernia appears medial to the point of pressure, it is likely to be direct. If no hernia appears, release the pressure and again get the patient to cough. If it appears, it is likely to be indirect. For smaller herniae it is possible to distinguish between direct and indirect by invaginating the scrotum with the little finger into the inguinal canal. Get the patient to cough. If the hernia is indirect, the impulse hits the tip of the finger; if direct, it hits the pulp. The difference, in fact, is academic since both will be carefully looked for at surgery.

Treatment

Uncomplicated. Elective herniotomy (i.e. excision of sac) in children. Herniotomy and herniorrhaphy (repair of the defect) in adults. There are three accepted methods of repair of inguinal hernia:

1. Lichtenstein repair – this is a tension-free mesh repair using polypropylene mesh.
2. Shouldice repair – this is a double-breasted repair of the transversalis fascia followed by suturing of the conjoint tendon to the inguinal ligament with non-absorbable sutures.
3. Laparoscopic – this may be via an extraperitoneal or intraperitoneal technique. NICE guidelines recommend this technique for bilateral or recurrent inguinal herniae.

Trusses may be used if surgery is contraindicated. A spring-loaded pad is applied to the defect after the hernia has been reduced. The patient should apply it after lying down and reducing the hernia. They are uncomfortable and unhygienic. Indications for a truss are rare.

Obstructed and strangulated herniae. These require emergency surgery, with resection of bowel if necessary followed by surgical repair.

Procedure

Repair of inguinal hernia

- Make an incision 2.5 cm above and parallel to the medial $2/3$ of the inguinal ligament.
- Divide the superficial fascia (Camper's and Scarpa's) ligating the superficial veins (superficial epigastric vein and possibly the superficial circumflex iliac vein in the lateral end of the incision.
- Expose the aponeurotic fibres of external oblique. Open the external oblique aponeurosis in the line of its fibres, extending the incision into the superficial inguinal ring.
- Dissect the ilioinguinal nerve off the spermatic cord and preserve it.
- Mobilize the cord. Check if there is a direct hernia (posterior to and separate from the cord). Carefully divide the layers of fascia covering the cord and check for an indirect sac. If indirect sac present, separate it carefully from the cord. Open the sac and reduce any contents. Twist the neck of the sac. Transfix and ligate the neck of the sac and excise redundant sac.
- Repair with Prolene mesh, attaching it to the pubic tubercle and inguinal ligament with a continuous Prolene suture and with interrupted sutures to the internal oblique and transversalis fascia, leaving an adequate opening for the cord to pass through.
- Close the external oblique with a continuous suture, making sure not to catch the ilioinguinal nerve.
- Close Scarpa's fascia and skin.
- Exert gentle traction on the testis to make sure that it is in the base of the scrotum.

Complications. Recurrence may occur but should be less than 2%. Other complications include infection, ilioinguinal nerve entrapment, and testicular ischaemia. Testicular ischaemia is rare after initial repair but occurs with a higher incidence after repair of recurrent herniae, possibly owing to cord damage.

Femoral hernia

The defect is in the transversalis fascia overlying the femoral ring at the entry to the femoral canal. The hernia passes through the femoral canal and presents in the groin, below and lateral to the pubic tubercle. It is more common in females and carries a higher risk of strangulation. Femoral herniae are often of the Richter type.

Symptoms and signs. A lump occurs below and lateral to the pubic tubercle. It may be reducible. It may not be noticed until it becomes tender and painful. This type of hernia should be carefully sought in the obese patient who presents with signs of intestinal obstruction without an obvious cause.

Treatment

Surgical repair. An incision is made directly over the swelling. The sac is opened, the contents reduced and the sac removed. The defect is repaired by inserting non-absorbable sutures between the inguinal ligament and the pectineal ligament, thus closing the femoral canal. If the hernia is strangulated or obstructed, a separate abdominal incision will be required to deal with the bowel. There is no place for a truss in the treatment of femoral hernia – it may, in fact, be dangerous by compressing the contents of an incompletely emptied sac against the pubic bone. This is one reason why it is necessary to distinguish accurately between inguinal and femoral herniae. Recurrence rate following surgery should be less than 3%.

Procedure

Repair of femoral hernia (low approach)

- Make an incision in the line of the groin crease over the hernial sac.
- Deepen the incision to identify the hernial sac.
- Ligate superficial veins as necessary.
- Expose the sac carefully defining the neck of the sac.
- Open sac, reduce any contents.
- Transfix and ligate the neck of the sac and excise the sac.
- Repair the femoral canal by suturing the inguinal ligament to the pectineal ligament without constricting the femoral vein.
- Place the left index finger over the femoral vein, insert a stitch into the inguinal ligament and the pectineal ligament, making sure that the most lateral stitch snugly fits around the index finger.
- Withdraw the index finger, allowing the vein to fill the space.
- Alternatively, the inguinal canal may be filled with a mesh plug which is tacked in place.
- Close the wound in layers.

Umbilical hernia

This occurs in children because of incomplete closure of the umbilical orifice – most close spontaneously during the first year of life. It is more common in black children. Surgical repair should only be carried out if the hernia has not disappeared by the age of 3 and the fascial defect is >1.5 cm in diameter.

Paraumbilical hernia

It occurs just above or just below the umbilicus, and is more common in females. Predisposing factors include multiple pregnancies and obesity. The neck of the sac is usually narrow and therefore, there is a high risk of strangulation. The most common content is omentum, followed by transverse colon and small intestine. Treatment is by excision of the sac and a two-layer overlapping repair (Mayo repair).

Epigastric hernia

This is usually a small protrusion through the linea alba in the upper part of the abdomen. Often, the hernia consists of extraperitoneal fat only, but it may contain omentum or small bowel. It may be extremely painful, probably because of trapping and ischaemia of extraperitoneal fat. Treatment is by simple suture of the defect with non-absorbable sutures.

Incisional hernia

This occurs through a defect in the scar of a previous abdominal incision.

Aetiology

- Age. Wound healing is poor in the older patient
- General debility, e.g. carcinomatosis, cirrhosis
- Obesity
- Postoperative wound infection
- Postoperative wound haematoma
- Raised intra-abdominal pressure postoperatively, e.g. coughing, straining, constipation, ileus
- Steroid therapy
- Type of incision. Midline vertical wounds have a higher incidence than transverse incisions. Incisional hernia is exceptionally rare through a Pfannenstiel incision
- Poor suturing technique. Rarely does a suture break.

Symptoms and signs. May occur up to 5 years postoperatively. A swelling protrudes through the wound. Many are large and involve the whole incision – consequently the neck of the sac is wide and the risk of strangulation rare. If the defect is small, there is a greater risk of strangulation.

Treatment

Small herniae. These may be repaired with interrupted non-absorbable sutures.

Large herniae. These may be very unsightly and noticeable through the clothes. If the patient is unfit for surgery, a corset may be worn. Surgical repair should otherwise be undertaken. The old scar should be excised and normal rectus sheath identified. The edges may then be approximated with non-absorbable sutures. Often to get an adequate repair the hernia is repaired in two layers overlapping. Very large defects may need interposition of foreign material, e.g. polypropylene mesh. The recurrence rate is high, being 10–20%.

Richter's hernia (→ Fig. 12.2)

Part of the circumference of the bowel becomes trapped in the defect. This is usually the antimesenteric border of the small bowel. A strangulated Richter's hernia may reduce spontaneously leaving a segment of bowel with a gangrenous area – this may subsequently perforate with resulting peritonitis.

Part of the circumference of the antimesenteric border of the bowel is trapped in the sac —

Figure 12.2 Richter's hernia.

Spigelian hernia

This is a hernia through the linea semilunaris at the lateral border of the rectus sheath. It occurs at a point a hand's breadth above the pubic symphysis at the level of the linea semicircularis (arcuate line of Douglas). This is the point at which the posterior rectus sheath becomes deficient and all aponeuroses of the abdominal muscles pass in front of the rectus muscle. Surgical repair is required.

Littre's hernia

This is a hernia that contains a Meckel's diverticulum in the sac.

Sliding hernia (hernia-en-glissade → Fig. 12.3)

The posterior parietal peritoneum 'slides' on the underlying tissue; therefore, the posterior wall of the sac is formed, not of peritoneum alone, but of sigmoid colon on the left and caecum on the right. These herniae occur in older patients, especially males with obesity and weak musculature. Diagnosis is made at surgery. Care needs to be taken when excising the sac.

Obturator hernia

This hernia occurs through the obturator foramen. It is commoner in elderly females. The diagnosis is usually made via a laparotomy for intestinal obstruction. It is difficult to feel the hernia as it occurs in the groin deep to pectineus. The hernia may cause pressure on the obturator nerve at the obturator foramen causing referred pain down the medial side of the thigh, especially if the hernia is strangulated (Howship–Romberg sign).

Lumbar herniae

These may occur through Grynfeltt's space (below the 12th rib) or Petit's triangle (just above the iliac crest). They usually contain extraperitoneal fat and are often mistaken for lipomas.

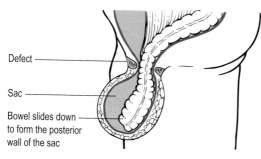

Defect —

Sac —

Bowel slides down to form the posterior wall of the sac

Figure 12.3 Sliding hernia. Part of the bowel wall (sigmoid colon or caecum) forms the posterior wall of the sac.

Internal herniae

Usually present with intestinal obstruction. They are often the result of iatrogenic causes such as defects left in the mesentery or following adhesions. Rarely, they may occur through the epiploic foramen of Winslow or into paracaecal or paraduodenal fossae.

OTHER CONDITIONS OF THE ABDOMINAL WALL

UMBILICUS

Discharge

Patent vitellointestinal duct

This may result in discharge of mucus or small bowel contents. It is usually associated with a Meckel's diverticulum and usually occurs in infancy.

Patent urachus

This may not present until early adult life or even old age and results from distension of the bladder usually because of outflow obstruction. Urine discharges through the umbilicus.

Abscess in a urachal cyst

This may discharge through the umbilicus.

Infection

This may occur deep in the umbilicus and cause discharge. It may be fungal. Inflammation of the umbilicus is called omphalitis.

Umbilical calculus

This is usually black in colour and composed of inspissated desquamated epithelium and may be associated with infection and discharge. This condition is not infrequently seen in the elderly and associated with poor hygiene.

Endometriosis

The umbilicus is usually painful and bleeds at the time of menstruation.

Mass

Umbilical hernia (see above)

Secondary carcinoma

This is rare and presents as an umbilical nodule (Sister Joseph's nodule). It may be associated with carcinoma of the stomach, colon, ovary or breast.

RECTUS SHEATH HAEMATOMA

This is due to tearing of the inferior epigastric vessels with haematoma in the posterior rectus sheath. It may occur in athletic, muscular young men during exercise or in thin elderly females. Occasionally it occurs during pregnancy. It may be also associated with disorders of coagulation or blood dyscrasias.

Symptoms and signs. Sudden onset of severe lower abdominal pain in the left or right lower abdomen. Occasionally its onset is slow and progressive. Examination in the early stages reveals a tender mass in the abdominal wall. Later bruising may be detectable in the suprapubic area.

Treatment. This is usually conservative. The acute pain and discomfort should disappear within a few days. In young patients with a rectus sheath haematoma on the right side, the symptoms and signs may be mistaken for acute appendicitis.

TUMOURS OF THE ABDOMINAL WALL

Most of these are benign lipomas. Most malignant tumours of the abdominal wall are metastatic. Musculoaponeurotic fibromatoses (desmoid tumours) may occur and are part of Gardner's syndrome (familial polyposis coli, osteomas, sebaceous cysts and desmoid tumours).

SWELLINGS IN THE GROIN AND SCROTUM

These are a common clinical problem. A list of conditions is shown in Table 12.1. They are discussed further in the relevant chapters.

TABLE 12.1 Lumps in the groin and scrotum	
Groin	Above the inguinal ligament: • sebaceous cyst • lipoma • direct inguinal hernia • indirect inguinal hernia • malgaigne's bulges (minor bilateral bulging of the inguinal canal – normal) • imperfectly descended testis • lipoma of the cord • hydrocele of the cord (rare) • hydrocele of the canal of Nuck (rare) Below the inguinal ligament: • sebaceous cyst • lipoma • femoral hernia • lymph nodes • saphena varix • femoral artery aneurysm (true or false) • imperfectly descended testis • neuroma of femoral nerve (rare) • synovioma of hip joint (rare) • obturator hernia (rare) • psoas abscess (rare)

Continued

TABLE 12.1 Lumps in the groin and scrotum—cont'd

Scrotum	• sebaceous cyst
	• indirect inguinal hernia
	• hydrocele
	• epididymal cyst (spermatocele)
	• epididymo-orchitis
	• testicular tumour
	• torsion of testes
	• varicocele
	• haematocele
	• sperm granuloma
	• torsion of testicular appendage

Acute abdomen

BASIC PRINCIPLES

Acute abdomen is the most common cause of emergency admission to a
surgical unit. The term 'acute abdomen' is difficult to define but it indicates
any non-traumatic disorder of acute onset in which the symptoms are
predominantly abdominal and for which in some cases, urgent surgery may be
indicated. In practice, it represents a spectrum of problems ranging from
sudden onset of severe abdominal pain with a life-threatening underlying cause
to minor abdominal symptoms of lengthy duration. The most important feature
of the acute abdomen is to sort out the severe causes in need of urgent surgery
(e.g. ruptured aortic aneurysm, perforated diverticulitis) from severe abdominal
pain that does not require surgery (biliary colic, ureteric colic, pancreatitis);
and also from those conditions that do not need urgent investigation and
treatment (e.g. mild gastroenteritis, constipation). Prompt diagnosis is essential.
A careful history and examination will indicate the cause of most acute
abdomens.

History

Age. Certain conditions are more likely to occur in certain age groups, e.g.
mesenteric adenitis in children, diverticulitis in the older patient.

Pain. This can be remembered from the mnemonic 'SOCRATES':

- Site: where did it start, has it moved?
- Onset: sudden, gradual
- Character: e.g. dull, vague, cramping, sharp, burning
- Radiation: e.g. loin to groin in ureteric colic
- Associated factors: e.g. vomiting, diarrhoea, fever, effect of movement, effect of
  micturition, etc.
- Timing: is the pain constant or intermittent; how long does the pain last?
- Exacerbations and relieving factors: what makes the pain better/worse?
- Severity.

Vomiting
- Did vomiting precede the pain?
- Frequency.
- Character, e.g. bile, faeculent, blood, coffee grounds.

Defaecation
- Constipation: absolute constipation with colicky abdominal pain, distension, and vomiting suggests intestinal obstruction.
- Diarrhoea: frequency, consistency of stools, blood, mucus, pus.

Fever. Any rigors.

Past history
- Previous surgery, e.g. adhesions may cause intestinal obstruction
- Recent trauma, e.g. delayed rupture of spleen
- Menstrual history, e.g. ectopic pregnancy.

Examination

General. Is the patient lying comfortably? Is the patient lying still but in pain, e.g. peritonitis? Is the patient writhing in agony, e.g. ureteric or biliary colic? Is the patient flushed suggesting pyrexia?

Pulse, temperature, respiration

Cervical lymphadenopathy. (e.g. mesenteric adenitis).

Chest. (e.g. referred pain from lobar pneumonia).

Abdomen

Inspection. Moves on respiration. Scars, distended, visible peristalsis (usually chronic obstruction in patient with very thin abdominal wall). Pain on coughing. Hernial orifices. Any obvious masses, e.g. pulsatile mass to suggest aortic aneurysm.

Palpation. Patient relaxed, lying flat, with arms by side. Be gentle and start as far from the painful site as possible. Check for guarding and rigidity. Rebound tenderness is unpleasant and should not be performed in the traditional manner of palpating the abdomen deeply and then suddenly withdrawing the examining hand. The presence of rebound tenderness can be inferred from more subtle signs such as percussing the abdomen, asking the patient to cough and asking whether bumps in the road during the ambulance journey were painful (hospitals always have speed bumps and can provide much information about an acute abdomen!). Check for masses, e.g. appendix mass, pulsatile expansile mass of aortic aneurysm. Check the hernial orifices.

Percussion. For example, tympanitic note with distension due to intestinal obstruction; dullness over bladder due to acute retention.

Auscultation. Take your time (30–60 s), e.g. silent abdomen of peritonitis, high-pitched tinkling bowel sounds of intestinal obstruction.

Rectal examination
This is just as important as the abdominal examination. It should be carried out in the left lateral position. Insert the well-lubricated gloved finger posteriorly into the sacral hollow. Move the finger around in the arc of a circle until it

impinges on the peritoneum of the rectovesical or rectouterine pouch. If the patient winces with pain when the finger impinges on the peritoneum, this is a sign of peritonitis in the most dependent part of the pelvis. The pain disappears when the finger comes off the peritoneum as it completes the circle and returns to the sacral hollow. The correct annotation of a positive rectal examination should be 'tender anteriorly'. 'Tender high up in the right' is inappropriate. There seems to be a misconception among medical students that you are feeling the area of the appendix. You are feeling for tenderness due to inflammation of the pelvic peritoneum caused by infected exudates draining to the most dependent part of the pelvis, i.e. the rectovesical or rectouterine pouch.

Vaginal examination

Discharge, tenderness associated with pelvic inflammatory disease, examine the uterus and adnexa, e.g. pregnancy, fibroids, ectopic pregnancy.

Investigations

- FBC: low Hb may indicate chronic bleeding; a raised white cell count with a neutrophil leukocytosis may indicate an inflammatory or infective process
- U&Es: fluid loss may result in renal impairment, vomiting may cause electrolyte abnormalities
- LFTs: may indicate gallstone pathology or hepatitis
- Amylase: a high amylase confirms the diagnosis of pancreatitis; a mildly raised amylase is also seen in ectopic pregnancy, perforated viscus, intestinal obstruction and intestinal ischaemia
- β-hCG: pregnancy/ectopic pregnancy – must be performed in all females of child-bearing age with iliac fossa pain
- CRP: inflammatory marker generally raised within 8 h of an inflammatory process – can be useful in difficult cases, e.g. suspected appendicitis of 12 h duration with a normal WCC and CRP is unlikely to be acute appendicitis
- ABG: generally only indicated in severely ill patients; it can give useful information on tissue perfusion by pH and lactate levels; PaO_2 and $PaCO_2$ can give important information for the anaesthetist prior to surgery
- CXR: exclude referred lesion, gas under diaphragm (→ Fig. 13.1)
- AXR: distended bowel with air/fluid levels, gallstones (10% are radio-opaque); calcified aorta, e.g. aneurysm; air in biliary tree (cholecystoduodenal fistula with gallstone ileus)
- USS: e.g. ovarian cyst, ectopic pregnancy, gallstones
- CT: useful in difficult cases – able to demonstrate free fluid, air, dilated bowel, pancreatitis
- KUB
- IVU for stones
- Angiography: e.g. acute GI haemorrhage of obscure cause, superior mesenteric embolus or thrombosis (duplex scanning may also be appropriate).

Figure 13.1 Gas (arrow) is seen under the right hemidiaphragm following perforation of a duodenal ulcer.

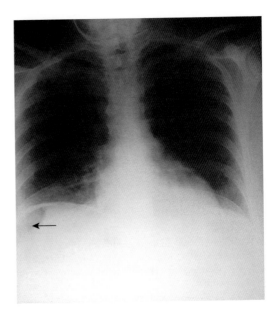

Causes

Some causes of the acute abdomen are shown in Table 13.1. These conditions are covered in the relevant chapters. (For information on the site of abdominal pain in relation to suspected pathology → Table 13.2.)

Diagnosis. Diagnosing patients with an acute abdomen is the 'bread and butter' of the on-call general surgeon. The legion of causes is almost impossible to remember. Furthermore, you will spend your entire life in the A&E department if you slavishly attempt to rule out all the causes of an acute abdomen. An easy method to classify patients with an acute abdomen is given below:

- Acute abdomen + shock, e.g. ruptured abdominal aortic aneurysm, pancreatitis
- Generalized peritonitis, e.g. perforated viscus
- Localized peritonitis, e.g. acute appendicitis
- Bowel obstruction
- Medical causes, e.g. lobar pneumonia.

These patients can then be divided into a number of management strategies. For example, not all patients with localized peritonitis need an operation. Indeed not all patients with pain and shock need an operation. An unnecessary laparotomy in pancreatitis can exacerbate the condition considerably.

TABLE 13.1 Causes of acute abdomen

Gastrointestinal	
Gut	Acute appendicitis
	Intestinal obstruction
	Perforated peptic ulcer
	Diverticulitis
	Inflammatory bowel disease
	Acute exacerbation of peptic ulcer
	Gastroenteritis
	Mesenteric adenitis
	Meckel's diverticulitis
Liver and biliary tract	Cholecystitis
	Cholangitis
	Hepatitis
	Biliary colic
Pancreas	Acute pancreatitis
Spleen	Splenic infarct and spontaneous rupture
Urinary tract	Cystitis
	Acute pyelonephritis
	Ureteric colic
	Acute retention
Gynaecological	Ruptured ectopic pregnancy
	Torsion of ovarian cyst
	Ruptured ovarian cyst
	Salpingitis
	Severe dysmenorrhoea
	Mittelschmerz
	Endometriosis
Vascular	Ruptured aortic aneurysm
	Mesenteric embolus
	Mesenteric venous thrombosis
	Ischaemic colitis
	Acute aortic dissection
Peritoneum	Primary peritonitis
	Secondary peritonitis
Abdominal wall	Rectus sheath haematoma
Retroperitoneal	Haemorrhage, e.g. anticoagulants

Management. Strategies include:

- Immediate operation – these patients will die unless taken to theatre immediately, e.g. ruptured abdominal aortic aneurysm.
- Preoperative preparation and operation urgently within 6 h – elderly patients may present with an acute abdomen and require urgent operation; however, preoperative dehydration and electrolyte abnormalities need to be corrected before going to theatre.
- Urgent operation (within 24 h) – certain conditions, particularly in young patients, may be dealt with on a routine emergency list, e.g. acute appendicitis, small bowel obstruction with no adverse symptoms (e.g. no fever, no leukocytosis, no peritonism).

TABLE 13.2 Site of abdominal pain in relation to suspected pathology

Whole abdomen	Generalized peritonitis and mesenteric infarction
Right upper quadrant	Acute cholecystitis Cholangitis Hepatitis Peptic ulceration
Left upper quadrant	Peptic ulceration Pancreatitis Splenic infarct
Right lower quadrant	Appendicitis Ovarian cyst Ectopic pregnancy Pelvic inflammatory disease Meckel's diverticulum Mesenteric adenitis Ureteric colic Rectus sheath haematoma Right-sided lobar pneumonia
Left lower quadrant	Sigmoid diverticular disease Ovarian cyst Ectopic pregnancy Pelvic inflammatory disease Ureteric colic Rectus sheath haematoma Left-sided lobar pneumonia
Radiating pain Back Groin	Peptic ulcer Pancreatitis Aortic aneurysm Acute aortic dissection Ureteric colic Testicular torsion

- Conservative treatment – numerous causes of an acute abdomen only require conservative treatment, i.e. nil by mouth, antibiotics (e.g. acute cholecystitis).
- Observation – many patients may have equivocal clinical signs but be in the early stages of a condition. Time is a great diagnostic tool and frequent re-examination may reveal evolving signs.
- Discharge.

Patients must be continually reassessed and evaluated as patients can move from one group to another; for example a young man admitted with RIF pain and booked for urgent operation within 24 h may perforate and thus display generalized peritonitis – in this instance the patient would require immediate operation.

Treatment
- Relieve pain
- Intravenous fluids and nasogastric suction
- Broad-spectrum antibiotics if peritonitis or sepsis
- Surgery if indicated.

Indications for surgery in the acute abdomen

There are no hard and fast rules but patients with the following symptoms will almost certainly require surgery:

- Localized peritoneal irritation with guarding or rigidity
- Spreading tenderness
- Tense or progressive distension
- Generalized peritonitis
- Shock with bleeding or sepsis
- Free gas on radiograph
- Mesenteric occlusion on angiography
- Blood, bile, pus or bowel contents on paracentesis.

MEDICAL CAUSES OF ACUTE ABDOMINAL PAIN

Occasionally, certain medical conditions may cause acute abdominal pain.

Referred pain

May be caused by degenerative disease of thoracic spine, herpes zoster, lobar pneumonia, pleurisy, MI.

Haematological

This may be due to sickle cell crisis.

Infective and inflammatory

These medical conditions are possible: tabes dorsalis, Henoch–Schönlein purpura.

Endocrine and metabolic

These conditions include uraemia, hypercalcaemia, diabetic ketoacidosis, Addison's disease, acute intermittent porphyria.

PERITONITIS

Peritonitis is an inflammatory or suppurative response of the peritoneal lining to direct irritation. It may be localized or generalized, bacterial or chemical. Localized peritonitis is due to transmural inflammation of a viscus, e.g. appendicitis, cholecystitis, diverticulitis. It may remain localized through being contained by omental wrapping or adhesion of adjacent structures. In many cases, however, it becomes generalized, spreading to involve the whole peritoneum. Sudden perforation of a viscus usually results in generalized peritonitis. With the latter the patient is seriously ill. Hypovolaemia results from massive exudation into the peritoneal cavity, and septicaemia may result if the cause is infective, e.g. faecal peritonitis from perforated diverticulitis. Chemical peritonitis results from gastric or pancreatic juice, bile, urine or blood in the peritoneal cavity. Bile causes little reaction if sterile but causes severe peritonitis if infected or mixed with pancreatic juice. Blood and urine cause little reaction if sterile but a severe reaction occurs if they are infective. (For a classification of peritonitis, → Table 13.3.)

TABLE 13.3 Causes of peritonitis

Acute	
Bacterial	Primary (rare):
	• streptococci, pneumococci
	• haematogenous spread
	• occurs in young girls, ascites, nephrotic syndrome and postsplenectomy
	Secondary (common):
	• related to perforation, infection, inflammation or ischaemia of GI or GU tract
Chemical	Gastric juice (e.g. perforated gastric ulcer)
	Pancreatic juice (e.g. acute pancreatitis)
	Bile (e.g. perforation of the gall bladder)
	Blood (e.g. ruptured spleen)
	Urine (e.g. intraperitoneal rupture of the bladder)
Chronic	Tuberculosis
	Starch (immunological reaction)

Symptoms and signs. These depend on the degree of peritonitis and the precipitating cause. They also relate to the abdominal signs from the original pathology and manifestations of systemic infection. Usually there is sudden onset of abdominal pain made worse by coughing and movement. Initially it may be localized (it may remain so in some cases) but often gradually spreads to involve the whole abdomen. Nausea, vomiting, fever, abdominal tenderness (localized or generalized), guarding, rigidity, distension, absent bowel sounds when ileus supervenes. Manifestations of systemic infection include tachycardia, sweating, rigors, tachypnoea, oliguria, disorientation, shock and Gram-negative septicaemia. In advanced cases, and with delay in presentation, renal, respiratory, and cardiac failure may result.

Investigations
- Hb
- PCV
- WCC
- U&Es: dehydration, ARF
- LFTs
- Amylase
- CXR: gas under diaphragm, small pleural effusion
- AXR: distended bowel (ileus), local ileus ('sentinel' loop – appendicitis, pancreatitis)
- USS: free fluid, localized collections
- CT – pancreatitis.

Complications
Systemic. Hypovolaemic shock, septic shock, ARDS, DIC, multiorgan failure, immunological failure.

Local. Intraperitoneal sepsis: residual abscesses, e.g. subphrenic or pelvic, wound infection, anastomotic breakdown, fistula formation, adhesions.

Prognosis. Overall mortality in generalized peritonitis is around 40%. Factors affecting mortality include age (elderly patients with faecal peritonitis have a high mortality), causation, duration of symptoms, degree of bacterial contamination, concomitant disease processes and organ failure.

Treatment. Principles of treatment involve the following:

Resuscitation. This requires pain relief with narcotic analgesics, i.v. fluids, NG aspiration, correction of electrolyte imbalance, catheterization. UO should be monitored and CVP (especially in elderly). Oxygen and antibiotics.

Treatment of causative lesion. In generalized peritonitis this almost invariably requires surgery. Acute pancreatitis is the exception. Principles of operative treatment involve removal of all infected material from the peritoneal cavity, correction of the underlying cause, and attempts to prevent complications. Swab for C&S. Thorough examination of the peritoneal cavity, debridement of serosal surfaces, removal of affected organ, e.g. appendicectomy, colectomy. Formation of stomas rather than anastomosis, which may leak in the presence of infection and unprepared bowel. Peritoneal lavage. Peritoneal drains. Occasionally, the abdomen should be left open and the exposed bowel covered with moist swabs (laparostomy).

Postoperative care. Attention should be paid to fluid and electrolyte balance. UO should be monitored. Antibiotic therapy, nutritional support and surveillance for sepsis. Ventilation may be necessary. CVVH or dialysis may be required for ARF.

INTRA-ABDOMINAL ABSCESSES

> An abscess is a localized collection of pus. Intra-abdominal abscesses can be divided into intraperitoneal and extraperitoneal. Following peritonitis pus may collect in either the subphrenic spaces, the pelvis or in locules between loops of bowel.

Intraperitoneal abscesses

These tend to arise in dependent areas of the abdomen where fluid may collect. They include:

- Subphrenic – occur following anastomotic leaks in gastric or hepatobiliary surgery, after splenic surgery, perforated peptic ulcer, acute cholecystitis and acute appendicitis
- Paracolic – occur with perforations secondary to inflammatory bowel disease, diverticulitis, malignancy or anastomotic leaks

- Right iliac fossa – occur with appendicitis, perforated peptic ulcer, inflammatory bowel disease
- Pelvic – as the most dependent part of the abdomen, pelvic abscesses are the most common type of intra-abdominal abscesses and can be caused by all the above plus gynaecological causes.

Extraperitoneal abscesses

These are much less common than intraperitoneal abscesses; they most frequently follow infections of organs in the retroperitoneum or where peritoneal organs have perforated into the retroperitoneum. Extraperitoneal abscesses are most commonly associated with:

- Pancreatitis
- Posterior perforation of duodenal ulcer
- Posterior colonic perforations
- Pyelonephritis
- Spinal infections, e.g. osteomyelitis.

Extraperitoneal abscesses can also present as a psoas abscess; these can occur primarily due to haematogenous spread, tuberculosis of the thoraco-lumbar spine or secondary to local infections, e.g. Crohn's disease.

Symptoms and signs. General signs include malaise, swinging pyrexia, tachycardia, localized pain and tenderness, prolonged ileus. Signs specific to the position of the abscess include:

- Subphrenic – chest pain, shortness of breath (secondary to basal atelectasis), shoulder tip pain (referred from diaphragmatic irritation), hiccups
- Pelvic – diarrhoea, urinary frequency, passage of mucus PR, boggy fluctuant mass on PR or PV examination
- Psoas – pain on extension of the hip (patients tend to hold their hip in flexion); palpable psoas abscess below the inguinal ligament.

Investigations
- Hb
- WCC
- ESR
- LFTs: occasionally raised
- Blood culture may be positive
- CXR: pleural effusion, raised hemidiaphragm, atelectasis
- AXR: ileus, air/fluid levels in abscess cavities (rare)
- USS
- CT
- Indium-labelled white cell scan.

Treatment. For well-localized, non-loculated abscesses, percutaneous drainage under US or CT control. If there are multiple abscesses or they are multiloculated, open drainage at laparotomy will be required.

Procedures

Laparotomy

The following description relates to laparotomy for peritonitis of unknown origin (rather than trauma).

- Incision – 'incision of indecision' approximately 10 cm centred on the umbilicus. Depending on the findings, the incision may then be extended up (bile) or down (faeces). The skin is incised with a knife and continued down to the linea alba with diathermy.
- Opening the peritoneum – the linea alba is opened along the length of the incision. Using two clips, the peritoneum is tented up and incised with scissors. The peritoneal opening is extended so that the operator and assistant can insert a finger and lift up the abdominal wall so that the remaining peritoneum may be incised under direct vision.
- Examination of the peritoneal cavity – once inside the abdomen, a thorough and stepwise search of its contents is undertaken as follows:
  — Liver from right to left (including gallbladder)
  — Spleen
  — Oesophagus, stomach from proximal to distal and then to the duodenum
  — Kocher's manoeuvre will be required to visualize the remainder of the duodenum and head of pancreas
  — The right kidney is palpated
  — The lesser sac will need to be opened to visualize the body and tail of the pancreas
  — The left kidney is palpated
  — Small bowel is examined from the ligament of Treitz to the ileocaecal valve taking care to examine both sides and the mesentery
  — As the small bowel is out of the abdomen the retroperitoneum can be palpated taking particular note of an aortic aneurysm
  — The caecum and appendix is then examined and follows onto the rest of the colon
  — Female reproductive organs
  — Hernial orifices.
- Abdomen closure – the commonest technique is to use loop PDS, one from the top of the incision and the other from the bottom and meeting approximately half way down (do not tie the knot at the umbilicus). The bites of linea alba should be 1 cm deep and 1 cm apart. The skin may be closed with clips or a subcuticular suture (clips are better after a contaminated procedure, as some clips may be removed in the postoperative period in the event of wound infection).

Perforated peptic ulcer

If the diagnosis is known preoperatively, then an upper midline incision may be used. If not an 'incision of indecision' may be performed and extended upwards if bile is seen.
The following are steps in the procedure:

- Perform a laparotomy as above. With a perforated viscus, a hiss of air will be heard as the peritoneum is incised.
- Send fluid for culture and sensitivity.
- Examine the duodenum (perforations are usually in D1) and stomach for perforations (if gastric ulcer then it will need to be biopsied to rule out malignancy).
- Using 3/0 Vicryl under run the ulcer with two or three sutures, starting 1 cm from the medial edge and exiting 1 cm from the lateral edge (take care not to catch the back wall). These sutures are then tied to approximate the edges of the ulcer. Do not tie the sutures too hard as the tissues will be friable and the suture will cut through. Do not cut the ends of the sutures at this point.
- Fashion a pedicle of omentum and lay across the perforation. Tie the sutures over the omentum to secure it in place.

- Wash out the abdomen thoroughly with copious amounts of normal saline, particularly above and below the liver and in the pelvis.
- Close the abdomen as for laparotomy.
- A drain is not usually needed.

Appendicectomy

Many appendicectomies are now performed laparoscopically. However, it is still important to understand the principles of open appendicectomy.

- A Lanz skin crease incision is made across McBurney's point (junction of the middle and outer third of a line joining the anterior superior iliac spine and the umbilicus).
- The incision extends down to the external oblique, which is incised in the line of the incision. The muscles can then be split in the direction of their fibres.
- The peritoneum is picked up between clips (once the second clip is applied, re-apply the first clip so as to drop any bowel that may have been picked up). Open the peritoneum in the line of the wound.
- Any free fluid is sent for culture and sensitivity.
- The appendix can be delivered into the wound by: (1) following the taenia coli down to the caecum where they converge on the appendix; (2) sweeping the finger from medial to lateral under the caecum and feeling for the inflamed appendix and pulling it up into the wound.
- Make a window in the mesoappendix at the point where the appendix meets the caecum. Place two clips across the mesoappendix and divide it. Suture ligate both ends.
- The base of the appendix is crushed with a haemostat. Another haemostat is placed below the crushed segment and the crushed segment is then ligated.
- Place another haemostat above the tie and divide the appendix with a knife.
- Place a seromuscular purse string suture around the base of the appendix and bury the stump by tying it.
- If the appendix is normal, look for another cause of abdominal pain, e.g. Crohn's disease, Meckel's diverticulum or ovarian pathology.
- Wash out the abdomen (especially the pelvis) with copious amounts of saline.
- Close the peritoneum with 3/0 Vicryl, the external oblique aponeurosis with 2/0 Vicryl and then close the skin with either clips or subcuticular suture.

Alimentary tract

OESOPHAGUS

> Most conditions of the oesophagus have dysphagia as a symptom. Dysphagia is difficulty in swallowing. It may result from local or general causes (→ Table 14.1).

Investigation of dysphagia

History

- May be an obvious cause, e.g. foreign body, ingestion of caustic substance
- May be a previous history of oesophagitis suggesting an inflammatory stricture
- Younger patients with history of dysphagia, worse for fluids than solids and no weight loss suggests achalasia
- Rapid onset of dysphagia in the elderly with weight loss suggesting malignancy
- The patient may be able to accurately locate the site and point at which the foods sticks, e.g. sternal notch with Plummer–Vinson syndrome, lower sternum with carcinoma at the cardia.

Examination.
There may be little to find. There may be evidence of weight loss and anaemia with malignant strictures. Koilonychia is associated with Plummer–Vinson syndrome. Glands may be palpable in the neck with carcinoma. The abdomen should be palpated to exclude liver secondaries. A lump may be palpable in the posterior triangle of the neck with pharyngeal pouch. This may gurgle when full of food.

Investigations

- Hb
- FBC

TABLE 14.1 Causes of dysphagia

Local	
In the lumen	Foreign body
In the wall	Congenital atresia
	Inflammatory stricture – reflux oesophagitis
	Caustic stricture
	Achalasia
	Carcinoma
	Plummer–Vinson syndrome (oesophageal web)
	Scleroderma
	Irradiation
Outside the wall	Mediastinal lymphadenopathy
	Bronchial carcinoma
	Retrosternal goitre
	Pharyngeal pouch
	Para-oesophageal (rolling) hiatus hernia
	Thoracic aortic aneurysm
	Dysphagia lusoria (vascular ring)
General	Myasthenia gravis
	Bulbar palsy
	Bulbar poliomyelitis
	Hysteria

- ESR
- U&Es
- LFTs
- CXR: mediastinal mass, bronchial carcinoma, thoracic aortic aneurysm, gas shadow behind heart with hiatus hernia
- Barium swallow and meal
- Fibreoptic oesophagoscopy (should not be used if pharyngeal pouch is suspected)
- Biopsy
- CT scan.

Treatment. Is dependent on the underlying cause.

FOREIGN BODY

This is usually accidental in children (small toys and coins), housewives (safety pins) and the elderly (false teeth). Deliberate swallowing occurs in the psychiatrically disturbed. Foreign bodies often impact at the narrowest parts of the oesophagus, i.e. at its commencement, where it is crossed by the left bronchus, and where it passes through the diaphragm. Smooth objects will usually pass into the stomach. Sharp and irregular objects impact.

Symptoms and signs. Usually painful dysphagia. Often no signs. Mediastinitis if perforation occurs.

Investigations
- CXR will show radio-opaque foreign body
- Air in mediastinum if perforation has occurred
- Barium swallow (Gastrografin if suspected perforation)
- Oesophagoscopy.

Treatment. Oesophagoscopy and removal. A flexible endoscope may be used in association with specially designed forceps for grasping foreign bodies. Thoracotomy with oesophagotomy may be necessary. Foreign bodies that pass through the oesophagus will normally be passed per rectum. Occasionally sharp objects may perforate the bowel wall. Initial treatment is by observation and serial radiograph to assess the passage of the foreign body. Failure to progress and development of tenderness are indications for surgery.

OESOPHAGEAL PERFORATION

> This may be caused by swallowed foreign bodies or corrosives; rupture at oesophagoscopy, dilatation or biopsy; penetrating wound, or following a violent vomit after a large meal (Boerhaave's syndrome).

Symptoms and signs. History of foreign body, corrosive ingestion, endoscopy, violent vomit. Sudden or gradual onset of pain in chest, neck and upper abdomen. Other symptoms are dysphagia, pyrexia, shock, cyanosis, surgical emphysema in suprasternal notch.

Investigations
- CXR: air in neck and mediastinum, pleural effusion
- Gastrografin swallow (not barium) will confirm the diagnosis and demonstrate the site.

Complication. Mediastinitis.

Treatment. Broad-spectrum antibiotics. Small perforations may be treated expectantly with i.v. fluids. Nil orally. Large perforations require surgical repair and drainage of the area.

INFLAMMATORY STRICTURE

> This may result from prolonged acid reflux with oesophagitis. Reflux occurs through an incompetent lower oesophageal sphincter. It is often associated with a sliding hiatus hernia. Other causes of reflux oesophagitis include: prolonged vomiting, prolonged nasogastric intubation, operations which destroy the cardio-oesophageal area, e.g. resection with gastro-oesophageal anastomosis, cardiomyotomy for achalasia. As a result of long-standing reflux, the lower oesophagus may come to be lined by columnar mucosa, an appearance known as Barrett's oesophagus.

Gastro-oesophageal reflux

Many patients with reflux do not have hiatus hernia. Some patients with a hiatus hernia do not reflux. Patients with reflux should have a 24-hour ambulatory oesophageal pH study prior to surgery. The test is positive if the pH is <4 for >4% of the 24-hour period.

Hiatus hernia

There are two types: sliding (90%) and rolling or paraoesophageal (10%). In the rolling type, the cardio-oesophageal mechanism is intact and therefore reflux does not occur. The stomach rolls up alongside the lower oesophagus pressing on it and causing dysphagia (→ Fig. 14.1).

Sliding hiatus hernia

The stomach slides through the hiatus and therefore the position of the cardio-oesophageal junction changes and reflux occurs (→ Fig. 14.1).

Symptoms and signs. Retrosternal burning pain worse on bending, stooping, or lying down. Heartburn. Acid regurgitation into mouth. Pain relieved by antacids. May radiate into jaw or left arm and simulate angina. Large herniae may cause cough, palpitations, or hiccups by mechanical effect. Oesophagitis may lead to ulceration and bleeding, the latter causing symptoms of anaemia. Stricture leads to dysphagia.

Investigations
- Hb
- FBC

Figure 14.1 (A) Sliding hiatus hernia. The stomach slides up into the chest. Reflux occurs. (B) Rolling (para-oesophageal) hernia. The stomach rolls up alongside the oesophagus and dysphagia occurs. The cardio-oesophageal mechanism is intact and therefore reflux does not occur.

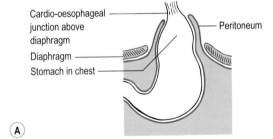

Sliding hiatus hernia

Cardio-oesophageal junction above diaphragm

Peritoneum

Diaphragm

Stomach in chest

(A)

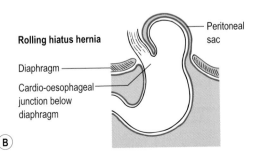

Rolling hiatus hernia

Peritoneal sac

Diaphragm

Cardio-oesophageal junction below diaphragm

(B)

Figure 14.2 Types of oesophageal stricture. (A) Peptic stricture associated with reflux. (B) Tortuous dilated oesophagus with 'rat's tail' stricture of achalasia. (C) The irregular 'shouldered' stricture of carcinoma.

- ESR
- U&Es
- LFTs
- Barium swallow: confirms hiatus hernia and also indicates reflux when patient is examined in the head-down position – stricture may be present ($\rightarrow$ Fig. 14.2)
- Upper GI endoscopy is the investigation of choice before barium studies which now rarely require to be done. Biopsy if stricture seen or diagnosis of oesophagitis is in doubt.

Treatment

Medical. Lose weight, loosen corset. Sleep propped up. Antacids. Proton pump inhibitors: omeprazole or lansoprazole are now the most effective treatment. Many patients obtain relief with this regimen.

Surgical. Indicated for failed medical treatment or complications, e.g. anaemia or severe dysphagia due to stricture. Surgery may also be indicated for young patients who do not want to take long-term acid-suppressant agents. There are several operations but a Nissen fundoplication ($\rightarrow$ Fig. 14.3) is the most commonly performed. The hernial defect is repaired and the mobilized fundus of the stomach is wrapped around the lower end of the oesophagus to provide an antireflux mechanism. This may be done by the 'open' or laparoscopic method.

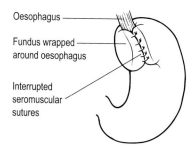

Oesophagus

Fundus wrapped around oesophagus

Interrupted seromuscular sutures

Figure 14.3 Nissen fundoplication. The fundus of the stomach is mobilized, wrapped around the lower oesophagus, and held with seromuscular sutures.

Rolling or para-oesophageal hiatus hernia
The cardia remains in its normal position and the stomach rolls up into the chest alongside the oesophagus. The cardio-oesophageal mechanism is intact and regurgitation does not occur (→ Fig. 14.1).

Symptoms and signs. Intermittent dysphagia due to a full stomach pressing on the adjacent oesophagus. Pain due to distension. Palpitations due to pressure on heart. Hiccups due to irritation of diaphragm. Respiratory embarrassment.

Investigations
● CXR: air/fluid level in mediastinum
● Barium meal
● CT scan.

Complications. Incarceration, gangrene, gastric volvulus.

Treatment. Unlike sliding herniae, rolling herniae should almost always be repaired. Nissen fundoplication with repair of the diaphragmatic defect is an appropriate procedure.

ACHALASIA

> This is due to failure of relaxation of the lower oesophageal 'sphincter'. It presents between 30 and 50 years and affects sexes equally. The cause is unknown but degeneration of Auerbach's plexus occurs.

Symptoms and signs. Intermittent dysphagia. Gets progressively worse. May be worse for liquids than for solids. Fluid regurgitation especially at night with aspiration pneumonitis. Retrosternal pain.

Investigations
● Barium swallow: dilated tortuous oesophagus above smooth tapering stricture ('rat's tail' appearance → Fig. 14.2)
● Oesophagoscopy: needs aspiration of stagnant food initially, exclude benign stricture or carcinoma.

Complications. Aspiration pneumonitis, oesophageal erosions. Carcinoma may develop even after treatment.

Treatment
Oesophageal dilatation. This is achieved using a pneumatic dilator introduced over a guide wire under radiological control. The success rate is over 50% but repeated dilatations are necessary.

Heller's operation (i.e. cardiomyotomy). The muscle layer is divided down to the mucosa over the lower end of the oesophagus and extended for about 1 cm on to the stomach. It is a similar principle to Ramstedt's operation for pyloric stenosis in infancy.

CARCINOMA OF THE OESOPHAGUS

This occurs most commonly in males. The commonest site is the lower third of the oesophagus followed by the middle third and upper third. Postcricoid carcinoma usually occurs in females and is part of the Plummer–Vinson syndrome. Achalasia of the cardia is also a predisposing cause. Squamous cell carcinoma occurs in the upper and middle thirds but adenocarcinoma may occur in the lower third associated with areas of gastric mucosa (Barrett's oesophagus) or by growth of a carcinoma of the cardiac area of the stomach into the oesophagus. Spread occurs by the following:

- Local invasion into surrounding structures, trachea, lung and aorta (massive haemorrhage may be terminal event)
- Lymphatic to paraoesophageal nodes, supraclavicular and abdominal nodes
- The blood stream to liver and lung.

Symptoms and signs. Dysphagia, usually rapid onset. Initially for solids then fluids. Weight loss, anorexia, anaemia. Palpable supraclavicular nodes, palpable irregular liver (secondaries).

Investigations
- Hb
- FBC
- ESR
- U&Es
- LFTs
- Barium swallow: 'shouldered' stricture ($\rightarrow$ Fig. 14.2)
- Upper GI endoscopy and biopsy
- CXR: mediastinal widening, secondaries in lung
- Bronchoscopy: to exclude invasion of oesophagus by primary lung tumour or vice versa, i.e. oesophageal tumour invading the bronchus with upper and middle third lesions
- USS of liver to exclude secondaries
- CT scan to define invasion and indicate operability
- Endoluminal ultrasound to determine staging
- PET to define invasion, spread, response to treatment.

Treatment. Resection. The stomach is mobilized and brought up into the chest and anastomosed to the remaining oesophagus in either the chest or neck. If the tumour is inoperable, an expandable metal stent may be placed through the tumour using a fibreoptic endoscope. Other methods of relieving dysphagia include laser therapy. Radiotherapy may be used for primary or palliative treatment of both squamous cell carcinomas and adenocarcinomas, the latter responding nearly as well as the squamous cell carcinomas. The best response is now with a combination of chemotherapy (cisplatin and 5-FU) and radiotherapy.

Prognosis. Prognosis is poor. Most patients survive less than 6 months if the primary is non-resectable. The 5-year survival following resection is less than 20%.

BARRETT'S OESOPHAGUS

Barrett's oesophagus refers to metaplasia of the cells in the lower oesophagus from squamous to columnar epithelium as a result of long standing acid reflux. OGD reveals areas of pink columnar mucosa replacing pearly white squamous epithelium. It occurs in 5–15% of patients with GORD. The risk of malignancy in patients with Barrett's oesophagus is 100 times higher than in the general population. Endoscopic surveillance with biopsy to identify dysplasia is required. Prevention involves treatment of GORD with proton pump inhibitors and anti-reflux surgery. Treatment of established dysplasia involves photodynamic therapy, radiofrequency ablation or endoscopic mucosal resection.

CORROSIVE OESOPHAGITIS

> The accidental or deliberate ingestion of corrosives causes severe oesophagitis. Common substances include caustic soda, bleach and sulphuric acid. Extensive damage occurs to the mouth, pharynx, larynx and stomach as well as to the oesophagus.

Symptoms and signs. History of ingestion. Burning pain from mouth to stomach. Fever. Shock. Respiratory distress if aspiration. Oedema of lips, lung, pharynx.

Investigations. Early endoscopy with fine fibreoptic endoscope to assess degree of damage.

Complications. Bleeding. Perforation. Stricture is a late complication.

Treatment
Emergency. Dilute acid (vinegar) or alkali (sodium bicarbonate) may be used to neutralize the ingested substance. *Never* induce vomiting. It may rupture the already damaged oesophagus.

Medical. Broad-spectrum antibiotics. Steroids. TPN.

Endoscopic dilatation of strictures. Gentle dilatation may be undertaken at 3–4 weeks.

Surgery. If a severe stricture develops, oesophageal replacement by interposition of a segment of colon is required. Stomach may also be used if that has been spared from the effects of the caustic injury. Surgery is also required if perforation occurs.

Prognosis. Appropriate early treatment of caustic burns usually gives good results. Extensive burns with strong acid or strong alkali progress to stricture formation and require surgery.

PLUMMER–VINSON SYNDROME (SYN. PATERSON–BROWN–KELLY SYNDROME, SIDEROPENIC DYSPHAGIA)

> This occurs in middle-aged females. It is an iron deficiency anaemia associated with a smooth tongue, koilonychia (spoon-shaped nails) and dysphagia. The dysphagia is due to the formation of a web in the upper oesophagus (postcricoid web). The condition is premalignant and carcinoma may develop in the upper oesophagus.

Treatment. Oesophageal dilatation if symptoms from web. Follow-up to check for developing carcinoma.

STOMACH AND DUODENUM

PEPTIC ULCERATION

> This occurs anywhere where pepsin and acid occur together. It is caused by an imbalance between secretion of acid and pepsin, and mucosal defence mechanisms. An acid environment and reduced mucosal defences provide ideal circumstances for pepsin to cause mucosal ulceration. If there is no acid, peptic ulceration cannot occur. Oversecretion of acid is associated with duodenal ulceration. Breakdown of the mucosal defences occurs in gastric ulceration. Exacerbating factors in peptic ulceration include stress, smoking, alcohol, NSAIDs, steroids, hyperparathyroidism, Zollinger–Ellison syndrome. Infection with *Helicobacter pylori* may impair mucosal defences and is associated with duodenal ulcer and gastritis and to a lesser extent, gastric ulcers. Common sites for peptic ulcer are the stomach and duodenum, the anterior and posterior walls of the first part of the duodenum and the lesser curve of the stomach being the most common sites. Less common sites include the oesophagus (Barrett's oesophagus), Meckel's diverticulum containing ectopic gastric mucosa and gastrojejunal anastomosis (after ulcer surgery).

Symptoms and signs
Duodenal ulcer (DU). Epigastric pain. May radiate through to back. Relieved by eating. Worse at night. Symptoms are periodic and last about 14 days and recur at 3–4-monthly intervals. They are often worse in spring and autumn. Vomiting is rare. If it occurs, pyloric stenosis should be suspected. Examination may reveal tenderness in epigastrium.

Gastric ulcer (GU). Epigastric pain. Not periodic. Food may precipitate pain. Pain may be relieved by vomiting. Patient may be afraid to eat and weight loss results. Examination reveals tenderness in epigastrium.

Investigations
- OGD and biopsy: risk of malignancy with GU; antral biopsy for mucosal urease test (CLO test)
- Serology for *H. pylori*
- Breath test
- Barium meal is rarely used nowadays but if a GU is diagnosed on a barium study, OGD and biopsy should be carried out
- Other routine investigations include Hb, FBC, U&Es, Ca, PO_4 and occasionally serum gastrin if Zollinger– Ellison syndrome is suspected.

Treatment
Medical
- Antacids, e.g. Mist. Mag. Trisil., relieve pain but are of limited value.
- Proton pump inhibitors reduce acid secretion by inhibiting the proton pump in parietal cells. Results in greater inhibition of acid than H_2 receptor antagonists. Omeprazole and lansoprazole may be used. First-line treatment is acid suppression with proton pump inhibitor plus eradication therapy for *H. pylori*,

i.e. triple therapy with omeprazole 20 mg b.d. plus two of the following three antibiotics: amoxicillin, clarithromycin, metronidazole. Check for eradication 6 weeks later by re-endoscopy and biopsy or breath test.

In addition to the above specific therapies, advice should be given regarding stopping smoking, stopping NSAIDs, and dealing with a stressful lifestyle.

Surgical. Indications are the following:

- Failed medical treatment (unusual nowadays).
- Complications – haemorrhage, perforation, pyloric obstruction. Operations in the past have included vagotomy and drainage and highly selective vagotomy. These operations are used rarely nowadays and the most common operation is pyloroplasty (Fig. 14.4) with oversewing of bleeding duodenal ulcer. Partial gastrectomy (Fig. 14.5) may be required for bleeding gastric ulcer.

Complications of peptic ulceration
Haemorrhage. Posterior duodenal ulcers erode the gastroduodenal artery. Lesser curve gastric ulcers erode the left gastric artery. OGD to locate the site of the ulcer.

Figure 14.4 (A) Truncal vagotomy and gastrojejunostomy. (B) Truncal vagotomy and pyloroplasty. The pylorus is opened longitudinally and sutured transversely thus destroying the pyloric sphincter.

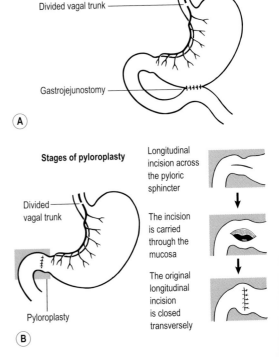

Divided vagal trunk

Gastrojejunostomy

(A)

Stages of pyloroplasty

Longitudinal incision across the pyloric sphincter

Divided vagal trunk

The incision is carried through the mucosa

Pyloroplasty

The original longitudinal incision is closed transversely

(B)

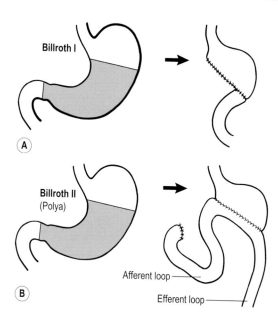

Billroth I

Billroth II
(Polya)

(A)

(B)

Afferent loop

Efferent loop

Figure 14.5 Types of partial gastrectomy. (A) Billroth I. The gastric remnant is anastomosed directly to the first part of the duodenum. (B) Billroth II (Polya). The duodenal stump is oversewn and continuity re-established by gastrojejunostomy.

A bleeding ulcer can be treated by injection, diathermy or laser coagulation at OGD. If the ulcer is not actively bleeding, a course of medical treatment may be given. The majority of patients stop bleeding spontaneously. If bleeding is massive or recurrent, surgery is required. The bleeding vessel in the base of the ulcer is oversewn to stop the bleeding. A GU is best excised or at least a biopsy should be taken to exclude malignancy. The pylorus is opened for treating a bleeding DU and is closed as a pyloroplasty. The patient is treated with long-term proton-pump inhibitors.

Perforation. Anterior DUs and GUs may perforate causing generalized chemical peritonitis. Surgery involves simple suture of the ulcer with reinforcement with an omental patch. A biopsy should be taken from the edge of a GU as there is a risk of malignancy. Check *H. pylori* status and eradicate if necessary. Long-term proton-pump inhibitors if chronic ulceration.

Pyloric obstruction. Late complication. Rare nowadays. Vomiting of large amounts of foul-smelling vomit often containing food eaten several days previously. Eructations of foul gas. Gastric succussion splash on examination. Empty stomach with wide-bore nasogastric tube. Confirm by OGD or contrast study. Surgical treatment is by gastrojejunostomy. Hypokalaemia and metabolic alkalosis may be present and require correction prior to surgery.

Obstruction of the mid-stomach may occur because of fibrosis of a large saddle-shaped ulcer astride the lesser curve. This gives rise to the 'hourglass' appearance on a barium study. It is largely of historical interest from the days when patients kept their ulcers a long time prior to consideration of surgery.

Zollinger–Ellison syndrome

Peptic ulcer disease caused by excessive production of gastrin. Peptic ulcers may occur in unusual sites, e.g. the third part of the duodenum. There is usually a gastrin-secreting pancreatic tumour (gastrinoma); 60% are malignant; 30% associated with MEN (Type I).

Symptoms and signs. Typical signs and symptoms of peptic ulcer. Diarrhoea may occur from overproduction of acid. Bleeding. Perforation. Recurrent ulcers after surgery for peptic ulcer. Ulcers resistant to medical treatment. May be family history of peptic ulcer.

Investigations
- Fasting serum gastrin: raised
- CT scan
- Angiography.

Treatment. Excision of tumour if spread to liver has not occurred. If tumour cannot be localized or has spread, acid secretion should be controlled by omeprazole. Rarely total gastrectomy may be needed to stop bleeding.

CARCINOMA OF THE STOMACH

> The incidence is declining but it remains a common tumour with a poor prognosis. Widespread geographical variations occur, the incidence being high in Japan and certain coastal countries where the intake of dietary nitrate is high. Eating smoked fish and highly spiced foods has been implicated. Other associations include blood group A (suggesting a genetic factor), pernicious anaemia, atrophic gastritis, previous gastric surgery and benign gastric ulcer.

Symptoms and signs. Onset silent and insidious. Vague dyspepsia, epigastric pain, weight loss, dysphagia (cardiac area), vomiting (pyloric area), anaemia, lassitude. Epigastric mass, hepatomegaly, ascites, left supraclavicular gland palpable (Virchow's node, Troisier's sign), gastric succussion splash, acanthosis nigricans.

Investigations
- Hb
- FBC
- ESR
- LFTs: alkaline phosphatase raised with liver secondaries
- OGD with biopsy
- USS: secondaries
- CT/PET scan for staging – may suggest linitis plastica which indicates generalized invasion of the whole wall of the stomach with cancer.
- Laparoscopy to exclude peritoneal metastases.

Treatment. This is surgical.

Attempt at cure. Wide excision of tumour usually with 5 cm margin and clearance of nodes. For distal tumours, partial gastrectomy (7/8) may suffice. For more proximal tumours, total gastrectomy. Over 60% are found to be incurable at laparotomy.

Palliative. Bypass gastrojejunostomy for antral tumours. Intubation via upper GI endoscopy with an expandable mesh stent.

Prognosis. In Japan, where screening programmes are undertaken because of the high incidence, the 5-year survival for early gastric cancer is around 90%. In the UK at least 60% of cases present too late for curative surgery. Overall about 20% survive 5 years. Radiotherapy is of no value.

GASTRIC SURGERY AND ITS COMPLICATIONS

> Carcinoma and complications of peptic ulcer are the commonest indications for gastric surgery. The operations of vagotomy, vagotomy and pyloroplasty, vagotomy and gastrojejunostomy and highly selective vagotomy are described but are largely of historical interest. Patients are still seen who have had these operations and have suffered the complications of them. Vagotomy is rarely, if ever, carried out nowadays.

Operations

Vagotomy *(Fig. 14.4)*

This reduces acid secretion from the stomach. It reduces gastric motility and therefore interferes with gastric emptying. A drainage procedure is therefore required.

Pyloroplasty *(Fig. 14.4)*

The pylorus is cut longitudinally and sewn up transversely. In this operation, vagotomy is designed to reduce acid secretion and thus allow the ulcer to heal. The pyloroplasty is performed to allow gastric drainage.

Gastroenterostomy *(Fig. 14.4)*

The most dependent part of the stomach is anastomosed to a loop of jejunum. This diverts acid away from the duodenum and allows the ulcer to heal. Vagotomy is carried out to reduce acid secretion and thus prevent stomal ulceration.

Highly selective vagotomy

The vagus is sectioned such that only the body of the stomach is denervated. The nerve of Latarjet to the pylorus is left intact, thus preserving motility of this region and allowing the stomach to empty without need for a pyloroplasty.

Gastrectomy *(Fig. 14.5)*

This may be partial or total. Partial gastrectomy usually involves removal of about 7/8 of the stomach. The gastric remnant may be reanastomosed directly to the first part of the duodenum (Billroth I) or the duodenal stump oversewn and the continuity re-established by a gastrojejunostomy (Billroth II or Polya gastrectomy. If partial gastrectomy is used for GU, the ulcer is removed together with the segment of stomach. For DU, removal of the bulk of the acid-secreting area of the stomach allows the ulcer to heal. The ulcer is not usually removed.

Complications

Recurrent ulceration
Symptoms are similar to those experienced preoperatively. Treatment is difficult. Zollinger–Ellison syndrome and hypercalcaemia should be excluded.

Epigastric fullness
Particularly after partial gastrectomy. Treatment is to take small meals frequently. The symptom tends to improve with time.

Bilious vomiting
Sudden emptying of the afferent loop with Billroth II. Associated biliary gastritis. May respond to metoclopramide. Severe cases need revisional surgery, e.g. Roux-en-Y anastomosis so that bile enters the GI tract lower down in the jejunum (→ Fig. 14.6).

Dumping
Early. Fainting, sweating and dizziness shortly after eating. May be a reflex caused by osmotic effect of large volumes of food 'dumped' into the jejunum. Less common after highly selective vagotomy. Patient may need to lie down and rest for half an hour. Symptoms may be improved by eating small dry meals frequently and avoiding heavy carbohydrate meals. Early dumping may subside spontaneously with time.

Late. Due to hypoglycaemia and occurs 1–3 h after a meal. Responds to glucose (sucking barley sugars).

Diarrhoea. This may be disabling after vagotomy. Codeine phosphate and small dry meals may help. The incidence is less after highly selective vagotomy.

Nutritional disturbances
Weight loss. May be due to reduced caloric intake or poor absorption.

Steatorrhoea. Due to poor mixing of food and enzymes, e.g. long afferent loop where food passes into the jejunum before it is adequately mixed with digestive enzymes coming from the afferent loop. Blind loop syndrome may be responsible,

Figure 14.6 Roux-en-Y conversion for bilious vomiting. The afferent loop is detached and reanastomosed lower down the jejunum.

Afferent loop

Efferent loop

Closure of site of detached afferent loop

Afferent loop anastomosed lower down in the jejunum

i.e. stasis in the long afferent loop with colonization with abnormal bacteria, which restricts digestion and absorption of food. Surgical correction of the afferent loop may be necessary.

Anaemia. Iron deficiency anaemia due to reduced hydrochloric acid, which is required for iron absorption. With total gastrectomy, megaloblastic anaemia may occur, owing to loss of intrinsic factor and subsequent B_{12} deficiency. Vitamin B_{12} injections are required.

Bolus obstruction. Destruction of the pylorus allows unmasticated food to pass into the small intestine. This may swell and lodge in the terminal ileum. This occurs particularly with orange pith and dried fruits. Patients should be warned not to eat these foods if the pylorus is not intact.

Carcinoma
May occur in the gastric remnant. This is rare.

UPPER GASTROINTESTINAL TRACT BLEEDING

This causes either haematemesis (vomiting of blood), melaena (passage of altered blood PR – usually black and tarry with a characteristic smell), or both. Causes include peptic ulceration, acute gastric erosions, oesophageal varices, oesophagitis, Mallory–Weiss syndrome, and carcinoma. Rarer causes include GIST, angiomatous malformations, haemobilia and bleeding disorders. Drugs that may precipitate bleeding include steroids, NSAIDs, and anticoagulants. Principles of treatment include replacement of blood loss, diagnosis of the cause and treatment of the condition.

Symptoms and signs. Clinically anaemic. With severe bleed, shock will occur. History of aspirin, NSAIDs, steroid or anticoagulant. Stigmata of liver failure. Abdominal mass.

Investigations
- Hb
- FBC
- U&Es
- LFTs
- Clotting screen
- Cross-match blood
- OGD
- Angiography if source of bleeding is obscure.

Treatment
- Bed rest, pulse, BP, CVP line. Infusion of crystalloid, colloid, blood.
- Treat shock.
- Catheterize.
- Establish diagnosis by endoscopy.
- Control varices with Sengstaken tube or injection.
- Give intravenous proton pump inhibitor.
- Eradication of *H. pylori*.

Indications for surgical intervention:
- Massive uncontrolled bleeding
- Rebleeding, especially if bleeding vessel or clot on ulcer has been seen at endoscopy
- More than 4 unit bleed in 24 h unless the cause is varices.

Interventional options are non-operative or operative:
Non-operative. Laser coagulation. Local cautery. Injection of adrenaline. Gastric hypothermia for gastric erosions. Varices may be treated by sclerotherapy. Octreotide infusion for varices. Angiomatous malformations may be treated by embolization.

Operative
- Peptic ulcer: oversewing of the ulcer + proton-pump inhibitors + eradication therapy for *H. pylori* if appropriate. Partial gastrectomy may be necessary
- Acute erosions: partial gastrectomy may be necessary
- Oesophageal varices: oesophageal transection. Portocaval or distal splenorenal shunting
- Carcinoma: partial or total gastrectomy.

Prognosis. The overall mortality for an upper GI bleed is 10%. Adverse prognostic factors include old age, shock at presentation, rebleeding and oesophageal varices.

OTHER CONDITIONS OF THE STOMACH AND DUODENUM

Stomach

Gastrointestinal stromal tumour (GIST)
Vary from benign (leiomyoma) to high grade malignant. Epigastric discomfort, indigestion, haematemesis or melaena due to ulceration of mucosa overlying tumour. Investigations include OGD and CT scan. Barium meal shows space-occupying lesion. Surgical excision is required. Imatinib (tyrosine kinase inhibitor) for incomplete removal or recurrence.

Lymphoma
Symptoms are those of peptic ulcer or gastric carcinoma. OGD and biopsy to confirm diagnosis. Treatment is by surgical resection followed by radiotherapy or chemotherapy; 50% of patients survive 5 years or more.

Duodenum
Other than peptic ulcer, conditions of the duodenum are rare. A duodenal diverticulum may occur on the medial wall near the ampulla of Vater. Most are asymptomatic. Rarely bleeding and perforation may occur. Symptomatic diverticulae should be excised. Tumours of the duodenum are rare. Adenocarcinoma does *not* occur in duodenal ulcers. Rarely, it may occur in other parts of the duodenum and if it arises near the bile ducts, may cause obstructive jaundice.

CONDITIONS OF THE SMALL BOWEL

Meckel's diverticulum

A remnant of the vitellointestinal duct of the embryo. Classically it occurs in 2% of patients, is 2 inches long, and 2 feet from the ileocaecal junction ('rule of 2 s'). It occurs on the antimesenteric border of the terminal ileum.

Symptoms and signs. Symptomless. Incidental finding at laparotomy. Symptoms typical of acute appendicitis may occur. Rectal bleeding (ectopic gastric mucosa). Rarely umbilical discharge (fistula), intestinal obstruction (due to entrapment around the band from the apex of the diverticulum to the back of the umbilicus), small bowel volvulus, or intussusception (ileo-ileal).

Investigations
● Technetium scan for GI bleeding may show gastric mucosa in a Meckel's
● Laparotomy is required for complications of Meckel's – the cause is not usually apparent until laparotomy is undertaken.

Treatment. Excision of the diverticulum.

Crohn's disease

This is dealt with in the section on inflammatory bowel disease.

Typhoid

Caused by *Salmonella typhi*. About 200 cases occur in the UK annually. It may occur in the immigrant population and in those who have travelled in countries where the disease is endemic. The organism enters Peyer's patches and may result in perforation or bleeding usually involving the ileum. This usually occurs during the third week of the disease. The patient shows signs of perforation with peritonitis. Surgical closure of the perforation is required. The bowel is very friable. Chloramphenicol i.v. is given for 2 weeks' postoperatively.

Tuberculosis

This may present as an acute abdomen in recent immigrants. It chiefly affects the terminal ileum and the ileocaecal region. Differentiation from Crohn's disease is essential.

Symptoms and signs. Ill patient: fever, diarrhoea, colicky abdominal pain. Weight loss. May be history of pulmonary TB. Mass in RIF. Chest signs.

Investigations
● CXR
● Mantoux
● Sputum culture
● AXR: small bowel obstruction
● Barium studies show thickening, ulceration and narrowing of terminal ileum
● USS: may show mass

- CT: may show abscess
- Diagnosis may be made only at laparotomy.

Treatment. Antituberculous therapy for 6 months to 2 years. Surgery is required if diagnosis is unclear, for perforation, abscess, bleeding or obstruction.

TUMOURS OF THE SMALL INTESTINE

> These form less than 5% of all tumours of the GI tract. Obstruction and bleeding are the usual symptoms.

Benign
These include adenomas, leiomyomas and lipomas. Obstruction, intussusception, or bleeding may occur. Polyposis of the small bowel (mainly jejunum) may occur in association with pigmentation of the lips and mouth (Peutz–Jeghers syndrome). Bleeding or intussusception may occur.

Malignant
Adenocarcinoma is rare and usually affects the jejunum. Bleeding and obstruction may occur. Lymphoma may present as intestinal obstruction or a palpable mass. Consider lymphoma in patients with coeliac disease. Palliation of these tumours is by radiotherapy or chemotherapy.

Carcinoid tumour
These occur most commonly in the appendix but can occur anywhere in the GI tract and occasionally in the lung. Those in the small bowel grow slowly but most of those greater than 2 cm have metastasized at the time of surgery. The tumours arise from argentaffin cells.

Symptoms and signs. May be none before metastases occur. Carcinoid syndrome is associated with liver metastases. Flushing (caused by alcohol, coffee), diarrhoea, bronchospasm, pulmonary stenosis. Loud borborygmi may be heard on auscultation. Hepatomegaly, palpable abdominal mass.

Investigations
- Raised 24-hour excretion of 5-HIAA
- USS
- CT.

Treatment. Resection of primary tumour. Partial hepatectomy if metastases confined to one lobe. Methysergide blocks 5-HT and may be beneficial in patients with metastases. Phenoxybenzamine may be helpful in reducing flushing. Other procedures include hepatic embolization, systemic chemotherapy and hepatic infusion chemotherapy.

Prognosis. Malignant carcinoid of the small bowel has a 25% 5-year survival.

SMALL BOWEL OBSTRUCTION

Mechanical obstruction of the small bowel may be simple (one point of obstruction) or closed loop (obstruction at two points enclosing a segment of bowel). If the bowel is viable, the obstruction is termed non-strangulating. If the blood supply is compromised, strangulating obstruction occurs with subsequent infarction of bowel. Strangulation occurs when the obstructing mechanism cuts off the mesenteric arterial blood flow, e.g. the neck of the sac with a loop of bowel trapped in a hernial sac, or the twist of a volvulus. Mechanical obstruction is more common in the small bowel than in the large bowel.

Causes. Causes may be found:

- in the lumen: gallstone ileus, food bolus (following pylorus-destroying operations, i.e. gastrojejunostomy or pyloroplasty)
- in the wall: congenital atresia, Crohn's disease, tumours, e.g. lymphoma or carcinoma
- outside the wall: herniae, adhesions, volvulus, intussusception.

Symptoms and signs. Colicky abdominal pain. The patient cannot get into a comfortable position. Vomiting. Constipation. Symptoms depend on whether the obstruction is high or low. High obstruction is characterized by early vomiting (bilious), and late constipation. Low obstruction is characterized by early constipation, and late vomiting (faeculent). Distension, marked with low obstruction, tympanitic abdomen, high-pitched tinkling bowel sounds. Hernial orifices should be carefully examined. Pyrexia, tachycardia, continuous pain and localized tenderness suggest actual or impending strangulation.

Investigations
- Hb
- FBC
- WCC with neutrophilia may indicate strangulation
- U&Es
- AXR: distended loops of small bowel in central abdomen (→ Fig. 14.7). Erect films show air/fluid levels. Absent or diminished colonic gas. Dilated proximal small bowel shows lines close together (valvulae conniventes) crossing completely the lumen of the bowel. These get progressively fewer the more distal the distended loop and are absent in the terminal ileum. Look for gas in the biliary tree (gallstone ileus with cholecystoduodenal fistula).

Treatment
Conservative
- Intravenous fluids and nasogastric aspiration
- Nil orally
- 2-hourly temperature and pulse
- Abdominal examination 8-hourly.

Some cases of simple mechanical obstruction, e.g. due to adhesions, will settle on this regimen.

Indications for surgery. Strangulating obstruction, e.g. a tender irreducible hernia, requires urgent surgery. If a conservative 'drip and suck' regimen has been

Figure 14.7 Small bowel obstruction. Distended loops of small bowel are visible in the central abdomen. These are identifiable as small bowel as the valvulae conniventes (arrows) cross the entire lumen.

undertaken for obstruction, surgery is indicated for signs of incipient strangulation (pyrexia, tachycardia, localized tenderness). Surgery is also required for simple obstruction that fails to settle, e.g. adhesions, gallstone ileus. At surgery, the affected bowel is inspected for viability. Indications of non-viability include:

● Absence of peristalsis
● Loss of normal sheen
● Loss of pulsation in bowel mesentery
● Colour: green or black bowel is non-viable and resection is required. Plum-coloured bowel may respond to wrapping for a few minutes in warm saline-soaked packs. If colour returns and it will transmit a peristaltic wave, it is viable.

Prognosis. Small bowel obstruction has a very low mortality rate if it is simple. Strangulating obstruction increases the mortality and if small bowel resection is required, especially in the elderly, the mortality rate may reach 25%.

APPENDICITIS

This is the commonest cause of the acute abdomen in the UK. It usually occurs when there is an obstruction in the lumen of the appendix either by a faecolith or foreign body or by enlargement of lymphoid follicles in its wall. It most often affects children, teenagers and young adults. It is rare at the extremes of life. In the infant, the lumen of the appendix is wide in relation to the remainder of the bowel and the diet is soft and hence, obstruction within the lumen is less likely. In the elderly, the lumen tends to be obliterated. Rarer causes of appendicitis include carcinoma of the caecum obstructing the appendiceal lumen, carcinoid tumour and obstructing fibrous bands. Occasionally a carcinoma obstructing the lumen of the appendix will cause it to distend and fill with mucus, i.e. a mucocele of the appendix.

Symptoms and signs. Central abdominal cramping or colicky pain. Nausea. Vomiting is uncommon. Occasionally the patient may pass a loose stool. Frank diarrhoea is uncommon. Central abdominal pain lasts approximately 8 h. It is followed by the development of a sharp, stabbing somatic type of pain in the RIF made worse by coughing or moving. Low-grade pyrexia (37.2–37.8°C). Flushed. Characteristic fetor (sweet faecal smell to breath). White furred tongue. Tachycardia (100 in first 24 h). Tender with guarding in RIF over McBurney's point. Examination PR: tender anteriorly in the rectovesical or rectouterine pouch.

> ⚠️ **In infants, diarrhoea and vomiting may be the only symptoms. This may lead to difficulty in diagnosis and confusion with gastroenteritis. In elderly patients there may be confusion and later, shock may develop.**

Investigations
- WCC: usually $>10 \times 10^9$/L with neutrophil leukocytosis
- USS: may show a mass or abscess; usefulness in early appendicitis depends on the experience of the ultrasonographer
- Diagnostic laparoscopy.

Differential diagnosis. In the classical case of acute appendicitis there are few conditions that enter into the differential diagnosis. These include mesenteric adenitis, Meckel's diverticulitis, Crohn's disease (regional ileitis), mesenteric embolus and right-sided colonic diverticulitis. All these conditions will initially cause central abdominal cramping pain with subsequent tenderness in the RIF.

In the atypical case, other causes of intra-abdominal pathology, urinary tract disease, gynaecological problems (see Ch. 22) and extra-abdominal conditions must be considered.

Abdominal disease. Cholecystitis, gastroenteritis, pancreatitis, perforated DU, intestinal obstruction, diverticulitis, non-specific abdominal pain.

Urinary tract. Acute pyelonephritis, renal colic, cystitis. An inflamed appendix adherent to the bladder may cause frequency and pyuria. Organisms will be absent on urinary microscopy.

Gynaecological causes. Salpingitis. Ectopic pregnancy. Degeneration of a fibroid. Mittelschmerz. Pelvic inflammatory disease.

Extra-abdominal causes. Referred pain from nerve roots, e.g. herpes zoster, degenerative and malignant disease affecting roots T11, T12. Referred pain from right lower lobar pneumonia. Referred pain from a right-sided testicular torsion.

Treatment. The treatment of acute appendicitis is appendicectomy. Prophylactic metronidazole by suppository should be given 1 h preoperatively to reduce the risk of wound infection.

Complications. Appendicitis may resolve spontaneously. The appendix may become surrounded by adjacent small bowel and omentum and give rise to an appendix mass. It may perforate giving rise to generalized peritonitis or it may perforate amidst local adhesions giving rise to an appendix abscess. Often it is difficult to diagnose appendicitis. If the symptoms have been present for 48 h ('48 h rule') and the diagnosis is truly appendicitis, then the patient should either have developed an appendix mass or generalized peritonitis. If neither of these two is present, then the diagnosis of appendicitis should be reviewed.

APPENDIX MASS

Omentum and small bowel adhere to the inflamed appendix. This usually happens 2–5 days after onset of initial symptoms. This should be initially treated conservatively. Mark out the size of the mass on the abdominal wall; i.v. fluids, analgesia, and antibiotics (cefuroxime and metronidazole) should be administered. If the mass resolves it is usual to carry out an interval appendicectomy after 3 months. If the mass gets bigger it is likely that an abscess is forming, i.e. the appendix has perforated within the appendix mass.

APPENDIX ABSCESS

If an appendix mass enlarges and the temperature fails to settle, an appendix abscess is developing. The patient may appear toxic with a tachycardia. An appendix abscess requires either surgical drainage and appendicectomy, or percutaneous insertion of a drain under ultrasound control. Interval appendicectomy is required subsequently.

Other complications include subphrenic abscess, pelvic abscess, paralytic ileus, septicaemia, portal pyaemia (rare). Long-term complications may be due to adhesions resulting in intestinal obstruction in a small proportion of patients. Tubal adhesions with infertility may occur in females.

Appendicitis in pregnancy

This is no commoner than at other times. Pain and tenderness are higher because of displacement of the appendix by the enlarging uterus. Prompt assessment and intervention are essential. There is a risk of abortion in the first trimester but if treatment is delayed until perforation occurs the risk is considerably higher (approximately 25%).

CONDITIONS OF THE COLON, RECTUM AND ANUS

COLONIC POLYPS

> A polyp is a sessile (broad-based) or pedunculated (on a stalk) protrusion from a body surface. In the colon, it is a lesion that projects into the lumen.

Hamartomas

Juvenile polyps

May occur in large or small bowel. Cause bleeding or obstruction. May auto-amputate in adolescence.

Peutz–Jeghers syndrome

Diffuse GI polyposis with mucocutaneous pigmentation of lips and gums. The polyps have no malignant potential. Surgery is indicated only for symptoms, i.e. obstruction or bleeding.

Neoplastic polyps

Adenomatous polyps and villous adenomas

These have malignant potential, especially the villous adenoma.

Familial polyposis coli

This is an autosomal dominant condition with multiple polyps involving colon and rectum. Duodenal adenomas may also occur and progress to malignancy. It first appears in adolescence. If untreated, malignancy will develop before the age of 40. Treatment is classically by subtotal colectomy with ileorectal anastomosis. However, now, most patients are offered restorative proctocolectomy with ileo-anal pouch. Ileorectal anastomosis is still a reasonable option. Occasionally, rectal polyps regress after this procedure. Regular (6-monthly) inspection of the rectum by sigmoidoscopy is undertaken and any polyps excised. Sulindac may reduce polyp formation. Recurrence is high with carcinoma developing in the rectum. Other operations include total colectomy with mucosal proctectomy, and ileo-anal anastomosis or in some cases panproctocolectomy with ileostomy. There is a need for upper GI surveillance as most of the mortality is from development of ampullary/duodenal carcinomas developing from duodenal adenomas.

Gardner's syndrome

A variant of familial polyposis, it is associated with desmoid tumours, osteomas of the mandible and multiple sebaceous cysts.

Inflammatory pseudopolyps

These may arise in ulcerative colitis. Lymphoid hyperplasia may also be apparent as a polyp.

Symptoms and signs of polyps. Passage of blood and mucus PR. Rarely obstruction or intussusception.

Investigations
- Sigmoidoscopy and biopsy
- Barium enema (→ Fig. 14.8)
- Colonoscopy.

Treatment. Pedunculated polyps or small sessile polyps may be removed at sigmoidoscopy or colonoscopy. If invasive carcinoma is found, colectomy is required.

COLORECTAL CANCER

Commonest GI cancer. Usually presents after middle life but can occur earlier. The highest incidence of colorectal cancer is seen in Western Europe and North America; the lowest incidence occurs in Asia and South Africa. The precise cause is unknown but environmental and genetic factors are important. Lack of dietary fibre, increased fat, increased bile acids, have been implicated. Other predisposing factors include inflammatory bowel disease, familial polyposis coli, colorectal polyps, and previous irradiation. Apart from familial adenomatous polyposis, there are other groups of patients who have hereditary predisposition to develop large bowel cancer.

There are two types of autosomal dominant hereditary non-polyposis colorectal cancer (HNPCC):

- Cancer family syndrome (CFS), which occurs with early onset at around 20–30 years and is associated with other adenocarcinomas especially endometrial carcinoma and breast carcinoma
- Hereditary site-specific colonic cancer (HSSCC), which shows the same characteristics as CFS except for the extracolonic carcinomas.

It has also been demonstrated that the frequency of colorectal cancer developing in first-degree relatives of patients with large bowel carcinoma is significantly higher than expected. The relative sites of distribution of carcinoma in the colon are rectum, 40%; sigmoid colon, 25%; descending colon, 5%; transverse colon, 10%; caecum and ascending colon, 20%.

Figure 14.8 A barium enema showing part of the sigmoid colon. A large pedunculated polyp is seen (arrow). There is also marked diverticular disease.

Symptoms and signs. Clinical features depend upon the sites. Right colon: anaemia, palpable mass, change in bowel habit. Left colon: change in bowel habit, lower abdominal colicky pain. Blood or mucus on or mixed with stool. With sigmoid cancers, spurious diarrhoea may occur. Rectal cancers present with frequency of defaecation because of tenesmus (a sense of incomplete evacuation). Blood and mucus PR. Patients may present with symptoms due to direct spread; sacral pain or sciatica due to direct invasion of the nerve. Jaundice due to liver or porta hepatis node metastases. Examination may reveal an abdominal mass or hepatomegaly. Examination PR may show blood on examining glove or mass may be palpable.

Some 25% of large bowel cancers present as emergencies. Obstruction may occur, e.g. small bowel obstruction with caecal cancers growing over the ileocaecal valve or obstruction occurring on the left side where the bowel lumen is narrow and the faeces more formed. Perforation may occur because of either direct perforation of the cancer or perforation of the caecum with a closed-loop obstruction where the ileocaecal valve is competent. Massive haemorrhage is rare.

Investigations
- Hb
- FBC
- U&Es (ureteric involvement)
- LFTs (liver secondaries, alkaline phosphatase raised)
- Sigmoidoscopy
- Biopsy
- Barium enema (5% of tumours are metachronous); 'apple core' lesion may be visible (→ Fig. 14.9)
- Colonoscopy
- USS: liver secondaries, ureteric obstruction
- CT/PET: secondaries.

Treatment (→ Fig. 14.10)

Elective
- Caecum and right colon: right hemicolectomy (see Procedures box, below)
- Transverse colon: extended right hemicolectomy
- Descending colon: left hemicolectomy
- Sigmoid colon: sigmoid colectomy.
- Rectum and rectosigmoid: anterior resection with primary anastomosis. If low rectal tumour, abdominoperineal excision of the rectum should be carried out with a permanent colostomy.

For any operation on the left side of the colon, the patient should be warned about a temporary defunctioning loop ileostomy until the primary anastomosis has healed.

Emergency. Correct fluid and electrolytes imbalance. In closed-loop obstruction a caecum of greater than 10 cm in diameter on AXR is an indication for urgent surgery, especially if it is tender. Right-sided tumours may be treated with right hemicolectomy with primary anastomosis. Lower left-sided tumours should be treated by resection of the tumour and Hartmann's procedure, i.e. closure of the rectal stump and fashioning of an LIF end colostomy. Continuity of the bowel is

Figure 14.9 A barium enema showing a colonic carcinoma. A typical 'apple core' lesion is visible (arrow).

re-established some weeks later. Some surgeons carry out an on-table colonic lavage with primary anastomosis covered by a loop ileostomy.

Prognosis. This is based on Dukes' classification, originally described for rectal cancer but now applied to all colorectal adenocarcinomas (→ Table 14.2).

Screening. Populations at risk include asymptomatic relatives of patients with colorectal cancer and patients who have large bowel polyps. Screening methods include regular rigid sigmoidoscopy, flexible endoscopic screening or screening for faecal occult bloods. Serum markers such as carcinoembryonic antigen (CEA) may also be used for follow-up after resection. Ultrasound may be used for liver surveillance following successful resection. If an isolated secondary occurs, liver resection may be carried out.

TABLE 14.2 Dukes' Classification[a]	
A	Confined to bowel wall; 80% 5-year survival
B	Through wall into surrounding tissue; 60% 5-year survival
C	Lymph node involvement; 30% 5-year survival
[a]If distant metastases are present, the 5-year survival is only 5%.	

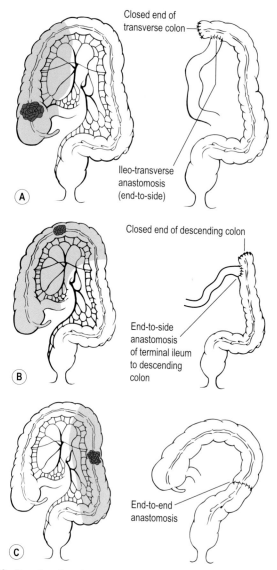

Figure 14.10 Operations for colorectal cancer. The diagrams indicate the extent of resection and the method of re-establishing continuity. (A) Right hemicolectomy. (B) Extended right hemicolectomy. (C) Left hemicolectomy.

(Continued)

Figure 14.10, cont'd (D) Sigmoid colectomy. (E) Anterior resection. (F) Abdominoperineal resection of the rectum with permanent colostomy. The shaded area is the area resected.

INFLAMMATORY BOWEL DISEASE

> The two main disorders are Crohn's disease and ulcerative colitis.

Crohn's disease

This is a chronic inflammatory disorder that may occur anywhere in the alimentary tract from the mouth to the anus. Common sites include the terminal ileum (regional ileitis), colon and rectum. Unlike ulcerative colitis the whole thickness of the bowel wall is involved. The aetiology is unknown. The disease occurs most commonly in the 15–35 age group. Familial clustering occurs. Malignancy may rarely occur in both the small and large bowel.

Symptoms and signs. Malaise, anorexia, fever, nausea, abdominal pain, weight loss, diarrhoea, rectal bleeding. Perianal inflammation with abscess, fissure, and fistulae formation may occur. Pallor, malnutrition, abdominal mass, perianal sepsis, fissures, fistulae, clubbing, erythema nodosum, pyoderma gangrenosum, uveitis.

Investigations
- Hb
- FBC
- ESR
- Folate
- B$_{12}$
- U&Es: electrolyte imbalances
- LFTs: albumin reduced
- CRP: elevated levels
- Radiographs – AXR: obstruction, perforation, toxic dilatation
- Small bowel enema and barium enema: skip lesions in small bowel, strictures (→ Fig. 14.11), 'rosethorn' ulcers, 'cobblestone' mucosa
- Sigmoidoscopy and biopsy
- Colonoscopy and biopsy
- USS
- CT: abscesses.

Complications. Extra-alimentary manifestations (see above). Toxic dilatation. Stricture. Internal fistulae. Haemorrhage. Abscess formation. Perianal complications. Gallstones. Renal calculi. Psychological problems. Risk of carcinoma.

Treatment

Medical. Correction of fluid and electrolyte imbalance. Nutritional support. Steroids: 40 mg daily of prednisolone in acute exacerbations. Rectal disease may respond to Predsol enemas. Mesalazine may help colonic disease and may reduce the frequency of relapses. Other drug therapies include azathioprine (useful as steroid-sparing drug in some cases), ciclosporin, metronidazole (especially for colonic disease with perianal sepsis). Antidiarrhoeal agents may be used for symptomatic control but should be stopped if obstructed symptoms occur.

Figure 14.11 Small bowel enema showing Crohn's disease. A stricture is seen in the terminal ileum (arrow).

Surgical. Indicated for toxic dilatation, acute haemorrhage, perforation, obstruction, abscess formation, fistula formation, failure of medical treatment, uncertainty of diagnosis, development and prevention of carcinoma. Surgery involves segmental resection of bowel, sparing as much bowel as possible. For short strictures stricturoplasty may be carried out. Proctocolectomy with ileostomy may be required. Unlike ulcerative colitis, surgery in Crohn's disease cannot be guaranteed to be curative.

Prognosis. Acute regional ileitis may be cured by right hemicolectomy. Colonic Crohn's often responds well to medical treatment but at least 50% of patients will require surgery at some time. The mortality rate is about 14% over 30 years. The disease pursues a course of remissions and exacerbations.

Ulcerative colitis

This is a chronic inflammatory disease that involves the whole or part of the colon. The inflammation is confined to the mucosa and nearly always involves the rectum, extending to involve the distal or total colon. The aetiology is unknown but immunological, dietary and genetic factors may be involved. The majority of cases present between 25 and 30 years. Familial clustering occurs. Malignant change occurs in the colon with time.

Symptoms and signs. Diarrhoea, rectal bleeding, abdominal pain, fever, weight loss. The disease may be acute and fulminant, intermittent or chronic. Pallor, malnutrition, abdominal tenderness, abdominal distension, erythema nodosum, pyoderma gangrenosum, arthritis, uveitis, jaundice (sclerosing cholangitis).

Investigations
- Hb
- FBC
- U&Es: dehydration and electrolyte imbalance in severe cases
- LFTs: hypoproteinaemia or abnormal because of complications of sclerosing cholangitis
- AXR: acute toxic dilatation, perforation
- Barium enema – double contrast (→ Fig. 14.12): loss of haustrations, mucosal distortion, colonic shortening, stricture due to carcinoma. Barium enema should not be performed on ill patients with toxic dilatation in case of perforation
- Sigmoidoscopy: red, inflamed mucosa, contact bleeding, pseudopolyps
- Biopsy
- Colonoscopy: assess extent of disease, exclude carcinoma.

Figure 14.12 Ulcerative colitis. There is shortening of the colon with loss of haustrations ('lead pipe' appearance).

Complications. Local complications include toxic dilatation, haemorrhage, stricture, perforation, and carcinoma. Extracolonic complications include seronegative arthritis (sacroileitis, ankylosing spondylitis), sclerosing cholangitis, chronic active hepatitis, uveitis, and amyloid.

Treatment

Medical. Acute severe ulcerative colitis is treated with i.v. fluids, blood transfusion, parenteral nutrition and parenteral steroids. This regimen is instituted usually for 5 days. Regular examination of the patient is undertaken. If the patient deteriorates or toxic dilatation or perforation supervene, urgent surgery is required.

In the less ill patient, oral steroids may be given until the disease is controlled. Those who respond to the above regimens may be treated with sulphasalazine or mesalazine orally to maintain the remission. Distal colitis and proctitis may be controlled by Predsol retention enemas for relapses and sulphasalazine for maintenance.

Surgical. Indications for surgery include acute toxic dilatation, perforation, failure to respond to medical treatment, chronic disease, severe arthritic symptoms, carcinoma. Surgery usually involves panproctocolectomy with ileostomy but other procedures now available include retention of the rectum with mucosal proctectomy or fashioning of an ileal pouch with maintenance of anal sphincters.

Prognosis. The mortality rate with toxic dilatation or perforation is around 5%. The risk of colorectal cancer increases after 10 years' duration of disease, being about 2% at 10 years and up to 30% at 30 years. The risk is greater in those with total colitis and severe disease. Dysplasia often precedes carcinoma. Colonoscopic surveillance should be carried out at least 2-yearly.

DIVERTICULAR DISEASE

Diverticulae are outpouchings of mucosa through the bowel wall associated with increased intraluminal pressure (pulsion diverticulae). They occur between the taenia coli where vessels penetrate the bowel wall. They occur most commonly in the sigmoid colon and descending colon but may occur anywhere in the colon. They are rare before the age of 40 but thereafter there is an increase in incidence with age such that about 40% of patients over 70 have them. Diverticular disease is rare in countries where there is considerable roughage in the diet and is largely a condition occurring in western civilized societies where the diet is refined.

Symptoms and signs. Diverticular disease may be asymptomatic (diverticulosis).

Acute diverticulitis. Gives rise to lower abdominal colicky pain with localizing somatic pain usually in the LIF. Diarrhoea, constipation, and abdominal distension may occur. Fever. Tender in LIF.

Chronic diverticular disease. May cause lower abdominal colicky pain, alternating constipation and diarrhoea and excessive flatus together with abdominal distension. There may be little to find on abdominal examination.

Investigations
- Hb
- FBC (WCC raised in acute but normal in chronic)
- Sigmoidoscopy to exclude carcinoma
- Barium enema (→ Fig. 14.13) or colonoscopy.

Differential diagnosis. Carcinoma of the colon. Crohn's disease. Ischaemic colitis.

Complications. Acute diverticulitis. Stricture formation. Perforation with either generalized peritonitis, paracolic abscess, or fistula formation (vesicocolic, vaginocolic, ileocolic). Haemorrhage. Large bowel obstruction.

Treatment

Uncomplicated, symptomatic diverticular disease. High-fibre diet. Antispasmodic, e.g. Colofac. Bulking agent, e.g. Fybogel.

Acute diverticulitis. Bed rest. Fluids only or nil orally. Analgesic. Antibiotics: cefuroxime and metronidazole i.v. When symptoms settle, treatment is as for uncomplicated symptomatic diverticular disease.

Perforation with generalized faecal peritonitis. Laparotomy. Peritoneal lavage. Resect perforated area. In case of sigmoid diverticulae treatment is by Hartmann's procedure (see Procedures box at end of chapter). Drain peritoneal cavity. Antibiotics as for acute diverticulitis. In the elderly, perforated diverticulitis with faecal peritonitis carries a high mortality.

Figure 14.13 Diverticular disease. A barium enema showing numerous diverticulae in the sigmoid colon.

Perforation with paracolic abscess. Percutaneous drainage followed by elective resection.

Perforation with fistula formation. This involves bladder, vagina or small bowel. A vesicocolic fistula presents with dysuria and pneumaturia (passing wind in urine), a vaginocolic fistula presents with the passage of faeces PV and ileocolic fistula with diarrhoea. Vesicocolic fistulae show gas in the bladder on a plain radiograph. Barium enema may show the communication. Primary resection and anastomosis is the treatment of choice for ileocolic and vaginocolic fistulae. Vesicocolic fistulae may be treated by defunctioning loop ileostomy followed by resection, followed by closure of the loop ileostomy. In an adequately prepared bowel, primary resection with end-to-end anastomosis of colon and closure of bladder with interposition of omentum between colonic anastomosis and bladder may be more appropriate treatment.

Haemorrhage. Usually self-limiting. May be profuse and require transfusion. Exact site may be difficult to establish. Angiography may be required. If haemorrhage is life threatening, total colectomy with ileostomy and preservation of rectal stump may be required. Continuity of the bowel is re-established subsequently.

Intestinal obstruction. Progressive diverticular disease causes stricture. Treatment is by resection with either a Hartmann's procedure followed by subsequent restorative surgery, or a primary anastomosis protected by a temporary defunctioning loop ileostomy.

VOLVULUS

> This is a twisting of a loop of bowel around its mesenteric axis. Partial or complete obstruction may result. Occlusion of the arteries at the base of the involved mesentery leads to gangrene and perforation. The sigmoid colon and caecum may be involved, the sigmoid being the more common.

Sigmoid volvulus

Middle-aged and elderly males are more often affected. The twist is usually anticlockwise. A large redundant sigmoid colon and constipation are predisposing factors.

Symptoms and signs. Sudden onset of lower abdominal colicky pain associated with gross abdominal distension. May be history of recurrent mild attacks associated with partial volvulus relieved by passage of large amounts of faeces and flatus. Distended tympanitic abdomen.

Investigations
● AXR: distended loop of bowel the shape of a 'coffee bean' arising out of the pelvis on the left side
● Barium enema may be helpful in doubtful cases – the barium column resembles a 'bird's beak' because of the way the lumen tapers towards the volvulus (→ Fig. 14.14).

Figure 14.14 Barium enema showing a sigmoid volvulus. A 'bird's beak' deformity is seen (arrow). In this case, barium has passed into the volvulus – often it does not.

Treatment. Decompression by sigmoidoscopy. A rectal flatus tube should be left *in situ* for 48 h. If the patient is fit, elective resection of the sigmoid is carried out at a later date. If decompression is unsuccessful or there are signs of gangrene or perforation, laparotomy with resection is undertaken, the two ends of the colon being brought out as a double-barrelled colostomy (Paul–Mikulicz procedure), which is later closed.

Caecal volvulus

This occurs when the caecum and ascending colon are excessively mobile, or if there has been a defect in rotation, the caecum retaining its mesentery.

Symptoms and signs. Sudden onset of abdominal pain, vomiting and constipation. Tympanitic mass in LUQ. Tender mass if impending infarction.

Investigations. AXR: dilated caecum in left upper quadrant.

Treatment. Laparotomy. If bowel is viable, untwisting with caecostomy. There is a high incidence of recurrence, however, and right hemicolectomy may be the best option. If caecostomy is carried out it may close spontaneously or may require subsequent closure. If the bowel is gangrenous at laparotomy, a right hemicolectomy is required.

Prognosis. The mortality rate is high, usually owing to delayed diagnosis.

Irradiation proctitis

This may complicate irradiation of pelvic lesions, e.g. cervix, uterus, bladder, prostate. Bleeding, diarrhoea and tenesmus may result. Later ulceration and stricture formation may also occur. Early symptoms appearing soon after irradiation may respond to steroid enemas. Diverting colostomy may be required for severe symptoms.

Angiodysplasia

Vascular anomalies that may be degenerative and may cause bleeding from the large bowel. This is most common in the elderly. It is commonest in the right colon.

Symptoms and signs. Bleeding PR, which may be torrential but is often repeated small bleeds.

Investigations
● Colonoscopy
● Selective mesenteric angiography in the actively bleeding phase.

Treatment. Coagulation under direct vision at colonoscopy. Embolization at angiography. Extensive areas require colectomy.

LARGE BOWEL OBSTRUCTION

> The major causes are carcinoma, diverticular disease and volvulus. In 20% of patients the ileocaecal valve is competent and decompression into the small bowel does not occur. Closed-loop obstruction therefore occurs, the caecum progressively distending. Ischaemia and perforation of the caecum may occur.

Symptoms and signs. Colicky abdominal pain, constipation, and vomiting (late). Constant severe pain suggests ischaemic bowel. Distended tympanitic abdomen. Obstructed bowel sounds. Rectum may be empty on examination PR.

Investigations
● Sigmoidoscopy: rectosigmoid lesions may be seen
● AXR: distended large bowel with air/fluid levels surrounding the abdomen like a picture frame (→ Fig. 14.15)
● Limited barium enema may show 'apple core' lesion
● Instant enema to exclude pseudo-obstruction.

Treatment. Drip and suck. Correct electrolyte imbalance. A caecum 10 cm or greater in diameter on radiograph is an urgent indication for surgery, especially if tender to palpation. Laparotomy with decompression of the obstruction. Right-sided lesions are treated by right hemicolectomy. Left-sided lesions may be treated by left hemicolectomy with covering loop ileostomy. Low left-sided lesions are treated by resection of the tumour with Hartmann's procedure. However, on-table

Figure 14.15 A plain AXR showing large bowel obstruction. (A) Supine film. The left colon is distended down to the pelvis where there is sharp 'cut-off' of the gas shadow. (B) Erect film. This shows air/fluid levels in the large bowel. Again the sharp 'cut-off' is seen in the pelvis. This represents the point of the obstructing lesion, which in this case was in the lower sigmoid colon.

lavage of the colon and primary anastomosis may be carried out in experienced hands with or without a defunctioning loop ileostomy. A carcinoma on the apex of the sigmoid loop may be treated by resection and a Paul–Mikulicz double-barrel colostomy. In a poorly patient a defunctioning colostomy or caecostomy may be carried out and elective resection delayed until a later date when the patient is fitter. Sigmoid volvulus may be treated by resection and a Paul–Mikulicz procedure. Colonic stenting may be carried out in those unfit for surgery.

Prognosis. The overall mortality rate approaches 15%. Perforation is the main cause of mortality.

ANAL CONDITIONS

HAEMORRHOIDS

> These are enlarged vascular cushions in the lower rectum and anal canal. They are not simply varicosities. At least 10% of the population will have symptomatic haemorrhoids at some time in their life. The classical position of haemorrhoids corresponds to branches of the superior haemorrhoidal artery occurring at the 3 o'clock, 7 o'clock and 11 o'clock positions with the patient in the lithotomy position.

Symptoms and signs. Asymptomatic. Rectal bleeding (on toilet paper or drips into toilet on defaecation). Prolapse. Itching. Piles are not painful unless they thrombose. First-degree piles remain in the rectum and manifest only by bleeding. Second-degree piles prolapse on defaecation but reduce spontaneously. Third-degree piles prolapse and require manual reduction. Check Hb if bleeding is prolonged or heavy. Examine abdomen to exclude other lesions. Digital rectal examination.

Investigations
- Sigmoidoscopy to exclude other lesions
- Proctoscopy to confirm presence of piles. Remember at least 10% of population will have piles. Abdominal pain is not associated with piles
- If there is any doubt as to the cause of bleeding, carry out colonoscopy.

Treatment
- Injection treatment: inject 2–3 mL of phenol in almond oil into the submucosa above the pile. This is suitable for first-degree and small second-degree piles.
- Other non-operative approaches include rubber band ligation, cryosurgery and photocoagulation.
- Large second-degree piles and third-degree piles require haemorrhoidectomy.
- Thrombosed piles may be treated by bed rest, analgesia and ice packs. The piles may thrombose with cure or remain as skin tags, which require subsequent excision. Some surgeons advocate emergency haemorrhoidectomy. Whatever treatment is used, subsequent regulation of bowel habit with high-fibre diet and bulk laxatives is required.

Complications of haemorrhoidectomy. Acute retention of urine. Haemorrhage (slipped ligature in the early postoperative period or secondary haemorrhage

8–10 days postoperatively). Stricture may occur with anal stenosis if too much skin has been excised.

Differential diagnosis. Perianal haematoma, rectal prolapse, fissure-in-ano, inflammatory bowel disease, anal polyp, carcinoma, proctalgia fugax.

RECTAL PROLAPSE

> This may be partial or complete. Partial prolapse involves the mucosa alone and prolapse is usually no more than a few centimetres. Complete prolapse involves all layers of the rectal wall and is most common in elderly females.

Symptoms and signs. Protruding mass from the anus, especially during defaecation. May reduce spontaneously. May need manual reduction and eventually becomes difficult to reduce. Blood and mucus PR from ulceration of exposed mucosa. Palpate prolapse between fingers. Mucosal prolapse reveals two layers of mucosa about 2–4 cm long with radial folds. Lax sphincter on examination PR. Complete prolapse is thick, up to 12 cm long and patient may be unable to contract sphincter muscles after prolapse reduced.

Differential diagnosis. Prolapsing haemorrhoids, polyps, intussusception.

Treatment. Mucosal prolapse usually responds to sclerosants injected submucosally as for piles. Excision of prolapsed mucosa may be necessary. Complete prolapse is treated by abdominal rectopexy. The rectum is mobilized and fixed to the sacrum usually by inserting a Teflon prosthesis to hold it in position (Ripstein procedure). Other procedures include excision of mucosa and longitudinal plication of the rectal muscle (Delorme procedure); and circumferential narrowing of the anus by inserting a suture subcutaneously around the anal orifice (Thiersch wire – although nylon rather than wire is used nowadays).

Complications. Abdominal rectopexy usually gives good results but residual incontinence due to chronic stretching of the sphincter may result. Thiersch wire procedure may result in infection and faecal impaction.

Rectal prolapse in children

Usually self-correcting. Parents require reassurance. Keep act of defaecation as short as possible and avoid straining. Repeat simple reduction is all that is required. A mild laxative may be necessary. In a few cases, subcutaneous injection of sclerosant may be required.

PERIANAL HAEMATOMA

Symptoms and signs. Acute perianal pain. Worse on sitting, walking and defaecation. Tense, smooth, tender blue lump at anal verge.

Treatment. Symptoms may subside spontaneously after 2–3 days during which time analgesia is given. If patient presents in acute phase, incision under LA should be carried out.

FISSURE-IN-ANO

> This is a tear at the anal margin due to passage of a constipated stool. The fissure is usually in the midline posteriorly but may occasionally be anterior. Multiple fissures may be due to Crohn's disease.

Symptoms and signs. Acute anal pain, severe on defaecation. Blood on toilet paper. Part the buttocks and the fissure may be apparent. Acute sphincter spasm. Examination PR impossible. Occasionally 'sentinel' pile. This is a skin tag at the anal verge external to the fissure.

Differential diagnosis. Crohn's disease, trauma (beware abuse in children), carcinoma, herpes, TB, syphilis and psoriasis.

Treatment
Conservative. If symptoms are relatively mild, LA gel or suppository may be applied. This is best applied some half hour before defaecation. Attention should be given to correcting constipation with a stool-softening laxative and high-fibre diet. An alternative treatment is to apply 0.2% GTN ointment locally, which relaxes the internal anal sphincter. This should be applied twice daily for 6 weeks. Many fissures heal with this regimen at the expense of headache due to absorption of GTN.

Surgical. Some 90% of acute anal fissures settle with conservative management. In those that do not, a lateral subcutaneous internal sphincterotomy should be carried out to relieve spasm and to allow the fissure to heal. A laxative and high-fibre diet should be taken in the postoperative period. Chronic fissures should be treated by lateral subcutaneous internal sphincterotomy. Recurrent fissures should be treated by excision of the fissure, which is sent for histological examination to exclude underlying causes, e.g. Crohn's, anal carcinoma.

ANORECTAL ABSCESSES (→ Fig. 14.16)

> These develop in tissue spaces adjacent to the anorectal area. They may be perianal (in a hair follicle, sebaceous gland or perianal haematoma), ischiorectal (in the ischiorectal fossa), intermuscular (between internal and external sphincters), or pelvirectal (spreading from a pelvic abscess – rare). In many cases, the infection may start in the anal crypt and spread along tissue planes.

Figure 14.16 The anatomy of anorectal abscesses.

Pelvirectal

Ischiorectal

Intermuscular (intersphincteric)

Perianal

Internal sphincter

External sphincter

Symptoms and signs. Constant, throbbing, perianal pain – worse on sitting. With pelvirectal abscesses, the pain may also be in the lower abdomen. Indurated tender mass perianally. Boggy mass on examination PR, in ischiorectal fossa or anteriorly if pelvirectal abscess. Fever.

Treatment. Prompt surgical drainage to prevent fistula formation. There is no role for antibiotics except in diabetics and the immunocompromised – and then only as an adjunct to surgery. Incision, curettage and packing are required.

Complications. Fistula-in-ano occurs in up to 30% of patients.

FISTULA-IN-ANO

> A fistula is an abnormal communication between two epithelial surfaces. In this instance, there is an internal opening in the anal canal and one or more external openings on the perianal skin. Most arise from delay in treatment, or inadequate treatment, of anorectal abscesses. Rarer causes include Crohn's disease, tuberculosis and carcinoma. It may be difficult to locate the internal opening. Application of Goodsall's rule ('if the external opening lies anterior to a line drawn transversely through the centre of the anus, the track passes radially through a straight line towards the internal opening. If the external opening is behind this line the track curves in a horseshoe manner to open into the midline posteriorly') (→ Fig. 14.17). Fistulae may be classified as subcutaneous, submucous, low anal (below puborectalis), high anal (opening in close relation to the anorectal junction) or pelvirectal (penetrating levator ani) (→ Fig. 14.18).

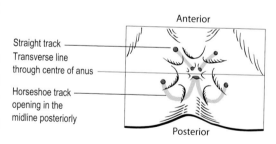

Straight track
Transverse line through centre of anus

Horseshoe track opening in the midline posteriorly

Anterior

Posterior

Figure 14.17 Goodsall's rule.

Pelvirectal

High anal

Low anal

Subcutaneous

Submucous

Figure 14.18 The anatomy of fistula-in-ano.

Symptoms and signs. History of abscess, which drains spontaneously or was surgically drained. Persistent drainage of pus, mucus, blood or faecal matter associated with perianal irritation and discomfort. Drainage may be intermittent if the fistula heals and opens recurrently. Single opening near anus. Examination PR reveals indurated track, pressure on which may cause discharge. Proctoscopy or sigmoidoscopy to define internal opening.

Investigations
- Fistulogram
- Endoanal ultrasound
- MRI.

Differential diagnosis. Pilonidal sinus, hidradenitis suppurativa, incontinence, Crohn's disease, trauma.

Treatment. The track is identified by probing and laid open under GA, so that it heals by granulation tissue from the base. With high fistulae or pelvirectal fistulae there is a danger to puborectalis when opening the track. Incontinence may result. Fortunately the latter types are rare but require specialist treatment, often by a two-stage operation.

PRURITUS ANI

> This is itching in the perianal area. It is a symptom of various conditions. Local causes include poor hygiene, sweating, fistula, haemorrhoids, neoplasia, warts, fungal infections, contact dermatitis (deodorants), worms, antibiotics (possibly via the complication of diarrhoea or fungal infection). General causes include diabetes mellitus, obstructive jaundice, Hodgkin's disease. Dermatological diseases include scabies, pediculosis, psoriasis and atopic eczema. The majority of causes are probably idiopathic or psychogenic. Often an 'itch/scratch' vicious circle is created and symptoms persist even after the initial cause has been eradicated.

Symptoms and signs. Worse at night whatever the cause. History of precipitating cause, e.g. antibiotics, diabetes, pruritus elsewhere. Perianal skin may be normal, or inflamed, moist or macerated. Examination PR and proctoscopy to exclude anal conditions, e.g. fistulae.

Investigations
- Hb
- WCC
- Blood sugar
- Perianal scrapings and microscopy for fungus.

Treatment. Specific for the underlying disease. Non-specific treatment includes advice on hygiene, diet, wearing loose underclothes, cleansing after defaecation with simple soap and application of glycerine and witch hazel. Application of hydrocortisone and LA cream may help. Occasionally the condition is difficult to treat.

SEXUALLY TRANSMITTED DISEASES

Condylomata acuminata (anal warts)
Caused by human papilloma virus. Usually sexually transmitted. Over 50% of patients admit to anal intercourse. May be few or a continuous carpet of warts extending into the anal canal. Symptoms include bleeding and pruritus. Small groups may be treated with topical podophyllin. Widespread lesions require surgical excision or diathermy. Recurrence is common.

Gonorrhoea
Gonococcal proctitis presents with pain, bleeding and purulent rectal discharge. Proctoscopy reveals ulcerated friable mucosa and pus in the rectal lumen. Culture confirms diagnosis. Treatment is usually by i.m. procaine penicillin and probenecid.

Herpes
Severe perianal pain, constipation, discharge and ulceration. Examination reveals vesicles and ulcers. Treatment is by topical or oral aciclovir.

Syphilis
Perianal or anal ulcers. May resemble anal fissure. Often painless. Diagnosis is confirmed by dark field examination of discharge and serology. Penicillin is treatment of choice. Contact follow-up is important.

AIDS
Anorectal manifestations include fissure, perianal sepsis, ulceration, fungal or viral infections, rectal lymphoma and Kaposi's sarcoma.

ANAL MALIGNANCIES

Anal tumours are rare and include epidermoid tumours, malignant melanoma, lymphoma (often in association with AIDS), and Kaposi's sarcoma (associated with AIDS). Adenocarcinoma occurs in the upper part of the anal canal but may spread across the dentate line and appear at the anal margin. The most common of the tumours is the epidermoid carcinoma (squamous cell carcinoma). Patients should be checked for a history of homosexuality with penetrative anal sex.

Symptoms and signs. Bleeding, pruritus, pain, discharge, palpable mass in anal canal. Patients may think they have haemorrhoids. Rectal examination may reveal visible tumour growing out of the anus. Hard, irregular, ulcerated mass. Palpable inguinal nodes. Hepatomegaly if secondaries.

Investigations
● Biopsy
● USS liver.

Treatment. Small, non-invasive lesions may be locally excised and treated with radiotherapy. Larger lesions invading the sphincters will require abdominoperineal resection, although recent evidence suggests survival rates may be as good with radiotherapy combined with chemotherapy.

Prognosis. A total of 50% of patients survive 5 years.

RECTAL BLEEDING

> Bleeding PR is a common clinical problem. The commonest causes are haemorrhoids, fissure-in-ano and colorectal cancer. Massive rectal bleeding may be due to diverticular disease, angiodysplasia, or a cause in the upper GI tract, e.g. peptic ulcer or an aorto-enteric fistula. If bright red rectal haemorrhage is coming from the upper GI tract, the bleeding is massive with rapid gut transit time and the patient will always be shocked. (For causes of rectal bleeding → Table 14.3.)

Symptoms and signs. Check colour and amount of blood. Bright red bleeding in small amounts usually indicates that the source is in the anal canal or rectum. Large amounts suggest diverticular disease or angiodysplasia. Bleeding from haemorrhoids may occasionally be considerable. Blood on toilet paper suggests haemorrhoids or fissure-in-ano. Dripping into the toilet at defaecation suggests haemorrhoids. Blood streaked on stools suggests rectosigmoid or rectal carcinoma. Blood and mucus on defaecation suggest rectal carcinoma. Blood, mucus and pus associated with abdominal pain, diarrhoea and fever, suggest colitis. Bleeding associated with change in bowel habit and abdominal pain suggests colonic cancer. Bleeding associated with pain on defaecation suggests fissure-in-ano or carcinoma of the anal canal. Check for abdominal pain, anal pain, change in bowel habit, abdominal distension. Symptoms of anaemia, weight loss, jaundice. Abdominal mass, e.g. colonic tumour, hepatomegaly (metastases). Abdominal tenderness, distended abdomen – shifting dullness (ascites) – obstructed bowel sounds. Inspection PR for piles, warts, fissure, tumour. Rectal mass (90% of rectal cancers can be felt on examination PR).

TABLE 14.3 Causes of rectal bleeding

Haemorrhoids
Fissure-in-ano
Carcinoma of anus
Colorectal carcinoma
Colorectal polyps
Diverticular disease
Inflammatory bowel disease
• Crohn's disease
• ulcerative colitis
Ischaemic colitis
Angiodysplasia
Irradiation colitis or proctitis
Rectal prolapse
Meckel's diverticulum
Intussusception
Mesenteric infarction
Aortoenteric fistula
Massive upper GI haemorrhage
Trauma
Bleeding diathesis

Investigations

- Hb
- FBC
- ESR
- U&Es (ureteric involvement with colorectal tumours)
- LFTs (liver metastases)
- Clotting screen
- Proctoscopy: haemorrhoids
- Sigmoidoscopy and biopsy
- Barium enema
- Colonoscopy
- Selective mesenteric angiography, preferably in bleeding phase
- Radiolabelled autologous red cells
- Technetium scanning (taken up by ectopic gastric mucosa in Meckel's)
- Gastroscopy if upper GI haemorrhage suspected.

Treatment. Principles of treatment include:

- Resuscitation if massive bleeding
- Diagnosis of the cause
- Definitive treatment of the cause.

The treatment of the various conditions is covered elsewhere in this book.

LIVER

> Diseases of the liver usually present to the surgeon as jaundice, hepatomegaly, or ascites. This section will deal only with liver disease as far as it concerns the surgeon. (For causes of hepatomegaly → Table 14.4.)

INFECTIONS IN THE LIVER

Abscess

This is rare and usually caused by pyogenic bacteria. Causes are due to the following:

- Portal pyelophlebitis secondary to acute abdominal infection, e.g. appendicitis, diverticulitis, peritonitis
- Biliary disease, e.g. cholecystitis, ascending cholangitis
- Trauma
- Direct extension from subphrenic abscess, empyema of gallbladder
- Septicaemia
- Infection of a liver cyst
- Rarely there is no cause, i.e. cryptogenic.

Symptoms and signs. Those of underlying disease. Fever, toxic, rigors, jaundice, upper abdominal pain, may be of acute onset with no apparent underlying cause. Tender hepatomegaly.

TABLE 14.4 Causes of hepatomegaly

Regular generalized enlargement without jaundice	Cirrhosis Congestive cardiac failure Reticuloses Budd–Chiari syndrome (hepatic vein obstruction) Amyloid
Regular generalized enlargement with jaundice	Viral hepatitis Biliary tract obstruction Cholangitis
Irregular generalized enlargement without jaundice	Secondary tumours Macronodular cirrhosis Polycystic disease Primary tumours
Irregular generalized enlargement with jaundice	Cirrhosis Widespread liver secondaries
Localized swellings	Riedel's lobe Hydatid cyst Amoebic abscess Primary carcinoma

Investigations
- WCC
- LFTs: abnormal
- Blood cultures positive
- USS
- CT
- Indium-labelled WC scan.

Differential diagnosis. Tumour, amoebic abscess.

Treatment. Multiple small abscesses require antibiotics, e.g. gentamicin and metronidazole. Prognosis is poor. These often complicate septicaemia in an immunocompromised patient. Solitary or multiple large abscesses may be treated by percutaneous drainage under US control. Occasionally open surgical drainage is required.

Amoebic abscess

Due to infection with protozoan parasite *Entamoeba histolytica*. More than 50% occur in the absence of amoebic dysentery. Abscesses may be single (common) or multiple. They may be small or very large containing up to 3 L of pus. They are more common in the right lobe of the liver. Cases in Europe occur in immigrants or those who have returned from areas where the disease is endemic.

Symptoms and signs. Insidious onset. Right hypochondrial pain. Malaise. Pyrexia. Weight loss. Occasionally rigors and diarrhoea. Jaundice uncommon.

Investigations
- USS
- CT.

Treatment. Metronidazole. Large cysts require percutaneous drainage and US control. Surgery is rarely required and usually only if cyst rupture has occurred.

Hydatid disease

Due to infection with an *Echinococcus granulosus* (tapeworm). The tapeworm develops in the dog intestine and ova are shed in the faeces. These contaminate grass or vegetables and are ingested by sheep, cattle or humans. The ova then pass to the liver via the portal circulation where they develop into hydatid cysts. These may also enter the kidneys and lungs. The disease occurs in sheep- and cattle-rearing countries of the world, e.g. Australia, Africa and Wales.

Symptoms and signs. Symptomless mass. Abdominal pain. Jaundice (due to pressure on ducts). Rupture into the peritoneal cavity results in peritonitis and shock.

Investigations
- AXR: calcified outline of cyst
- Hydatid serology
- USS
- CT.

Treatment. Medical treatment is by albendazole. This may result in shrinkage in some cases but usually surgery is indicated. Care must be taken to avoid spilling cyst contents into the peritoneal cavity as anaphylactic shock may occur. The cyst is usually aspirated under direct vision and a scolicidal agent injected into the cyst, e.g. hypertonic saline. The cyst is then carefully excised and the cavity closed. Albendazole is given pre- and postoperatively.

LIVER TUMOURS

Secondary tumours are common arising from the GI tract, lung and breast. More than 25% of patients who die of malignant disease have liver secondaries. Primary tumours are rare. The commonest malignant primary tumours are hepatocellular carcinoma and cholangiocarcinoma. Benign tumours are rare and include adenoma and cavernous haemangioma.

Primary malignant tumours

Hepatocellular carcinoma

About 50% of these carcinomas occur in patients with cirrhosis. It is common in Africa and the Far East, and more common than cholangiocarcinoma. It is associated with hepatitis B, the contraceptive pill, aflatoxin, anabolic steroids.

Symptoms and signs. Pre-existing cirrhosis. Abdominal pain. Weight loss. Fever. Ascites. Jaundice. Hepatomegaly.

Investigations
- Hb
- ESR
- LFTs abnormal
- α-fetoprotein raised (mainly in cirrhotics)

- CXR: raised diaphragm, lung secondary
- USS
- CT
- PET
- Liver biopsy under US control
- Arteriography prior to resection to assess resectability and blood supply.

Treatment. Surgical resection if confined to one lobe. Liver transplantation. Chemotherapy directly into hepatic artery.

Prognosis. Small tumours confined to one lobe treated by hepatic lobectomy have a good prognosis. Otherwise the prognosis is poor, death usually occurring within 1 year.

Cholangiocarcinoma

The tumour arises from the cells of the intrahepatic bile duct system. It is less common than hepatocellular carcinoma. There is an association with primary sclerosing cholangitis, liver fluke infestation and anabolic steroids.

Symptoms and signs. Usually presents with jaundice.

Investigations
- Hb
- LFTs: bilirubin ↑, alkaline phosphatase ↑
- USS
- CT
- Liver biopsy under US control
- ERCP.

Treatment. Rapid, direct, and lymphatic spread makes surgical cure rare. Surgical resection with hemihepatectomy is sometimes possible. Palliation of jaundice via surgical bypass or endoscopic stenting. Rarely liver transplantation may be feasible.

Prognosis. Bad. Most patients are dead within 6 months.

Hepatic metastases

Common. More than 90% of patients with hepatic metastases have metastatic disease elsewhere.

Symptoms and signs. Those of the primary tumour. Previous surgery for primary. Anorexia, vomiting, weight loss, cachexia. Upper abdominal pain or discomfort. Jaundice. Ascites. Hard, irregular, palpable liver.

Investigations
- Hb
- LFTs: alkaline phosphatase ↑, bilirubin ↑, albumin ↓
- CEA for colorectal secondaries
- USS
- CT (→ Fig. 14.19)
- Biopsy under US control.

Treatment. Younger patients with metastases from colorectal cancer, confined to one lobe of the liver and up to four in number, should be treated by partial

Figure 14.19 CT scan of abdomen. Numerous liver metastases are seen in both the right and left lobes of the liver.

hepatectomy. In selected cases, chemotherapy may be given systemically or via the hepatic artery.

Prognosis. Depends upon the type of metastatic tumour. Most patients survive less than 2 years but there is a 35–40% 5-year survival rate for patients with colorectal secondaries that are completely resected.

PORTAL HYPERTENSION

> Portal hypertension occurs when portal venous pressure equals or exceeds 15 mmHg (20 cm water). Collateral channels open up between the portal and systemic circulations, the clinically most important of these being at the gastro-oesophageal junction, leading to the development of oesophageal varices which may be responsible for torrential bleeding. Other consequences of portal hypertension include splenomegaly, ascites (in hepatic and posthepatic forms) and the manifestations of hepatic failure (encephalopathy).

Causes

Prehepatic. Congenital malformations, neonatal umbilical sepsis. Exchange transfusion via umbilical catheter. Tumour.

Hepatic. Cirrhosis, schistosomiasis.

Posthepatic. Budd–Chiari syndrome (obstruction of the hepatic veins which may be due to idiopathic hepatic vein thrombosis, congenital obliteration, or blockage of the hepatic vein by tumour), constrictive pericarditis.

Symptoms and signs. Jaundice. Mental changes. Flapping tremor. Coma. Haematemesis and melaena. Ascites. Spider naevi, liver palms, clubbing, gynaecomastia, testicular atrophy, caput medusae. Peripheral oedema. Leukonychia. Dupuytren's contracture. Xanthoma. Kayser–Fleischer rings. Bruising.

Investigations
- Hb
- FBC
- LFTs
- Coagulation screen
- OGD.

Treatment of bleeding oesophageal varices

Acute bleed. Resuscitate. CVP monitoring. Blood transfusion. FFP. Platelets. Urgent endoscopy to confirm diagnosis. Inject the varices with sclerosant at the time of endoscopy. If a good view cannot be obtained because of gross bleeding, the following measures should be undertaken:

- Tamponade with a Sengstaken–Blakemore tube
- Administer vasopressin i.v. to lower portal venous pressure
- Administer i.v. metoclopramide – constricts lower oesophageal sphincter and empties stomach of blood
- Somatostatin may be beneficial by reducing portal venous pressure.

The control of bleeding by tamponade is temporary while the next stage of treatment is planned. Usually this is sclerotherapy, which is effective in 90% of patients. Patients who fail to respond should be considered for oesophageal transection or shunting.

Definitive treatment after bleeding
- Chronic injection sclerotherapy. The varices are injected at monthly intervals until they are obliterated. Endoscopic follow-up is carried out on a regular basis. Complications of this technique include ulceration, stricture, and dysphagia.
- Portosystemic shunting. Splenoportogram and CT are carried out to assess the patency of the portal vein. Shunts may be portocaval, mesocaval, or splenorenal. They may be carried out as an emergency to lower portal pressure but it is rare to do so since the advent of injection sclerotherapy. Shunting is usually carried out in the elective stage when there have been previous bleeding episodes. For a successful shunt operation, hepatic function needs to be reasonably good. Jaundice, hypoalbuminaemia, ascites, and encephalopathy indicate a bad prognosis with shunt operations. Liver transplantation is preferable except when the obstruction is prehepatic with good liver function.

Prophylaxis. Many patients with varices never bleed. If varices are known to be present, oral β-blockade with propranolol significantly decreases the incidence of bleeding and rebleeding.

Prognosis. Up to 40% of patients having their first variceal bleed will die. Long-term survival after portocaval shunt operations is poor. The 5-year survival after portocaval shunting for alcoholic liver disease is about 45%. Some degree of encephalopathy develops in 14–30% of patients.

EXTRAHEPATIC BILIARY SYSTEM

CHOLELITHIASIS (GALLSTONES)

This is common and present in 10% of the population over 50. It is more common in females, especially in multiparous women. Obesity, drugs, contraceptive pill, clofibrate, haemolytic disorders, ileal disease (resection, Crohn's disease) are aetiological factors. Factors that may produce lithogenic bile include increased cholesterol content, reduced bile acids, biliary stasis. Classically three types of stone are described:

● Cholesterol stones: (may be solitary), cholesterol 'solitaire' – radiolucent
● Pigment: occur with haemolysis – small, black, irregular and friable – radiolucent
● Mixed: often faceted – contain calcium, pigment, and cholesterol – 10% are radio-opaque (→ Fig. 14.20).

About 80% of stones are asymptomatic. Symptoms are related to the complications they cause.

Figure 14.20 Gallstones. An incidental finding on barium enema. There are several radio-opaque gallstones in the right hypochondrium.

Complications
Gallbladder. Acute cholecystitis, chronic cholecystitis, acute-on-chronic cholecystitis. Empyema (pus in the gallbladder). Mucocele (mucus in the gallbladder). Carcinoma. Perforation of gallbladder.

In the ducts. Obstructive jaundice, cholangitis, pancreatitis.

In the gut. Gallstone ileus (associated with cholecystoduodenal fistula).

Acute cholecystitis

Gallstones are the most common cause. Rarely, acalculous cholecystitis may occur. Sometimes it is associated with typhoid fever. Most cases are in fact acute-on-chronic, many patients having demonstrated symptoms of chronic cholecystitis in the past.

Symptoms and signs. Nausea, fever, vomiting. RUQ pain radiating under ribs to right scapula. Tender with guarding R hypochondrium. Positive Murphy's sign.

Investigations
- Hb
- WCC
- LFTs
- USS.

Treatment. Nil orally; i.v. fluids. NG suction. Analgesia (usually pethidine). Antibiotic (usually cefuroxime i.v.). Symptoms usually settle in 48–72 h. Elective cholecystectomy is usually carried out 3 months later. Emergency cholecystectomy may be required if symptoms do not settle on conservative management.

Chronic cholecystitis

Virtually always associated with gallstones. Repeated episodes of infection cause chronic thickening and fibrosis.

Symptoms and signs. Flatulent dyspepsia. The classical case is the middle-aged obese female who gets upper abdominal discomfort and distension relieved by belching. Intolerance of fatty food. Often little to find on clinical examination.

Investigations. USS.

Treatment. Cholecystectomy. This may be by the open or laparoscopic technique. Unfit patients may be placed on a low-fat diet to control symptoms or treated by extracorporeal shock wave lithotripsy if suitable. Dissolution of stones which are small and non-radio-opaque in a functioning gallbladder may be attempted with chenodeoxycholic acid given orally.

Biliary colic

This is a symptom rather than a complication of gallstones. It is produced by impaction of a stone in the neck of the gallbladder or in the cystic duct. The stone may either fall back into the gallbladder or pass through the cystic duct into the CBD, whence the pain abates.

Symptoms and signs. Sudden onset of severe pain across the epigastrium (it is not confined to the RUQ). Severe spasms of colic against the background of continuous severe pain. The patient rolls around in agony and cannot get into a comfortable position. Tachycardia, sweating, and vomiting. Examination may reveal rigidity in the upper abdomen (beware making a diagnosis of peritonitis – in peritonitis the patient does not roll around but remains still). An attack may last 2–4 h. Following an attack, jaundice may occur owing to the passed stone impacting in the CBD.

Treatment. Pethidine i.m. Subsequent investigations for gallbladder disease and cholecystectomy if appropriate.

Mucocele

This may follow an attack of biliary colic. Stone impacts in neck of gallbladder. Bile absorbed. Mucus secretion continues.

Symptoms and signs. Previous history of biliary colic. RUQ discomfort. Occasionally patient feels lump. Large, tense globular mass in RUQ.

Investigations. USS.

Treatment. Cholecystectomy.

Empyema

This follows an attack of cholecystitis. Infection develops after impaction of a stone in the neck of the gallbladder. Obstruction leads to stasis, overgrowth of bacteria and the gallbladder fills with pus.

Symptoms and signs. Attack of acute cholecystitis or biliary colic. Fever, toxicity. RUQ pain. Tender mass in RUQ.

Investigations
- WCC
- USS.

Treatment. Give i.v. fluids. NG suction. Antibiotics – cefuroxime and metronidazole. Cholecystectomy. Occasionally there is so much inflammation that it is impossible to safely carry out cholecystectomy. Drainage of the gallbladder with formation of a cholecystotomy may be appropriate in these circumstances. Cholecystectomy may be undertaken at a later date.

Perforation of the gallbladder

This is rare and usually presents either as generalized biliary peritonitis or leakage of pus from a perforated empyema. Infected biliary peritonitis has a high mortality especially as this condition is most common in the elderly. Treatment involves laparotomy, peritoneal lavage, cholecystectomy and antibiotics (usually gentamicin and metronidazole).

Carcinoma

Associated with long-standing gallstone disease and is commoner in females. Local invasion of the liver and bile ducts occurs. Jaundice occurs owing to direct extension into the bile duct together with secondaries in the nodes at the porta hepatis. Small tumours may be an incidental finding at cholecystectomy for gallstones. In the latter case, long-term survival may be expected. Many cases present late when local spread and lymph node metastases have occurred. In this case, prognosis is poor – 90% of patients surviving less than 1 year.

Cholangitis

This is a serious condition caused by complete or partial biliary obstruction in association with ascending infection of the biliary tree. It may be complicated by septicaemia and liver abscesses.

Symptoms and signs. Fever, rigors, jaundice (Charcot's biliary triad).

Investigations
- WCC
- Blood cultures
- USS
- MRCP.

Treatment. Antibiotics – cefuroxime/metronidazole/gentamicin. Acute suppurative cholangitis may occur with pus under tension in the biliary tree. Urgent decompression of the bile ducts via a cannula inserted endoscopically via the ampulla of Vater may be required.

Gallstone ileus

This results from a fistula occurring between the fundus of the gallbladder and the adjacent duodenum. A stone passes through the fistula and may impact in the terminal ileum causing obstruction to the small bowel.

Symptoms and signs. Colicky abdominal pain, vomiting and distension. History of flatulent dyspepsia. The diagnosis should be suspected in middle-aged to elderly females with symptoms of small bowel obstruction in the absence of a hernia or previous abdominal surgery to suggest adhesion formation.

Investigations. AXR: dilated loops of small bowel, air in the biliary tree (→ Fig. 14.21A). CT, dilated small bowel, gallstone in lumen, air in biliary tree (Fig. 14.21B).

Treatment. Laparotomy. Removal of stone from small bowel lumen by 'milking' through ileocaecal valve or removal by enterotomy. Cholecystectomy at a later date if symptoms referable to gallbladder continue.

Acalculous cholecystitis

Acute cholecystitis without gallstones may occur in a variety of conditions. It may be due to infection, e.g. typhoid, or may occur following sepsis, burns, TPN, multiple injuries, in the puerperium and after unrelated surgery. Treatment is the same as for calculous acute cholecystitis.

Non-surgical treatment of gallstones

Oral dissolution therapy. Suitable for small radiolucent stones in a functioning gallbladder. A combination of chenodeoxycholic acid and ursodeoxycholic acid is given orally. Side-effects include diarrhoea, pruritus and transient rise in serum transaminases. Treatment must be continued for months. Recurrence rates are high.

Extracorporeal shock wave lithotripsy. Suitable for medium-sized, radiolucent stones in a functioning gallbladder. Concurrent treatment with chenodeoxycholic acid and ursodeoxycholic acid is required. Treatment by this method requires further evaluation. Biliary colic may occur as fragments are passed through the cystic duct.

Figure 14.21 (A) Plain AXR showing gallstone ileus. In this case, a large non-radio-opaque stone was obstructing the upper jejunum. Only one small loop of distended bowel is seen in the abdomen (large arrow). Gas is clearly seen in the biliary tree (small arrow) indicating the presence of a cholecystoduodenal fistula. (B) CT abdomen showing gallstone ileus. A large gallstone (large arrow) is seen in a dilated loop of small bowel. Gas is seen in the intrahepatic biliary tree (small arrow).

Endoscopy. Stones in the CBD may be treated by endoscopic sphincterotomy and stone extraction. This treatment is suitable for the elderly, unfit patient with a gallstone impacted in the CBD. It allows jaundice to settle even if there are residual stones in the gallbladder; no further treatment is required if they remain asymptomatic. It is useful also for removing retained stones missed at cholecystectomy and exploration of the common bile duct, or recurrent stones forming in the CBD.

Treatment of asymptomatic gallstones. These may be seen on AXR or USS carried out for other conditions, or they may be discovered at laparotomy for another condition. In the younger patient, cholecystectomy is advisable to prevent the complications and to offset the long-term complication of carcinoma. In the elderly and unfit, no treatment is advised.

OBSTRUCTIVE JAUNDICE

Jaundice occurs when the serum bilirubin exceeds 40 mmol/L. Posthepatic obstructive jaundice occurs because of obstruction of the extrahepatic biliary tree.

Causes
In the lumen. Gallstones (common), roundworms (rare), blood clots in haemobilia.

In the wall. Congenital biliary atresia, traumatic stricture, sclerosing cholangitis, cholangiocarcinoma, choledochal cysts.

Outside the wall. Carcinoma of the head of the pancreas, carcinoma of the ampulla of Vater, malignant nodes in the porta hepatis.

Symptoms and signs. Previous history of cholecystectomy. Previous history of malignancy. Painless jaundice suggests malignancy. Jaundice preceded by severe upper abdominal pain suggests gallstones. Gradual onset of jaundice associated with dark urine and pale stools. Pruritus. Smooth palpable liver. Palpable gallbladder (carcinoma of pancreas or ampulla of Vater – Courvoisier's law states that 'if in the presence of jaundice the gallbladder is palpable, the cause of the jaundice is unlikely to be due to stones'). The reason for this is that with gallstone disease the gallbladder is usually fibrotic and unable to distend and thus become palpable.

Investigations
- Hb
- FBC
- ESR
- U&Es
- LFTs: bilirubin and alkaline phosphatase markedly raised
- PT: may be clotting defect due to poor absorption of vitamin K
- USS: may show dilated ducts and site of obstruction, gallstones in gallbladder; the technique is poor for the lower end of the bile duct and head of pancreas as gas may obscure view
- CT: shows intrahepatic lesions, demonstrates invasion of adjacent structures
- MRCP

Figure 14.22 ERCP. A gallstone (arrow) is seen in the dilated bile duct.

- ERCP (→ Fig. 14.22): possible to carry out biopsy, defines level of lesion, allows stenting and relief of jaundice
- PTC (→ Fig. 14.23) if ERCP impossible
- Liver biopsy.

Treatment. Check PT. Correct any clotting problem with parenteral vitamin K. Give mannitol and i.v. fluids preoperatively to prevent hepatorenal syndrome. Prophylactic antibiotics. Subsequent treatment depends on the cause of jaundice:

Gallstone in CBD. Explore duct at time of cholecystectomy or remove at ERCP and sphincterotomy.

Congenital biliary atresia. (→ Ch. 20).

Traumatic stricture. Needs bypass via Roux loop of intestine anastomosed to the proximal dilated duct.

Sclerosing cholangitis. Hepaticojejunostomy, i.e. anastomose a loop of jejunum to a dilated duct at the hilum of the liver. Stenting by endoscopic retrograde route or percutaneous transhepatic route may be of benefit. The prognosis is poor.

Figure 14.23 A percutaneous transhepatic cholangiogram. At least two stones (arrows) are seen within a grossly dilated bile duct. There is free flow of contrast into the duodenum.

Cholangiocarcinoma. Primary resection is rarely possible and has a high mortality. Stenting combined with radiotherapy produces a few long-term survivors.

Choledochal cyst. Excision of cyst with Roux-en-Y choledochojejunostomy.

Carcinoma of the head of the pancreas or ampulla of Vater. Attempted curative resection may be carried out via a pancreaticoduodenectomy (Whipple's operation). Relatively few tumours are curable. Recurrence rates are high. If the tumour is inoperable as judged by invasion of adjacent structures on CT, or because of liver metastases, stenting may be carried out. If the tumour is found to be inoperable at laparotomy a 'triple bypass' is carried out (→ section on pancreas).

Nodes at the porta hepatis. Stenting is the treatment of choice. Adjuvant radiotherapy may help depending upon the type of tumour invading the nodes.

Complications of surgery on the jaundiced patient. Coagulation disorders. Renal failure. GI tract haemorrhage (stress ulcers). Delayed wound healing.

PANCREAS

PANCREATITIS

Inflammation of the pancreas may be divided into acute and chronic. Acute pancreatitis is a condition presenting with acute onset of abdominal pain associated with raised levels of pancreatic enzymes in the blood and urine. The gland normally returns to functional and anatomical normality after the cause is treated. Recurrent attacks may occur (relapsing acute pancreatitis). Chronic pancreatitis is a continuing inflammatory disease characterized by irreversible functional and anatomical abnormalities in the gland, resulting in fibrosis of the gland and pancreatic insufficiency.

Acute pancreatitis

Aetiological factors include biliary tract disease (60%), alcohol (20%). Other causes include hyperlipidaemia, hyperparathyroidism, viral infections (mumps, Coxsackie virus), hypothermia, trauma, postoperative, drugs (steroids, oestrogen-containing contraceptives, azathioprine, thiazide diuretics), familial, scorpion bites, idiopathic, autoimmune (polyarteritis nodosa), post-ERCP, pancreatic carcinoma.

Symptoms and signs. Severe epigastric pain radiating through to back. Nausea, vomiting, shock. Tender in epigastrium initially spreading to whole abdomen. Abdominal distension. Absent bowel sounds. Bluish discoloration in flank (Grey Turner's sign) or periumbilical area (Cullen's sign) – due to haemorrhagic pancreatitis with spread of blood retroperitoneally to these areas.

Investigations
- Hb
- PCV
- WCC ↑
- U&Es
- LFTs: bilirubin ↑, mild derangement of others
- Amylase raised >1000 u/L
- Ca^{2+} ↓
- Blood sugar ↑
- ABG
- PO_2 ↓
- ECG changes may occur, diminished T waves. Beware the patient with haemorrhagic pancreatitis who presents late and in whom the amylase is normal because of extensive destruction of the pancreas
- AXR: absent psoas shadows, 'sentinel loop' adjacent to pancreas because of local ileus
- CXR: small pleural effusions
- CT: necrosis, abscess, assessment of severity.

Complications. ARF. ARDS. Gastric erosions (haematemesis and melaena). DIC. Psychosis. Diabetes. Local complications include pancreatic necrosis, abscess formation, pseudocyst formation. Relapsing acute pancreatitis. Chronic pancreatitis.

Differential diagnosis. Perforated peptic ulcer. Acute exacerbation of peptic ulcer. Cholecystitis. Mesenteric infarction. MI.

Treatment

Mild case. N/G suction. Give i.v. fluids. Nil orally. Analgesia (pethidine), antibiotics (cefuroxime and metronidazole). Careful monitoring of urine output. Monitor WCC, blood sugar, U&Es, LFTs, calcium, ABG.

Severe case. Best treated in ITU. Severity is indicated by Ranson's criteria:

- At presentation, age >55, WCC >16 × 10^9/L, glucose >11 mmol/L, LDH >350 IU/L, AST >200 IU/L
- During first 48 h: PCV: fall >10%, urea >16 mmol/L, Ca^{2+} <2 mmol/L, PaO_2 <8 kPa, base deficit <4. The more criteria present the greater the mortality.

Treatment involves nil orally, NG suction; i.v. fluids (crystalloid, colloid, blood), catheterize and measure urine output hourly, analgesia (pethidine), antibiotics (i.v. cefuroxime and metronidazole or i.v. imipenem), early enteral feeding (in severe cases this may reduce mortality), peritoneal lavage ('prune juice' peritoneal fluid indicates severe haemorrhagic pancreatitis), H_2 receptor antagonists as prophylaxis against gastric erosions, inotropic support (dopamine, dobutamine), calcium gluconate for hypocalcaemia, O_2 by mask, ventilation if ARDS, dialysis if ARF. ERCP if common bile duct stones, i.e. jaundice with deranged liver function tests and dilated common bile duct.

Indications for surgery
- Uncertainty of diagnosis.
- Deterioration of patient's condition. Drainage of abscesses or removal of necrotic pancreas may be required. Fat necrosis may be seen at laparotomy. Drainage of pseudocyst. Early cholecystectomy if gallstones are the cause.

Prognosis. Mortality rate overall is about 10%. With acute haemorrhagic pancreatitis it exceeds 30%.

Chronic pancreatitis

Chronic alcoholism is responsible for most cases. A few cases result from hypercalcaemia, hyperlipidaemia or familial predisposition. Direct trauma with subsequent duct stricture is responsible for a few cases. Damage to acini occurs with destruction of the parenchyma, fibrosis and ductal stenoses with dilatation beyond.

Symptoms and signs. Upper abdominal pain often radiating through to the back. Weight loss. Nausea, vomiting, steatorrhoea. 30–40% develop diabetes. A few patients may become addicted to narcotic analgesics because of the severity of the pain. Upper abdominal tenderness. Occasionally jaundice if CBD obstructed.

Investigations
- AXR: speckled pancreatic calcification
- Blood glucose may be raised
- Ca may be raised
- Lipid profile (hyperlipidaemia)
- Amylase elevated during exacerbations

- USS: cystic change and duct dilatation
- CT
- MRCP/ERCP: assess duct dilatation and stenoses.

Treatment

Medical. Stop alcohol. Low-fat diet. Pancreatic extracts given orally (Pancrex or Creon). Treat diabetes mellitus. Fat-soluble vitamins. Adequate analgesia. Coeliac plexus blockade may be necessary.

Surgical. Largely carried out for pain. Decompression of the duct by endoscopic sphincterotomy and insertion of pancreatic duct stent at ERCP. Longitudinal pancreaticojejunostomy may be carried out. Other operations include resection of the head, body and tail or whole gland. If total pancreatectomy is required, brittle diabetes results – consider isolating the islets cells from the pancreas and carrying out autotransplantation.

Prognosis. Depends upon ability to abstain from alcohol – 25% of patients die within 15 years. Some patients have a miserable life with narcotic addiction, diabetes mellitus and malnutrition.

Pancreatic cysts

True cysts are rare, and may be associated with congenital polycystic disease, retention cysts, hydatid disease and tumour (cystadenoma and cystadenocarcinoma). Pseudocysts are more common and are a consequence of acute pancreatitis, pancreatic trauma or, rarely, posterior perforation of a gastric ulcer.

Pancreatic pseudocyst

This is a collection of fluid in the lesser sac.

Symptoms and signs. Pancreatic trauma. Acute pancreatitis. Perforated posterior GU. Rarely no history. Development of a tender epigastric mass. Fever, weight loss, nausea and vomiting.

Investigation

- WCC
- Amylase
- Bilirubin occasionally elevated
- USS
- CT: collection of fluid in lesser sac.

Complications. If left, some cysts may absorb spontaneously. Rarely infection, rupture, or haemorrhage into the cyst may occur.

Treatment. Drainage under USS control. If it recurs, laparotomy with drainage of the cyst into the posterior wall of the stomach may be required (cystogastrostomy).

TUMOURS OF THE PANCREAS

Carcinoma of the pancreas

Adenocarcinoma of the pancreas is increasing in frequency in the age range 40–60 years. It is rarely curable because of local invasion or lymph node metastases before it has been detected. Early diagnosis is difficult. Some 60% occur in the head of the pancreas, 25% in the body and the remainder in the tail. Risk factors include diabetes mellitus, alcoholism, cigarette smoking. It is more common in workers in the chemical industry.

Symptoms and signs. Epigastric pain. Deep, boring back pain. Jaundice (head of pancreas, secondaries in porta hepatis). Weight loss, fatigue, malaise, indigestion, pruritus. Palpable epigastric mass. Palpable gallbladder (Courvoisier's law – 'if in the presence of jaundice the gallbladder is palpable, the cause of the jaundice is unlikely to be stones'). Hepatomegaly. Thrombophlebitis migrans. Rarely splenomegaly due to splenic vein thrombosis from direct invasion of latter. Virchow's node.

Investigations
- Hb
- FBC
- ESR
- LFTs
- Blood sugar
- FOBs positive
- USS: often small mass obscured by bowel gas
- CT scan (→ Fig. 14.24) degree of invasion, metastases, guided biopsy
- PET scan: invasion, metastases
- MRCP/ERCP: duct obstruction and may show tumour.

Treatment
- Pancreaticoduodenectomy (Whipple's operation) for carcinoma of the head of the pancreas (→ Fig. 14.25). This involves a partial gastrectomy, partial

Figure 14.24 CT scan of the upper abdomen. There is a carcinoma in the pancreas (arrow).

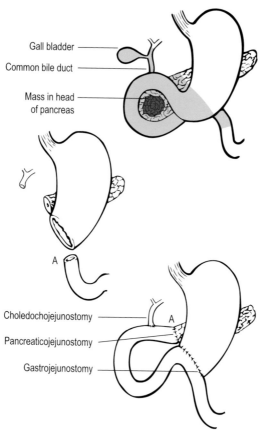

Gall bladder

Common bile duct

Mass in head of pancreas

A

Choledochojejunostomy

Pancreaticojejunostomy

Gastrojejunostomy

Figure 14.25 Pancreaticoduodenectomy (Whipple's operation). The shaded area is excised.

pancreatectomy, and distal choledochectomy and cholecystectomy. Continuity is re-established via a Roux-en-Y choledochojejunostomy, pancreaticojejunostomy and gastroenterostomy. Operative mortality is high. Relatively few cases are suitable for this operation and the cure rate is very low.

- Total pancreatectomy for extensive tumour.
- Tumours in the tail may be treated by distal pancreatectomy.
- Palliative decompression and relief of jaundice can be treated by 'triple bypass', i.e. cholecystojejunostomy (to drain bile past the obstruction from gallbladder to jejunum), jejunojejunostomy (to prevent food passing up into the

Figure 14.26 Triple bypass for carcinoma of the head of the pancreas.

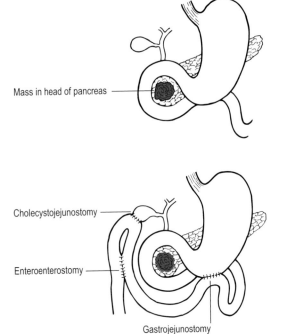

Mass in head of pancreas

Cholecystojejunostomy

Enteroenterostomy

Gastrojejunostomy

gallbladder), and gastrojejunostomy (to ensure adequate drainage of food from the stomach should the tumour invade the duodenum) (→ Fig. 14.26).
- As the prognosis is poor and many cases are inoperable at presentation, endoscopic stenting to relieve the jaundice is becoming the treatment of choice.

Prognosis. Many patients are dead within 6 months of presentation. Even with apparently operable lesions, only 5–10% of patients survive 5 years.

Endocrine tumours of the pancreas
Rare. Include gastrinomas (see Zollinger–Ellison syndrome, above), insulinomas and, more rarely, glucagonomas and VIPomas.

Insulinoma
Some 80% are solitary benign tumours of the β cells; 10% are malignant and 10% are multiple. They produce insulin and the symptoms are related to this.

Symptoms and signs
Related to cerebral glucose deprivation. These include weakness, sweating, palpitations, memory lapse, bizarre behaviour, coma. Hypoglycaemic episodes are usually precipitated by fasting and relieved by food.

Related to GI tract. These are hunger, abdominal pain and diarrhoea. Symptoms relieved by eating. Often excessive appetite with weight gain. The classical diagnostic criteria are known as 'Whipple's triad':

- Attacks are precipitated by fasting
- Blood sugar is low during an attack
- Symptoms are relieved by the administration of glucose.

Investigations
- Fasting blood sugar
- Plasma insulin
- Glucagon provocation test: infuse glucagon i.v., an elevated insulin level is diagnostic
- CT scan to localize tumour
- Rarely, selective angiography may be required
- Intraoperative ultrasound.

Treatment. Because of malignant potential, treatment should be surgical exploration and excision.

SPLEEN

SPLENOMEGALY

The spleen must be enlarged to about three times its normal size before it becomes clinically palpable. The lower margin may feel notched to palpation. It may become so large that it is palpable in the RIF. Massive splenomegaly in the UK is likely to be due to CML, myelofibrosis or lymphoma. Splenomegaly may lead to hypersplenism, i.e. pancytopenia as cells become trapped in an overactive spleen and are destroyed. Anaemia, infection, or haemorrhage may result. (For causes of splenomegaly → Table 14.5.)

Indications for splenectomy

These are: trauma; as part of other operative procedures, e.g. radical gastrectomy, splenorenal shunting; haematological disease, e.g. haemolytic anaemia, ITP; tumours; cysts; occasionally for diagnosis.

Effects of splenectomy

Haematological
- Leukocytosis
- Thrombocytosis – platelet counts rise after splenectomy and may reach 1000×10^9/L. Peak rises usually at 7–10 days. There is little evidence to support an increased risk of thromboembolic disease. Full anticoagulation is not indicated, although prophylactic aspirin may be given if the platelet count is very high.
- Abnormal blood film
  — nuclear remnants (Howell–Jolly bodies)
  — denatured haemoglobin (Heinz bodies)
  — iron granules (Pappenheimer bodies).

TABLE 14.5 Causes of splenomegaly

Infective	
Bacterial	Typhoid
	Typhus
	Tuberculosis
	Septicaemia
	Abscess
Viral	Glandular fever
Spirochaetal	Syphilis
	Leptospirosis
Protozoal	Malaria
Parasitic	Hydatid cyst
Inflammatory	Rheumatoid arthritis
	Sarcoid
	Lupus
	Amyloid
Neoplastic	Leukaemia
	Lymphoma
	Polycythaemia vera
	Myelofibrosis
	Primary tumours
	Metastases
Haemolytic disease	Spherocytosis
	Acquired haemolytic anaemia
	Thrombocytopenic purpura
Storage diseases	Gaucher's disease
Deficiency diseases	Pernicious anaemia
	Severe iron deficiency anaemia
Splenic vein hypertension	Cirrhosis
	Splenic vein thrombosis
	Portal vein thrombosis
Non-parasitic cysts	

Immunological. Splenectomy removes secondary lymphoid tissue. The spleen is a major site of phagocytosis, antibody production ($\downarrow$ IgM), opsonization of bacteria. It is also a major reservoir for lymphocytes.

Post-splenectomy management

Patients who have undergone splenectomy are more susceptible to infection from capsulated organisms, e.g. *Streptococcus pneumoniae*, *Haemophilus influenzae* and *Neisseria* species. Infections with these organisms can lead to overwhelming post-splenectomy infection. This has an insidious presentation with a prodromal illness, confusion, nausea and collapse; >50% are due to *Strep. pneumoniae*. The risk is greatest in young children. In patients in whom splenectomy is a planned procedure, vaccination against pneumococcal infections should be given prior to splenectomy. In children prophylactic penicillin should be given for at least 2 years post-splenectomy and some authorities recommend continuing until 18 years old. In patients having emergency splenectomy the procedure should be covered with penicillin; some authorities recommend that this should be continued for 2 years. Vaccination should be administered postoperatively. A polyvalent pneumococcal vaccine (Pneumovax) is given. Protection lasts 4–5 years after which revaccination is advisable. Vaccination against *H. influenzae* type B (HiB) and meningococci A and C should also be given. Patients should also be informed of the increased risk of infection in areas where malaria is endemic.

Rupture of the spleen (→ Ch. 4)

Spontaneous rupture

May occur when the spleen is the site of disease, e.g. infectious mononucleosis, malaria, lymphoma, leukaemia, typhoid. In any disease where there is splenomegaly trivial trauma may cause splenic disruption.

Procedures

Right hemicolectomy

- Make a midline incision centred on umbilicus.
- Carry out a laparotomy. Check for liver metastases.
- Incise the lateral peritoneal attachment of the right colon and mobilize it from the posterior abdominal wall.
- Identify and preserve gonadal vessels, the ureter and second part of the duodenum.
- Mobilize the hepatic flexure by dividing the greater omentum from the right extremity of the transverse colon.
- Once the right colon is mobilized identify the ileocolic and right colic vessels. Ligate and divide them close to their origins so as to remove any affected lymph nodes.
- Mobilize the terminal ileum up to 15 cm from the ileocaecal valve.
- Divide the transverse colon and terminal ileum between clamps.
- Close the end of the transverse colon with either staples or two layers of PDS sutures.
- Close the end of the terminal ileum in similar fashion.
- Re-establish continuity by side-to-side ileo- transverse anastomosis using a staple gun or PDS sutures.
- Bring out a drain through a separate stab incision in the abdominal wall.
- Close the abdomen in layers.

Hartmann's procedure

- Long midline incision.
- Carry out a full laparotomy to determine the nature of the lesion, e.g. malignancy or diverticular disease.
- Depending on the degree of contamination, consider resection and primary anastomosis with covering loop ileostomy. If not feasible, proceed to Hartmann's procedure.
- Mobilize left colon to sacral brim.
- Identify ureter and gonadal vessels.
- Ligate inferior mesenteric artery, preserving left colic artery.
- Ligate inferior mesenteric vein.
- Carry out radical excision if carcinoma, i.e. ligating inferior mesenteric artery close to aorta.
- Resect specimen.
- Oversew or staple rectal stump.
- Create a site for colostomy.
- Construct colostomy in left iliac fossa.
- If contamination, carry out copious lavage with normal saline.
- Insert drain through a separate stab incision to pelvis.
- Close incision.

Peripheral vascular disease

ARTERIAL

History
Peripheral vascular disease usually affects the lower limb but may affect the upper limb, GI tract, cerebral vessels and renal vessels. Risk factors include smoking, hypercholesterolaemia (family history), hypertension, diabetes and thrombophilia.

Clinical features
Features of the history depend on the system involved.

Limbs
Intermittent claudication is the classic symptom of peripheral vascular disease involving the lower limb. It is a pain in the muscle due to ischaemia brought on by exercise and relieved by rest. It is consistently brought on by the same degree of exercise. It is typically cramping in nature and is most common in the calf (superficial femoral artery disease) or buttock (aorto-iliac disease). It can vary with temperature, e.g. it is worse in the cold and it is more severe when going uphill. The main differential diagnosis is spinal claudication (pain is present at rest and is relieved by leaning forward, i.e. it may be better going uphill) and venous claudication (the pain is 'bursting' and takes longer to go at rest). Any sudden deterioration in the claudication distance requires urgent assessment. More severe disease may result in the complaint of 'rest pain'. This is a constant pain, typically in the feet and occurring at night while in bed (due to ↓ cardiac output therefore ↓ BP and peripheral vasodilation, all of which leads to decreased blood supply). It is relieved by hanging the leg out of bed or walking. Gravity increases the blood flow and hanging the leg out of bed cools it and therefore decreases metabolism and hence requires less blood flow. Eventually gangrene, i.e. tissue necrosis, may supervene. Males with aorto-iliac disease may complain of buttock claudication and impotence (Leriche's syndrome).

Other systems
A history should be sought for symptoms involving other areas of the vascular system, e.g. cardiac (MI, angina); GI system (upper to central abdominal cramping pain coming on about 20 min after a large meal – 'mesenteric angina');

cerebrovascular: (1) carotid (anterior circulation): stroke, TIAs, transient blindness, i.e. amaurosis fugax; (2) vertebral (posterior circulation): dizziness, drop attacks, bilateral blindness, diplopia, vertigo, problems with stance/gait; and renal (hypertension).

Examination

The patient's limb should be examined in a warm room.

Inspection

Check the colour of the limb. An ischaemic limb may be as white as marble (acute ischaemia) or show varying degrees of pallor, purple/blue cyanosis or a red shiny appearance (chronic ischaemia). Look for scars from previous vascular procedures. In the male, the ischaemic leg is typically hairless. The vascular angle (Buerger's angle) is the angle to which the leg must be raised before it becomes white. Normally the straightened leg can be raised to 90° and the toes will stay pink. In a severely ischaemic leg elevation to 15° may cause pallor. Following elevation, the limb is placed in the dependent position and in the presence of severe ischaemia a purple/red colour occurs as the foot is reperfused. In a normal limb, the veins should be full even when the patient is horizontal. In the ischaemic foot, veins will be collapsed and look like pale blue gutters in the subcutaneous tissue. This is the sign of guttering of the veins. Inspect the pressure areas (heel, tips of toes, ball of foot, head of fifth metatarsal) for signs of trophic changes, ulceration or gangrene; inspect between the toes.

Palpation

Check the skin temperature. Check the capillary refilling time, i.e. press the tip of the nail or pulp of the toe or finger for 2 s and observe the time taken for the blanched area to turn pink. In the normal digit this should occur immediately. Delay (>2 s) will occur in the ischaemic digit. Palpate and record all the pulses. They should be assessed for strength (assessed as normal, weak or absent). Pulses should be recorded as shown in Table 15.1 and the presence of any aneurysmal dilatation noted.

TABLE 15.1 Tabulation of pulses

Pulses	R	L
Radial	++	++
Brachial	++	++
Subclavian	++	++
Carotid	++ (bruit)	++
Femoral	++	++ (bruit)
Popliteal	+	−
Posterior tibial	−	−
Dorsalis pedis	−	−

++, normal volume; +, diminished volume; −, absent.

Auscultation

Listen along the course of all the major arteries for bruits. Listen to the arteries in the neck, the abdomen and the groin. Measure the BP in both arms to exclude subclavian disease. The Ankle-Brachial Pressure Index (ABPI) should be measured in the lower limb.

Procedure

How to perform ABPIs

The ABPI provides a measure of the severity of peripheral vascular disease. A ratio of 0.9–>1 is considered normal; 0.5–0.9 equates to the presence of intermittent claudication and <0.5 is defined as critical ischaemia. ABPIs are measured by placing a cuff around the patient's ankle and using a hand-held Doppler probe, the dorsalis pedis (DP) and/or posterior tibial (PT) pulses are detected. The cuff is then inflated above the systolic pressure and deflated until the signal returns. This is repeated for both DP and PT pulses. Brachial artery pressure is then measured and the ratio calculated. In diabetic patients, the arteries may be incompressible and lead to falsely elevated levels.

ARTERIAL OCCLUSIVE DISEASE

Acute arterial occlusion

This is defined as a deterioration in the blood supply of the leg that leads to rest pain or signs of severe ischaemia of less than 2 weeks' duration. This may range from a patient without PVD who has an embolic occlusion and presents with a dramatically ischaemic limb to a patient with chronic PVD who develops severe new onset rest pain.

Causes

Embolus. This may come from the heart (left auricular thrombus in AF, mural thrombus following MI, vegetation secondary to valvular lesions, atrial myxoma) or it may come from proximal atherosclerotic plaques or from thrombus within aneurysms.

Thrombosis. This usually occurs in an area of arteriosclerotic narrowing due to plaque rupture. There is usually a history of claudication or rest pain prior to the acute event. It may also occur with popliteal aneurysm, a blocked bypass graft and thrombotic conditions, e.g. antiphospholipid syndrome.

Trauma. This may be: penetrating trauma; a result of arterial catheterization or angioplasty; following a limb fracture, e.g. popliteal artery damage following supracondylar fracture of the femur; brachial artery damage following a supracondylar fracture of the humerus in a child; accidental intra-arterial injection, e.g. a misplaced injection in an intravenous drug abuser.

Symptoms and signs

Acute embolus in a normal limb. The classical symptoms are the six 'Ps': pain, pallor, paraesthesia, paralysis, pulselessness and perishing cold. Not all these symptoms are present in every case and the most reliable of these signs are paralysis and paraesthesia. In a patient with an embolic source of occlusion and with no previous PVD and thus no preformed collateral circulation, the ischaemia is sudden and profound and muscle may only survive for 6 h from the onset of symptoms. It is therefore necessary to establish the exact time of onset of symptoms.

Acute-on-chronic ischaemia in a limb with PVD. In contrast, a patient with chronic limb ischaemia may not present so acutely and the limb will certainly survive longer periods of ischaemia. In either group, the presence of sensory changes or calf tenderness on squeezing or passive dorsiflexion of the foot and toes indicates impending muscle infarction and requires immediate revascularization. After 6 h there is vasodilatation and release of deoxygenated blood as a result of tissue hypoxia. This leads to a more mottled appearance that still blanches on pressure. At this stage, the leg may be saved by prompt surgery. After 12 h, the arteries and veins thrombose, capillaries rupture and there is fixed staining that does not blanch. At this stage, the limb is unsalvageable and revascularizing the limb is inappropriate and may lead to mortality due to release of potassium, lactic acid, etc.

Investigations
- FBC
- U&Es
- Glucose
- Clotting screen
- Cross-match
- CXR
- ECG
- Duplex Doppler
- Angiography (catheter angiogram or CT/MR angiogram) – only indicated in patients who do not have an immediately threatened limb
- Echocardiogram – usually performed at a later date to identify cardiac sources of emboli.

Treatment. Initial management involves ABC – patients may be compromised secondary to arrhythmias or other cardiac events and often have significant co-morbidities. Anticoagulate with heparin. Administer analgesia. Administer oxygen via facemask.

The further management depends on the clinical condition of the limb. Options include:

Embolus in a normal limb. The diagnosis is clinical (angiogram is unnecessary) and the patient should be taken to theatre immediately for embolectomy.

Thrombosis in a limb with PVD. In these patients the presentation may not be as dramatic. Angiography can provide much information about the cause of ischaemia. Treatment options include: surgical thrombectomy; bypass grafting; thrombolysis – provided that the limb will survive for at least 12 h to give time for clot dissolution.

In all patients, fasciotomy should be considered to prevent compartment syndrome after revascularization. In some patients where ischaemia is considered irreversible, a primary amputation may be performed. However, in some cases with major co-morbidities, terminal care may be more appropriate.

Prognosis. Ideally, surgery should be undertaken within 6–8 h of onset of symptoms if a good result is to be obtained. Delay in treatment increases the incidence of amputation and mortality. The mortality from embolic episodes is 20–30% irrespective of the treatment of the emboli. The mortality is more a consequence of the co-morbid conditions or the cause of the emboli.

Chronic arterial occlusion

Lower limb (aorto-ilio-femoral disease)

Causes. Invariably due to arteriosclerosis, usually consequent on smoking. Arteriosclerosis may involve the arteries of the lower limb singly or in combination. Typical patterns include aorto-iliac disease, isolated iliac stenoses and superficial femoral occlusion. Other causes include multiple recurrent small emboli, vasculitis, fibromuscular dysplasia, Buerger's disease, cystic adventitial disease (especially in the young), popliteal entrapment (especially in the young), polycythaemia and Takayasu's disease (rare).

Symptoms and signs. Intermittent claudication affecting the calf (block in the superficial femoral artery), the thigh (block in the external iliac artery) or buttock (block in the lower aorta or common and internal iliac arteries). Occlusion of the aortoiliac segment associated with buttock claudication and impotence is known as Leriche's syndrome. Rest pain may develop involving an aching pain in the toes and forefoot that appears when the patient lies horizontal. It is relieved by hanging the foot over the side of the bed. Ischaemic ulcers and gangrene may supervene. Ischaemic ulcers tend to develop at pressure areas, e.g. bunion area, tips of toes, lateral aspect of head of fifth metatarsal and around the heel. The foot may be cold, pale and show venous guttering and dependent rubor. Absent or reduced pulses. Palpable thrills. Bruits.

Investigations
- Haemoglobin
- FBC
- ESR
- U&Es
- Glucose
- Lipids
- CXR
- ECG
- Treadmill test to assess claudication distance
- Duplex ultrasound – non-invasive; gives information about the degree of stenosis by visual estimation and velocity measurement
- ABPIs, i.e. ankle–brachial ratio. Normally, this is between 1 and 1.2. Pressures around 0.8 are compatible with claudication and pressures around 0.4 with rest pain. Pressures below 0.4 indicate severe ischaemia and are usually associated with ulceration and gangrene
- CT/MRI angiogram (Figs 15.1, 15.2) – non-invasive but does not allow intervention
- Angiography(by direct arterial puncture) – invasive and thus has complications (haematoma, dissection, emboli, false aneurysm, contrast reaction and contrast nephrotoxicity) but allows therapeutic interventions to be performed (see below).

Figure 15.1 MRA aorta and iliac vessels. There is a tight stenosis at the origin of the left external iliac artery (large arrow) involving the origin of the internal iliac artery which is occluded. There is also a stenosis at the origin of the right external iliac artery (small arrow).

Figure 15.2 MRA femoral vessels. There is a block in the left (superficial) femoral artery in the adductor canal (arrow). The distal artery fills via numerous collaterals.

Treatment

Medical. Mild to moderate claudication that is not disabling does not require surgical treatment. Advice is given to patients to lose weight, stop smoking, exercise regularly within their claudication distance. Advice is also given on foot care, particularly chiropody. Antiplatelet agents should be given, usually aspirin, but in patients who will not tolerate aspirin, an alternative antiplatelet agent should be prescribed, e.g. clopidogrel. Correct any cholesterol or triglyceride abnormality with a statin. There is clear evidence that cardiac events can be reduced by up to one-third by reducing low density lipoproteins/cholesterol by one-third, regardless of the baseline cholesterol, down to a total cholesterol of 3.5 mmol/L by use of a statin. Control hypertension. Nicotine patches to help stop smoking. Drugs such as naftidrofuryl and cilostazol have been used and may increase pain-free walking distance. Infusions of Iloprost (a prostacyclin analogue) are occasionally used in critical ischaemia with no hope of reconstruction but are rarely helpful. Regular patient follow-up is required. Patients should be encouraged to seek medical advice if claudication suddenly deteriorates or rest pain develops.

- *Endovascular.* Intervention consists of angioplasty ± stenting. Intervention may be divided into supra-inguinal and infra-inguinal:
  — *Supra-inguinal.* Angioplasty of aorto-iliac disease is relatively straightforward and results in good patency rates. The use of stents is generally reserved for sub-optimal angioplasty (i.e. residual pressure gradient across the stenosis) or a technical complication such as dissection.
  — *Infra-inguinal.* Endovascular intervention is not as successful for infra-inguinal disease. For femoro-popliteal disease, the long term patency rates are lower. However, lesions in the superficial femoral and popliteal artery are often suitable for intervention. Stents are not generally used unless due to procedural complications. In critical ischaemia sub-intimal angioplasty can be used to recanalize occluded vessels with good rates of limb salvage.

Chemical lumbar sympathectomy with injection of phenol under radiological guidance can occasionally be used in patients with unreconstructable disease in an attempt to control pain.

Surgical. Surgical options include endarterectomy, bypass (supra-inguinal and infra-inguinal) and primary amputation.

- *Endarterectomy.* Performed for flow limiting common-femoral/profunda femoris origin disease. This essentially involves dissecting out the occluding plaque and closing the vessel with or without a patch to allow increased blood flow.
- *Bypass*:
  — *Supra-inguinal.* Surgical methods of treating aorto-iliac disease include aorto-bifemoral bypass, ilio-femoral bypass or femoro-femoral cross over grafts (for unilateral iliac occlusion).
  — *Infra-inguinal.* There are numerous options. These include femoro-popliteal bypass (above or below knee) and femoro-distal bypass (to posterior tibial, anterior tibial, dorsalis pedis or peroneal arteries). Ideally reversed vein should be used, usually the great saphenous vein, as is offers better patency rates and lower risk of infection. If vein is unavailable then prosthetic material such as ePTFE may be used. They may be used with a collar/cuff of vein at the anastomosis to improve patency, i.e. Miller cuff, Taylor patch or St Mary's boot.
- *Amputation.* Areas of tissue loss may be amputated after arterial reconstruction has been performed and the tissues have demarcated. However, in some cases of critical ischaemia where reconstruction is not an option and pain is uncontrolled or the leg is not viable, the only option is primary amputation.

Prognosis. The majority of patients with intermittent claudication are managed conservatively with <7% progressing to critical ischaemia. Patients with critical ischaemia have a poor prognosis, 50% dying within 5 years.

Upper limb

Causes. The upper limb is significantly less affected by peripheral disease with most episodes of acute ischaemia being secondary to emboli. Thoracic outlet syndrome (see below) may be responsible for claudication or rest pain. Distal arterial disease may be due to embolization from an area of dilatation or frank aneurysm just beyond the subclavian artery compression.

Symptoms and signs. Emboli usually lodge in one of three sites in the brachial artery: (1) proximally at the origin of the profunda brachii; (2) at the mid-arm level at the origin of the superior ulnar collateral artery and (3) distally at the brachial bifurcation. It is rare for emboli to lodge in the subclavian or axillary arteries. Symptoms and signs are similar to those in the lower limb, as are the initial investigations.

Treatment. Analgesia. Oxygen. Intravenous heparin 5000 units. Embolectomy in the acutely ischaemic limb. Thrombolysis. Conservative management with an i.v. heparin (the rich collateral circulation in the upper limb means that the limb is not always acutely threatened).

CEREBROVASCULAR DISEASE

Some 80% of strokes are ischaemic and 20% are haemorrhagic. Atherosclerosis is the commonest cause and usually affects the internal carotid artery just distal to the common carotid bifurcation. Disruption of a plaque at this point can lead to thrombus formation and secondary embolism, leading to a stroke or TIA. A stroke is defined as a focal neurological deficit of >24 h of presumed vascular origin. A TIA has a similar definition but lasts <24 h. In practice, TIAs often last <30 min.

Symptoms and signs. These may be classed as carotid (anterior circulation) or vertebrobasilar (posterior circulation).

- Carotid. Paralysis or numbness of the contralateral arm or leg or temporary loss of vision of ipsilateral eye (amaurosis fugax). Dysphasia
- Vertebrobasilar. Bilateral motor/sensory signs, dysarthria, bilateral visual loss, balance problems, nystagmus and homonymous hemianopia. The presence of a carotid bruit has no real clinical relevance as it can be present with a non-significant stenosis and absent with a severe stenosis. Examination may reveal reduced carotid pulses or bruits over the carotid artery.

Investigations
- FBC
- U&E
- Cholesterol
- Clotting screen
- Glucose
- Thrombophilia screen (younger patient)

- Autoimmune screen (younger patient)
- ECG. Arrhythmias may cause embolic strokes.
- Echocardiogram – if embolic source is suspected
- CT scan – identify cerebral infarcts or haemorrhage or rare causes of CVA, i.e. cerebral tumour or abscess
- Duplex. Identification of significant stenosis of the internal carotid artery on the affected side (remember right-sided symptoms would be from a left carotid stenosis and vice versa). If an internal carotid artery is occluded, then surgery is pointless
- Carotid angiography – rarely performed nowadays as small risk of stroke associated with the procedure
- MR angiogram (Fig. 15.3) – largely replaced carotid angiography in the assessment of internal carotid disease.

Treatment. Management depends on two factors, i.e. degree of stenosis and whether it is symptomatic or asymptomatic. Patients with a carotid stenosis of <50%, whether symptomatic or not, should be managed medically. Patients with a symptomatic stenosis >50% are generally best treated by carotid endarterectomy.

Figure 15.3 MRA carotid artery. (A) Common carotid artery. (B) Internal carotid artery. (C) External carotid artery. (D) Vertebral artery. There is a tight stenosis (arrow) of the internal carotid artery.

Asymptomatic patients with stenosis >60% are best treated by carotid endarterectomy. Another group of asymptomatic patients that often require intervention are patients undergoing coronary artery bypass grafting. In these patients, a high grade stenosis (i.e. >90%) or a combined stenosis (right and left carotid) >150% are indications for treatment.

Medical. Medical management of internal carotid artery stenosis consists of:

- Risk factor modification – control BP, control diabetes, stop smoking, treat high cholesterol.
- Statins are used to treat high cholesterol but also reduce the number of strokes and major cardiovascular events even with normal cholesterol.
- Anti-platelet drugs – treatment with aspirin alone, in combination with dipyridamole or clopidogrel alone are acceptable treatment.

Endovascular. Recent trials have suggested higher rates of stroke with internal carotid stenting. As such, most centres would reserve its use for patients unfit for carotid endarterectomy or with contraindications to carotid endarterectomy such as previous neck radiotherapy or neck scarring around the operative site.

Surgical. Operative treatment of carotid artery stenosis is carotid endarterectomy. This involves opening the artery longitudinally and creating a subadventitial plane to remove the arteriosclerotic plaque. The operation may be performed under GA or with a local anaesthetic regional cervical block. A carotid shunt (taking blood from common carotid to internal carotid) may be used. Generally, all GA cases will use a shunt while cases performed under LA will use a shunt selectively depending on the patient's neurological condition after the application of clamps. A Dacron patch is used to close the arteriotomy after endarterectomy to prevent later stenosis.

Complications of carotid endarterectomy include bleeding, infection (very rare but catastrophic given the presence of a prosthetic patch), MI, stroke (in the region of 2–4% risk and may occur via embolism caused by dissection technique or postoperative thrombosis secondary to an intimal flap), nerve damage (marginal mandibular nerve, hypoglossal, vagus, superior laryngeal and recurrent laryngeal).

RENOVASCULAR DISEASE

Hypertension may be caused be renal hypoperfusion with release of renin from juxtaglomerular cells with activation of angiotensin. The most common causes are arteriosclerosis and fibromuscular dysplasia of the renal arteries. Arteriosclerosis usually involves the origin of the artery and occurs in the older patient. Fibromuscular dysplasia affects the middle to distal part of the artery and usually occurs in the younger patient. Renal artery stenosis has been shown to increase 5-year mortality in patients with peripheral vascular disease and in coronary artery disease it has been shown to double the risk of death, despite coronary revascularization.

Renal artery stenosis is an important, and potentially correctable, cause of renal failure in the older patient. The diagnosis of renal artery stenosis is frequently made following a deterioration of renal function in patients commenced on angiotensin-converting enzyme (ACE) inhibitors or angiotensin II receptor (AR) blockers.

Symptoms and signs. Hypertension – either symptomatic or picked up on routine examination, e.g. insurance medical. Rapid onset or accelerated hypertension. Hypertension in a young adult or child. Hypertension refractory to treatment. Sudden deterioration in renal function. Deterioration in renal function after ACE inhibitors or AR blockers. Occasionally it may be picked up on an IVU when a non-functioning or poorly functioning kidney is noted. It may be picked up when there is a small kidney on CT or the presence of a bruit in the flank. Flash pulmonary oedema.

Investigations
● Duplex scanning
● CT/MR angiography
● MAG3 scan with and without captopril – this can demonstrate any difference between the two kidneys and if this is exacerbated by an ACE inhibitor.

Treatment. A stenosis of >50% is considered significant and critical if >70%. Treating the stenosis is no guarantee that either hypertension or renal failure will improve. Current indications for intervention include: ↓ renal function or ↑ BP despite maximum medical treatment; flash pulmonary oedema; rapid onset renal failure; renal failure in patients with cardiac disease while taking ACEI or AR blockers; loss of renal mass on conservative treatment; progression of stenosis.

Treatment options include medical, radiological and surgical.

Medical. Control BP. Antiplatelet drugs. Statins. Good diabetic control. Lifestyle changes, i.e. stop smoking. Diet.

Endovascular. Options include angioplasty alone or with stenting. Offers good results, particularly with fibromuscular dysplasia.

Surgery. Occasionally indicated. Options include bypass, endarterectomy and patch, nephrectomy + bench surgery and auto-transplantation. Nephrectomy (if kidney unsalvageable).

VISCERAL ISCHAEMIC DISEASE

Visceral ischaemic disease covers a number of conditions including acute mesenteric ischaemia, chronic mesenteric ischaemia and acute mesenteric venous thrombosis.

Acute mesenteric ischaemia

This carries a very high mortality rate as a result of late diagnosis and due to its relative rarity. Causes are generally embolic or as a result of in situ thrombosis on an underlying stenosis. Less common causes include non-occlusive infarction (due to low flow states, i.e. hypotension and inotropes), vasculitis, fibromuscular dysplasia, aortic dissection and thrombosis of visceral arterial aneurysm.

Symptoms and signs. Embolus classically presents as acute severe abdominal pain with few clinical signs. Vomiting or diarrhoea, which may be bloody. There may be a history of atrial fibrillation, sepsis, oral contraceptive, 'mesenteric claudication' (chronic mesenteric ischaemia), portal hypertension. The pain experienced is usually out of proportion to the early physical findings. Subsequently, the patient will develop fever, abdominal tenderness, distension and ultimately peritonitis and shock.

Investigations
- FBC
- WCC ↑
- HCO_3 ↓
- Serum lactate ↑
- Serum amylase may be raised with infarcted bowel (confusion with acute pancreatitis)
- AXR – may not be helpful or show air/fluid levels
- CT with i.v. contrast may show signs of bowel ischaemia
- Angiography (duplex ultrasound for the diagnosis of acute mesenteric ischaemia is highly unreliable)
- Laparotomy provides the diagnosis in most cases.

Treatment. Urgent laparotomy. Venous thrombosis (see below) without infarction requires anticoagulation. If the patient does not improve within 12 h, a 'second look' laparotomy may not be required to assess intestinal viability.

In the case of arterial occlusion, there is extensive irreversible ischaemia if surgical treatment may be possible. If the length of non-viable bowel is not excessive, then surgical resection with stoma and mucous fistula may be appropriate. Patients are left with a short segment of bowel and consequent metabolic problems. If no pulse is present in the superior mesenteric artery, then an embolectomy should be performed. If a tight stenosis is found to be present at the origin of the superior mesenteric artery, bypass grafting or endarterectomy should be carried out.

Chronic mesenteric ischaemia

Visceral occlusion is usually due to arteriosclerosis. In practical terms the superior mesenteric artery is most often involved.

Symptoms and signs. Cramping upper abdominal pain approximately 30 min after a meal ('mesenteric angina'). This usually lasts 1–3 h. Patients always have weight loss because of 'food fear' due to the pain caused by eating. Frequently they also have diarrhoea. An upper abdominal bruit may be audible. Occlusive vascular disease is likely elsewhere.

Investigations
- Duplex scanning
- MR angiography.

Treatment. Treatment is by endovascular techniques or surgery. Endovascular treatment involved angioplasty ± stenting. Surgery involves endarterectomy with patching or bypass from aorta to distal superior mesenteric artery using either reversed vein or Dacron.

Acute mesenteric venous thrombosis

This is less catastrophic than acute arterial occlusion. Presentation may be more prolonged over several weeks; 75% of cases are due to hypercoagulability, intra-abdominal sepsis and portal hypertension.

Symptoms and signs. Abdominal pain which may get worse after eating and over time. Diarrhoea. Vomiting.

Investigations
- Duplex Doppler
- CT with contrast.

Treatment. Treatment depends on the clinical condition of the patient. If the patient has peritonitis then a laparotomy should be performed and any non-viable bowel resected and any source of intra-abdominal sepsis addressed. However, if the patient is stable then it may be managed conservatively with heparin and lifelong warfarin therapy. If CT shows no intra-abdominal cause, a thrombophilia screen should be carried out prior to commencing anticoagulation.

ANEURYSMS

An aneurysm is an abnormal dilatation of an artery. Aneurysms may be true or false (see below). A true aneurysm contains all layers of the vessel wall and appears as either a fusiform or a saccular dilatation. True aneurysms are commonest in the infrarenal aorta, iliac vessels, common femoral and popliteal arteries. A false aneurysm may occur anywhere and is usually the result of trauma. (For Classification of aneurysms → Table 15.2.)

Aortic aneurysms

An aorta may be aneurysmal from the ascending aorta to the aortic bifurcation. Aortic aneurysms can be divided into thoracic (→ Ch. 9), thoracoabdominal or abdominal alone. Abdominal infrarenal aortic aneurysm is the most common type.

Aetiology. Aneurysms are due to degeneration of the arterial media, particularly a reduction in elastin. The exact aetiology of aortic aneurysms is unknown but contributing factors include: (1) elastin degradation due to increased levels of metalloproteinases; (2) flow dynamics –the infrarenal aorta is a common site as pulse pressure here is maximal due to tapering calibre and reflected waves from the bifurcation; (3) hypertension – involved in formation but also rate of expansion; (4) atherosclerosis – not causally linked but often also present; (5) collagen defects, e.g. Marfan's disease and Ehlers Danlos syndrome; (6) genetic association – 25% of first degree relatives will develop an aneurysm; (7) smoking – associated with more rapid expansion; (8) association with emphysema and inguinal hernias; this may relate to a collagen defect but the exact link is unclear.

TABLE 15.2 Aetiology of aneurysms

True	
Congenital	Berry aneurysm of circle of Willis
	Aneurysmal varix associated with arteriovenous fistula
Acquired	Trauma: irradiation
	Infection: syphilis, mycotic aneurysm
	Degeneration: arteriosclerosis, cystic medical necrosis
False	Trauma

Symptoms and signs. Often asymptomatic and picked up on abdominal examination for other conditions or ultrasound scanning for other conditions. Symptomatic ones often cause backache by pressure on the adjacent lumbar vertebral bodies or abdominal pain. Examination reveals a pulsatile abdominal mass just above the umbilicus. Look for other peripheral artery aneurysms (especially popliteal).

Investigations

- USS to assess the maximum diameter of the aneurysm, and relationship to renal arteries
- CT scan
- Investigations to assess patient's fitness for surgery – FBC, U&E, clotting studies, ECG, chest X-ray, lung function tests, ABGs, echocardiogram.

Complications. These include:

- Rupture with retroperitoneal haemorrhage or intraperitoneal haemorrhage, or into the IVC (AV fistula)
- Distal emboli
- Severe back pain due to erosion of the lumbar vertebral bodies
- Thrombosis with distal ischaemia.

Treatment. Once diagnosed, the investigations depend upon the size of the aneurysm. If <5 cm, then the patient is kept under surveillance. Surveillance is yearly if <4.5 cm and 6-monthly if >4.5 cm. Once over 5 cm, the patient undergoes a number of investigations to assess suitability for surgery. The threshold for treatment remains a diameter of >5.5 cm. Once 6 cm the annual risk of rupture is around 10–20%. If the patient is frail with poor morbidity, no treatment may be appropriate. For those suitable for treatment, either endovascular repair (EVAR) or open repair may be undertaken. EVAR is not suitable for all aneurysms but confers a much lower earlier mortality than open repair and may be attractive for high risk cases. Open repair involves an in-lay Dacron graft or a Dacron Y graft to the iliac arteries or femoral arteries. Mortality for elective surgery should be <10%. Mortality rate is more related to MI and CVA than to direct complications of surgery to the aneurysm.

Ruptured aortic aneurysm (→ Fig. 15.4)

Classically, the patient presents with severe abdominal pain radiating to the back or iliac fossa and is associated with collapse or a hypotensive episode. A pulsatile mass may be palpable. Intraperitoneal rupture is instantly fatal; retroperitoneal rupture may tamponade the bleeding allowing the patient to reach hospital. Patients with ruptured aneurysms survive to reach hospital because of vasoconstriction, abdominal tamponade, development of a prothrombotic state and the development of 'controlled' hypotension. The infusion of even modest amounts of crystalloid or colloid rapidly upsets that fine balance. If the patient requires significant volumes of fluids to maintain blood pressure on the way to hospital or in the emergency room, then it is very unlikely that that patient will survive surgery. A patient who is conscious and talking has an adequate blood

Figure 15.4 CT scan of the abdomen showing a large leaking abdominal aortic aneurysm. Note the areas of calcification in the wall of the aneurysm. There is evidence of leakage to the left of the aneurysm (arrow).

pressure. Rarely the aneurysm may rupture to the right into the IVC causing a massive AV fistula with severe heart failure and massive lower limb oedema.

Investigations. If the diagnosis is clinically obvious, the patient is transferred immediately to the operating theatre for repair. If the diagnosis is in doubt and time allows, a CT scan should be performed (USS will show an aneurysm but *not* a rupture).

Treatment. Emergency repair should be undertaken once blood is available. Open repair is with an in-lay Dacron graft or a Dacron Y graft. Some centres are performing emergency EVAR with good results. The postoperative mortality is between 30% and 50%. Postoperative morbidity is high and results from haemorrhage, ARDS, ARF, multi-organ failure, MI, stroke, and colonic ischaemia. Late complications include graft infection, often with aorto duodenal fistula and life-threatening haemorrhage. This requires graft removal and bilateral axillofemoral grafting. However, extra-anatomical bypass is becoming less popular as they reinfect. *In situ* replacement with vein graft (femoral vein) or antibiotic-soaked graft (rifampicin).

Inflammatory aneurysm

Around 5% of aneurysms are described as inflammatory. This inflammation extends through all layers of the aorta. It obscures tissue planes and makes operative dissection particularly challenging. In severe cases, the inflammation may extend into the retroperitoneum to involve the IVC and ureters (ureters may require preoperative stenting).

Iliac artery aneurysm

These may involve the common iliac and internal iliac artery. The external iliac is almost never involved. They are usually present in association with aortic aneurysm. Aneurysms of the internal iliac are a particular challenge as operative access is difficult. They may rarely occur in isolation. Management options include:

- Surgical repair using a Dacron graft
- Endovascular stenting
- For internal iliac artery aneurysms, ligation if there is a patent internal iliac artery on the opposite side.

Femoral aneurysms

These usually involve the common femoral artery.

Symptoms and signs. Usually asymptomatic pulsatile mass in the groin. May be associated abdominal aortic aneurysms. Symptoms include compression of local structures, thrombosis and ischaemia, distal emboli and rupture. False aneurysms are common in the femoral artery and may result from:

- percutaneous catheterization for angiography; stab wounds
- previous surgery, especially with prosthetic grafts (infection).

Treatment. Small true aneurysms (<2.5 cm) may be treated expectantly unless symptomatic. Rapidly expanding true aneurysms require surgery. Stenting may be carried out but surgery is the preferred method of repair. Iatrogenic false aneurysms are being increasingly treated by compression therapy, usually with an ultrasound scan probe and thrombin injection.

Popliteal aneurysm

This is the commonest site for aneurysms after the aorta. Of patients with AAA, 10% have a popliteal aneurysm; 40% of patients with a popliteal aneurysm have an AAA. They are bilateral in 50% of cases.

Symptoms and signs. Pulsatile mass in the popliteal fossa. If a medical student can palpate a popliteal pulse easily, it may be aneurysmal. Complications include thrombosis with compromise of the distal circulation and distal embolism, compression of local structures, e.g. popliteal vein with DVT and rupture (rare).

Treatment. Treatment is considered when the size is >2 cm. Surgery is the preferred method of treatment but endovascular stenting may be considered for high risk patients. Stenting is carried out using a special prosthesis that allows bending at the knee. Surgical repair is either by an exclusion bypass (with ligation of the popliteal artery above and below the aneurysm) or an in-lay graft.

Visceral artery aneurysms

Aneurysms may arise from the splenic artery, hepatic artery, superior mesenteric artery or renal arteries.

Symptoms and signs. Visceral aneurysms may produce abdominal or flank pain. Renal artery aneurysms may cause haematuria or hypertension. Diagnosis is confirmed by ultrasound scanning and arteriography.

Prognosis. Splenic artery aneurysms may affect women during the child-bearing years. Rupture is an uncommon but major complication and tends to occur in the third trimester of pregnancy and is associated with a high mortality rate. If splenic artery aneurysms are picked up incidentally and are >2.5 cm, then treatment should be considered. Treatment is often possible with embolization under angiographic control. Hepatic artery aneurysms are prone to rupture. The mortality rate for surgery on visceral aneurysms is high, particularly if they rupture.

False aneurysms

A false aneurysm is a pulsating haematoma, the cavity of which is in direct continuity with the lumen of an artery. It is contained by a fibrous capsule consisting of adventitia and surrounding tissues rather than the layers of the vessel wall. False aneurysms can result from trauma, occur at the site of anastomosis, maybe secondary to i.v. drug abuse or iatrogenic following insertion of percutaneous catheters, i.e. at angiography. As flow through the defect continues, the aneurysm will slowly expand and may be extremely rapid if infection is present, e.g. in intravenous drug abusers. Presentation is with a pulsatile mass, usually in the groin, or with rupture. Diagnosis is usually via duplex ultrasound. Management depends on the cause and size of the aneurysm:

- If <2 cm, they will usually spontaneously thrombose
- Compression with an ultrasound probe until thrombosed. This may be combined with an injection of thrombin
- Surgical exploration and repair of defect
- Anastomotic false aneurysm may require revision (provided no infection is present)
- In IVDUs infection is often present and this may have destroyed the femoral vessels. Here, the only option is to ligate all vessels. This is associated with a high rate of limb loss or disabling claudication.

OTHER VASCULAR PROBLEMS

Thromboangiitis obliterans (Buerger's disease)

This affects small vessels of the extremities. It occurs almost exclusively in young males who are heavy cigarette smokers. It may be associated with migratory thrombophlebitis.

Symptoms and signs. Claudication in the muscles of the foot. Digital pain, cyanosis, coldness progressing to necrosis and gangrene. Ankle and wrist pulses disappear first and the proximal pulses remain normal. Progressive digital ischaemia occurs with eventual loss of feet and hands.

Investigations. Arteriography reveals discrete foci of occlusions alternating with apparently uninvolved arterial segments in the distal circulation.

Treatment. It is essential to stop smoking to avoid progression of the disease. Sympathectomy is only of temporary benefit – if the patient continues smoking, amputation is necessary for rest pain or gangrene. Reconstructive surgery is rarely possible because the disease involves the small distal vessels. Repeated prostacyclin infusions (Iloprost) may be beneficial.

Raynaud's phenomenon

This is a vasospastic condition of diverse aetiology. The following conditions have been implicated:

- Systemic diseases or conditions, e.g. collagen diseases (scleroderma), cryoglobulinaemia, myxoedema, macroglobulinaemia
- Compression syndromes, e.g. carpal tunnel syndrome, cervical rib, thoracic outlet syndrome
- Occupational trauma, e.g. vibration-induced white finger (pneumatic drill, chainsaw, grinders), piano playing, typing, cricket.

Symptoms and signs. Sequential changes of pallor, cyanosis and rubor, particularly after exposure to cold. This represents vasoconstriction followed by reflex vasodilatation. In severe long-standing cases tissue necrosis may occur involving non-healing ulcers and gangrene of the extremities. Tissue necrosis always denotes underlying pathology, i.e. the patient has secondary Raynaud's as opposed to primary Raynaud's disease.

Investigations
- FBC
- Platelets
- ESR
- CXR (cervical rib)
- Cold agglutinins
- Serum protein electrophoresis
- Autoantibody screen
- Rheumatoid factor
- LE cells
- Arteriography.

Treatment
- Treatment of underlying disorder, e.g. excise cervical rib
- Avoidance of cold exposure – heated gloves and boots
- Stop smoking
- Advice from Raynaud's and Scleroderma Association
- Drugs, e.g. calcium channel blockers (nifedipine), naftidrofuryl, i.v. prostaglandins (Iloprost)
- Plasmapheresis
- Sympathectomy (relatively ineffective)
- Very rarely amputation may be required.

Diabetic foot

Contributory factors include microangiopathy, peripheral neuropathy, impaired immunity, impaired tissue metabolism, and the glucose-rich environment, which favours bacterial overgrowth.

Symptoms and signs. The patient may present with either a neuropathic foot or an ischaemic foot with signs of both large and small vessel disease. The neuropathic and ischaemic elements frequently co-exist.

The neuropathic foot is warm, dry with palpable pulses. Calluses may be present, as may painless penetrating ulcers at pressure points and sites of minor injury. Painless necrosis of the toes may occur. Spreading infection can occur along plantar spaces. There is usually general loss of pain and thermal sensation. In severe cases, Charcot's joints may result.

The ischaemic foot is cold with absent pulses, calluses, painful ulcers, claudication and rest pain.

Investigations
- FBC
- U&E
- Glucose
- HbA_{1c}
- Blood culture if systemically unwell
- X-ray foot for osteomyelitis
- Duplex ultrasound
- ABPIs to assess extent of vascular disease.

Treatment
Neuropathic foot
- Control diabetes
- Stop smoking
- Lose weight
- Refer for chiropody to remove calluses
- Treat infections with antibiotics. Antiseptics and dressings may be required for ulcers
- Remove necrotic tissue
- Ray amputations with filleting out of dead tissue until healthy bleeding tissue is obtained
- Weight-bearing areas should be protected by specialized footwear.

Ischaemic foot
- Control diabetes
- Stop smoking
- Lose weight
- Chiropody
- Treat infection with antibiotics
- MRA with a view to possible arterial reconstruction or angioplasty
- Major amputations, e.g. below knee or above knee; minor amputations are rarely successful when the major element is ischaemic.

Thoracic outlet syndrome
This represents a variety of symptoms related to arterial, venous and nerve compression as they exit from the chest. Compression usually occurs in the area bounded by the clavicle, the first rib and the scalenus anterior muscle. Causes include:

- An anatomically tight thoracic outlet and compression occurs between 1st rib and clavicle

- Hypertrophy of the scalene muscles
- Cervical rib (present in <1% of population)
- Fibromuscular band (from C7)
- Clavicle or 1st rib fractures or exostoses.

Symptoms and signs

Neurological. More common cause. Presents with sensory and motor deficit in the distribution of C8/T1. Symptoms can be exacerbated by movement or arm position and tend to be worse at night.

Arterial. Less common. Claudication or rest pain. Distal arterial disease may be due to embolization from an area of dilatation or frank aneurysm just beyond subclavian artery compression. Raynaud's phenomenon may be present.

Venous. Venous hypertension – compression of subclavian vein or axillary vein thrombosis (Paget–von Schrötter syndrome).

Investigations

- CXR: cervical rib (the CXR should include the thoracic inlet and the total number of ribs on a particular side counted – if there are 13, then a cervical rib is present)
- Duplex Doppler – in positions of provocation, e.g. with the arm raised above the head, will give more functional information about the impingement on the subclavian artery than will angiography
- MRA: to assess vessel compression (with stress views) – subclavian artery stenosis or constriction by fibrous band
- Venography: compression of subclavian vein or subclavian vein thrombosis
- Nerve conduction studies to distinguish from carpal tunnel syndrome.

Treatment. With minimal neurological symptoms, shoulder girdle exercises may be appropriate. For severe compression, surgical decompression of the thoracic outlet with division of fibrous bands or removal of the first rib or cervical rib if present. Aneurysms may need to be resected and repaired. For patients presenting with primary axillary vein thrombosis (Paget–von Schrötter syndrome), treatment is with a combination of thrombolysis, anticoagulation and early decompression of the thoracic outlet.

Arteriovenous fistula

Two types exist:

- *Congenital* – May present as multiple small lesions. Present from birth. Clinically manifest 10–20 years. May enlarge to involve most of the limb
- *Acquired* – Due to trauma, e.g. stabbing, arteriography, iatrogenic for dialysis. Usually history of trauma and typically single communication.

Symptoms and signs. Pain and swelling in area of fistula. Enlarged tortuous arteries and veins. Increased skin temperature. Elongation of limb. Venous hypertension distally. Ischaemia distally. Palpable thrill. Continuous machinery bruit.

Investigations

- CXR for cardiomegaly
- Limb radiograph for bone elongation
- Duplex Doppler – non-invasive

- MRI: this will show the true extent of the lesion, which is nearly always more extensive than appears to be the case clinically
- Arteriography: this should only be performed if consideration is being given to embolization.

Complications. Cosmetic, haemorrhage, thrombosis, distal ischaemia, venous hypertension in limb, high output cardiac failure (Branham's sign – compression of the fistula results in a fall in the heart rate).

Treatment. Not all arteriovenous fistulae require treatment. Small peripheral fistulae may be observed and frequently will never cause difficulties. Indications for intervention include haemorrhage, expansion, severe venous or arterial insufficiency, cosmetic deformity and heart failure. Most fistulae are now managed by embolization under radiographic control. Simple ligation of feeding vessels should never be performed. Recurrence is inevitable and when recurrence does occur, previous ligation means that it is difficult to perform angiography and embolization. Embolization and excision may be required for very large lesions.

Vascular access for haemodialysis

Vascular access may be obtained either by a dual lumen catheter placed in a central vein (internal jugular, femoral or subclavian) or the creation of an arteriovenous fistula. Dual lumen catheters are often the first-line management for patients presenting with acute renal failure (as many as 30% of patients with renal failure present in the acute stage). Central lines may be tunnelled and used long term in some patients who have no alternative route for vascular access. Preferred long-term route for haemodialysis is via an arteriovenous fistula. This is created by anastomosing a superficial vein to a nearby artery. Flow in the vein significantly increases and over the next 4–6 weeks the veins will dilate and become suitable for needling. The most common form of fistula is the radiocephalic fistula created between cephalic vein and radial artery either at the anatomical snuff box or at the wrist. The fistula is usually created initially in the non-dominant arm (so as to be accessible for the patient to needle). In the event of failure of a radiocephalic fistula, or lack of suitable veins to create one in the first place, fistulae may be performed at the elbow (brachiocephalic fistula, brachiobasilic fistula) or ePTFE grafts may be placed in the forearm in either straight or looped configuration or as a loop in the thigh.

Complications
- Immediate – bleeding
- Early – infection and thrombosis
- Late – steal syndrome (the hand becomes ischaemic as blood is diverted into the fistula and away from the arteries supplying the hand); aneurysmal varix formation; high output cardiac failure; venous hypertension.

AMPUTATIONS

Indications for amputation
- Vascular, e.g. severe rest pain with arteries unsuitable for reconstruction, gangrene
- Trauma

- Infection, e.g. gas gangrene, osteomyelitis
- Tumour, e.g. osteogenic sarcoma, soft tissue sarcomas, subungual melanoma
- Useless limb, e.g. poliomyelitis, severe brachial plexus lesions associated with vascular damage.

Principles of amputation

- Select the appropriate level. Must be adequate circulation at that level to ensure healing. Tissues must show healthy bleeding at time of surgery
- Amputation level must take into account the fitting of a prosthetic limb
- Assess joints. Contractures or arthritis may influence the amputation level.

Preparation for amputation

A major amputation is a disfiguring operation. Fully explain the operation to the patient who may take a while to accept that it is necessary. Preoperative physiotherapy and occupational therapy should be undertaken and a visit made to the Limb Fitting Centre. Ensure that the patient is pain-free. Epidural anaesthesia may be useful in this context. Give antibiotic (penicillin) with induction of anaesthesia, which is prophylactic against *Clostridium perfringens* (gas gangrene).

Types of amputation

Minor

This involves simple amputation at the base of the digit, or 'ray' amputations where, e.g. in the foot, the metatarsal head and tendons are removed. This type of amputation is useful in diabetics, Buerger's disease and severe Raynaud's. Occasionally for ischaemia of all toes, transmetatarsal amputation may be undertaken. This requires a long plantar flap of skin to be successful. The indications are as above.

Major

Below-knee amputation. This provides the patient with the best chance of mobilizing with a prosthesis. Healing can be expected in 80% of patients. Below knee amputation is suitable in diabetics with a palpable popliteal pulse, Buerger's disease and in some patients with arteriosclerosis. Contraindications include ischaemia extending to involve the posterior skin flap, fixed flexion contractures and occlusion of the profunda femoris artery. The standard tibial stump is 8–12 cm long and the fibular is transected slightly higher. A long posterior flap with muscle is fashioned and this is folded over to cushion the bone end. Function is variable, less than half the patients being independently mobile at 2 years.

Gritti–Stokes amputation. This amputation involves opening the knee joint, transecting the femur just above the femoral condyles and folding the anterior portion of the patella over the end of the femur. It is claimed to result in less blood loss than above knee amputation, to provide a better lever in bed bound patients and, in bilateral amputees, provides a more stable sitting position.

Above-knee amputation. This is a common amputation in patients with arteriosclerosis. The stump of the femur is 25 cm long measured from the greater trochanter. Equal anterior and posterior myoplastic flaps sutured over the bone end.

Less-frequently performed amputations. These include Lisfranc (tarsometatarsal disarticulation), Chopart's (tarso-tarsal disarticulation) and Symes (ankle disarticulation). They are rarely used and are of historical significance only. Disarticulation at the hip and hindquarter amputations are usually performed for major trauma or malignancy, although they are sometimes used for vascular disease (aorto-iliac).

Postoperative care

Pain relief. The aim is to prevent breakthrough pain rather than treating pain once it occurs.

Care of the good limb. This involves physiotherapy. It is important to avoid pressure ulcers by nursing on sheepskin or air bed.

Physiotherapy. Build up muscle power and coordination. Start as soon as the patient is comfortable and continue in gymnasium. The aim is to prevent contractures and ensure rapid mobilization with prosthesis.

Prosthesis. Measure patient as soon as stump shrinks and volume of stump is stable.

Complications

Early. These include haemorrhage, haematoma, abscess, gas gangrene, wound dehiscence, ischaemic flaps and fat embolism.

Late. These include pain, sinus formation, osteomyelitis, neuroma, phantom limb and ulceration of the skin (pressure from prosthesis or continuing ischaemia).

VENOUS DISORDERS

VARICOSE VEINS

These are dilated tortuous veins. They are divided into primary and secondary.

Primary varicose veins are the most common and are often familial. They are possibly due to weakness of the superficial vein wall that allows dilatation of the valve ring allowing the valve to become incompetent with retrograde flow. This then leads to increased venous pressure and further valve failure. Other contributory factors include prolonged standing, family history, hormonal factors (more common in pregnancy – progesterone has an effect on the vein wall), ageing.

Secondary varicose veins may be classified as follows:
- Obstruction to venous outflow, e.g. pregnancy, fibroids, ovarian cysts, abdominal lymphadenopathy, pelvic cancer, iliac vein thrombosis or retroperitoneal fibrosis
- Valve destruction, e.g. DVT
- High flow and pressure, e.g. AV fistulae.

Symptoms and signs. Tortuous dilated veins of the great or small saphenous system. Aching discomfort worse towards the end of the day, relieved by sitting with legs elevated. May present with complications (see below). Examine the patient standing up and assess the site and size of the veins. Palpate for defects in the fascia. Check the state of the skin and subcutaneous tissue. Carry out Trendelenburg's test to assess the site of incompetent perforating veins. This is carried out with the patient supine, the leg being elevated and the tourniquet applied just below the saphenofemoral junction. The patient then stands erect for 30 s. If the saphenous vein fills rapidly from below with the tourniquet in place, the perforators lower down the legs are incompetent. If the long saphenous vein fills rapidly from above following removal of the tourniquet, the valve at the saphenofemoral junction is incompetent. Repeat at different levels down the leg to determine the level of incompetent perforators.

In practice, Trendelenburg's test is rarely used nowadays and has been replaced by hand-held Doppler machine (see below). If a swelling is apparent over the saphenofemoral junction (saphena varix), the diagnosis should be confirmed by placing the hand over the swelling and tapping the varicose veins lower down the legs. A palpable thrill at the groin will confirm the presence of a saphena varix. Auscultation over the veins should be carried out to exclude arteriovenous fistulae. Perthes test may be performed to exclude deep venous obstruction (tourniquet applied below the saphenofemoral junction and the patient has to exercise on the spot. Severe 'bursting' pain indicates obstruction of the deep venous system.) but this is usually assessed by duplex Doppler nowadays.

Investigations. Diagnosis usually made on clinical grounds with hand-held Doppler assessment. In difficult or recurrent cases, Duplex ultrasound may be used. If a secondary cause is suspected, then abdominal ultrasound can be performed.

Procedure

How to perform hand-held Doppler assessment of varicose veins

The patient is examined with the legs exposed from the groin downwards. The leg to be examined is turned outwards with the legs slightly apart. For SFJ incompetence, the femoral artery is located and the probe moved medially, squeezing and releasing the calf until antegrade blood flow is heard in the femoral vein (a 'whoosh' on compression but not on releasing). Move the probe inferomedially to identify the great saphenous vein. If there is reflux, this should be heard as a 'whoosh' with calf compression and a further 'whoosh' on releasing (lasting >1 s). The small saphenous vein can also be examined and this is done about 10 cm above the knee. The probe is moved from posterior to anterior while squeezing the calf. The saphenopopliteal junction is identified by turning the patient to face away from you, the popliteal artery is identified in the knee crease and moving medially, will identify the popliteal vein and lateral to it will be the small saphenous vein. Compression of the calf again allows determination of antegrade flow and any reflux.

Complications. Superficial thrombophlebitis. Haemorrhage. Varicose eczema. Varicose pigmentation due to haemosiderin deposition. Lipodermatosclerosis. Chronic venous ulceration. Long-standing venous stasis ulcers may become malignant (Marjolin's ulcer).

Treatment. Mild varicosities – compression stockings and periodic elevation of the legs. Small varicosities below the knee are suitable for injection with a sclerosing agent and compression bandaging worn for 2 weeks. This treatment can also be used for remaining varicosities after surgery. Surgery is indicated for saphenofemoral incompetence, saphenopopliteal incompetence, or thigh perforators. Mark out the varicose veins prior to surgery. Surgery includes

saphenofemoral disconnection and stripping for incompetence of the great
saphenous vein. Stripping is generally only performed to knee level.
Saphenopopliteal disconnection can be used for varicosities involving the small
saphenous system. Stripping is not performed, as this will risk damage to the
sural nerve. Stab avulsions through tiny incisions at previously marked sites are
used for residual veins. Compression bandaging is required postoperatively.
Encourage early mobilization. Walk for 5–10 min every hour during the day.
Sit with legs elevated postoperatively. Endoluminal techniques are being
increasingly used, which result in quicker recovery and reduced postoperative
pain. Techniques include laser and radiofrequency ablation.

DEEP VEIN THROMBOSIS (DVT)

This is a major cause of morbidity and mortality after surgery and trauma. It may occur
spontaneously with high oestrogen contraceptive pill. HRT may be an aetiological factor.
Only about 25% of DVTs cause symptoms and signs, others being silent. Pathological
features (Virchow's triad) leading to DVT include:

- Changes in the constituents of the blood
- Changes in the blood flow
- Changes in the vessel wall.

Predisposing factors include trauma and surgery, previous DVT, malignant disease,
prolonged bed rest, cardiac failure, oestrogen-containing oral contraceptive pill,
pregnancy, pelvic masses, obesity, dehydration, certain blood disorders, e.g.
polycythaemia, thrombophilia (protein C, protein S, anti-thrombin III deficiency; factor V
Leiden). In a UK study of all admissions to a district general hospital, 10% of all deaths
were due to pulmonary embolism. In addition, up to 30% of patients in hospital have
asymptomatic non-occlusive calf vein thrombosis.

Symptoms and signs. Swelling of the leg, tenderness of the calf muscles,
increased temperature of the leg. Homans' sign (calf pain on passive dorsiflexion
of the foot) is insensitive, non-specific and potentially dangerous. Occlusion of
the iliofemoral segment produces gross swelling of the whole limb, which is
painful and white (phlegmasia alba dolens). Complete blockage of the iliofemoral
segment with extension of thrombosis into venules and capillaries causes extreme
pain with bluish discoloration and impending venous gangrene (phlegmasia
caerulea dolens).

Investigations

- D-Dimer (cleavage fragment from formed thrombus – can be elevated in
  malignancy, infection and postoperatively)
- Duplex ultrasound
- Venography – very rarely indicated nowadays.

Treatment. The aims of treatment are to prevent propagation of the clot, minimize
the risk of pulmonary embolism (PE) and to reduce the chance of developing post-
thrombotic syndrome in the future.

Prevention. General measures include adequate hydration, avoiding calf pressure,
and early postoperative mobilization. Some authorities recommend stopping oral

contraceptives at least 6 weeks prior to surgery, while others merely recommend heparin prophylaxis. The case for stopping HRT is controversial. Patients at special risk should be treated as follows:

- Low molecular weight heparin, e.g. subcutaneous Clexane 20 mg daily
- Calf compression devices used intraoperatively
- Graded compression stockings, i.e. thromboembolic deterrent (TED) stockings. These should be worn preoperatively, intraoperatively and postoperatively until the patient is mobilizing satisfactorily.

Therapeutic. Once the diagnosis has been confirmed, then anticoagulation is commenced. This may be with i.v. unfractionated heparin or treatment dose of low molecular weight heparin. This is then converted to oral warfarin and maintained at an INR of 2–2.5 for 3–6 months. Limb elevation when resting. Calf exercises. Compression stockings. Surgery or an endovascular approach may be required. A reduction in post-thrombotic syndrome has been shown following early recanalization leading to preservation of valvular competence. However, in UK practice, it is usually only used if there is an extensive iliofemoral DVT in a young patient with a mechanical cause for the DVT or with a threatened limb with impending venous gangrene. Techniques used include:

- Catheter directed thrombolysis – catheter is directed into the thrombus for local delivery of thrombolytic agents
- Percutaneous mechanical thrombectomy – device used that actually breaks down the thrombus (may be combined with thrombolysis)
- Surgical thrombectomy – surgical removal of the thrombus.

In some cases, anticoagulation may fail, be contraindicated or result in complications. In these cases, an IVC filter may be required to prevent PE. Indications for a filter include:

- Contraindication to anticoagulation, e.g. risk of bleeding
- Thromboembolic event despite adequate anticoagulation
- Complication of anticoagulation, e.g. bleeding
- Inability to achieve adequate levels of anticoagulation
- Free-floating IVC thrombus.

CHRONIC VENOUS INSUFFICIENCY

This is caused by persistent and sustained ambulatory venous hypertension. Causes include:
- Muscle pump dysfunction, e.g. fused ankle in arthritis or neurological impairment after CVA
- Abnormal valve function which may be primary (affecting both the superficial and deep veins) or secondary after DVT with destruction of deep valves (known as post-phlebitic limb)
- Congenital valve absence (very rare).

Along with changes in the large veins that result in venous hypertension, there are several abnormalities at the microcirculatory level. These include:

- White blood cell trapping. WBCs become trapped in capillaries and cause endothelial activation and release of inflammatory cytokines which increase vascular permeability and contribute to the presence of a fibrin cuff together with release of proteolytic enzymes and free radicals. In addition they cause tissue ischaemia by blocking capillaries.
- Fibrin cuff. An increase in venous pressure is transmitted to the capillaries and opens endothelial pores resulting in molecules such as fibrinogen moving into the interstitial space. This polymerizes to fibrin and may act as a barrier to oxygen diffusion causing local tissue ischaemia.

Symptoms and signs

- Peripheral oedema. This gets worse towards the end of the day and tends to settle with elevation
- Varicose veins
- Venous eczema and brawny induration of the skin
- Venous pigmentation associated with haemosiderin deposits in the tissues
- Venous stasis ulceration, which is common in the area of the medial malleolus
- There is often severe pain associated with the swelling and ulceration
- Venous claudication. This indicates obstruction of the deep venous system. It is described as a 'bursting' pain which comes on with exercise and takes 10–20 min to settle.

Investigations

- Hand-held Doppler – to assess superficial venous incompetence and can allow assessment of arterial system (via ABPIs)
- Duplex Doppler – allows assessment of both superficial and venous systems
- Venography (rarely used).

Treatment. Difficult to treat and patient rarely gets complete relief.

Medical. Advise patient to avoid long periods of standing and to sit with legs elevated. Graduated compression stockings or 4-layer bandaging (ensure ABPI >0.8 before using compression). Treat venous stasis ulcers by reducing swelling of the leg by bandaging, excision of necrotic tissue and control of any cellulitis with antibiotics. Clean ulcers with normal saline, osmotic preparations, or enzymatic preparations. Emollients for venous eczema.

Surgery. Options for surgical intervention include:

- Superficial venous surgery. As for management of varicose veins and includes ligation of the SFJ and stripping of the GSV. Useful in isolated superficial reflux or combined deep and superficial reflux. Has been shown to aid healing of ulcers
- Perforator vein surgery. Involves use of an endoscope to locate and ligate venous perforators. Has been shown to achieve good rates of ulcer healing
- Deep vein surgery. Rarely indicated. Options include veno-venous bypass, vein transposition and vein valve transplantation
- Ulcer debridement and skin grafting
- Amputation. Carried out if ulceration becomes complicated or is intractable.

SUPERFICIAL THROMBOPHLEBITIS

This is characterized by a local inflammation of a segment of superficial vein. The vein is tender, red and feels like a 'cord'. The causes are shown in Table 15.3. Treatment is usually symptomatic and depends on the underlying cause. However, when it involves the great saphenous vein at the saphenofemoral junction, this has a risk of thromboembolism and is treated as for a DVT with anticoagulation or urgent ligation.

LYMPHOEDEMA

This is a condition of localized fluid retention and tissue swelling due to hypoplasia or obstruction of lymphatics. It may be primary or secondary.

Primary

Primary lymphoedema can be classified into two subsets: isolated, where the condition is not inherited and familial where there is a definite inherited trait. Further subdivisions can then be made according to the age of onset. Congenital hereditary lymphoedema presents at birth or within the first 2 years of life. Milroy's disease is an autosomal dominant familial form of congenital lymphoedema. Lymphoedema praecox occurs at puberty or shortly afterwards. Lymphoedema tarda occurs after the age of 30. However, lymphoedema presenting for the first time in later life should prompt a search for underlying malignancy, especially pelvic.

Secondary

Lymphatic obstruction may occur secondary to other disease processes, e.g. secondary neoplasms in lymph nodes, infection in lymph nodes, e.g. filariasis (common worldwide, rare in UK) or may occur following surgical removal of lymph glands, i.e. block dissection or radiotherapy.

TABLE 15.3 Causes of superficial thrombophlebitis

Varicose veins
Occult carcinoma:
- bronchus
- pancreas
- stomach
- breast

Mondor's disease – superficial thrombophlebitis on chest wall
Buerger's disease
Polycythaemia
Local bacterial infection
Polyarteritis
Iatrogenic – intravenous infusions
Drug abuse
Idiopathic

TABLE 15.4 Causes of swelling of the leg

Local	
Acute swelling	Trauma
	DVT
	Cellulitis
	Allergy
	Rheumatoid
	Ruptured Baker's cyst
Chronic swelling	Venous:
	• varicose veins (uncomplicated varicose veins rarely cause leg swelling)
	• obstruction to venous return, e.g. pregnancy, pelvic tumours, IVC
	• obstruction, post-phlebitic limb
	Lymphoedema
	Congenital malformations, e.g. arteriovenous fistulae
	Paralysis (failure of muscle pump)
	Dependency
General	Congestive cardiac failure
	Hypoproteinaemia, e.g. liver failure
	Nephrotic syndrome, malnutrition
	Renal failure
	Fluid overload
	Myxoedema

Symptoms and signs. There is progressive swelling of one or both extremities, usually beginning around the ankle but often involving the whole extremity. The scrotum may be involved. Oedema is non-pitting and does not settle with elevation. Often the leg aches and feels tight but there is no pain. Minor trauma will cause cellulitis. Need to differentiate from other causes of leg swelling (→ Table 15.4).

Investigations. Lymphoedema is essentially a clinical diagnosis and no further investigations are required in the great majority of patients. Where investigations are necessary, the following may be used:

● Lymphoscintigraphy
● Lymphangiography (used rarely). Isotope lymphoscintigraphy is easy to perform and less traumatic for patients than lymphangiography
● CT scan to exclude pelvic malignancy.

Treatment. It is important that lymphoedema is differentiated from other causes of lower limb swelling. Treatment is either medical or surgical. The aim of treatment is to control the oedema and to prevent infection. Compression stockings or compression devices (Flowtron therapy) are the mainstay of treatment. Check ABPIs before applying compression. Compliance is essential. Diuretics are contraindicated in lymphoedema. Avoid prolonged standing. Massage. Exercise. If any breaks in the skin occur, e.g. insect bites or minor trauma, antibiotics should be prescribed. Cellulitis and fungal infections should be treated promptly. Occasionally, surgical treatment is helpful but does very little to improve the cosmetic appearance. Surgery is only suitable for a minority of patients. The choices include reduction procedures (excess tissue is removed and the defect either closed directly or skin grafted) or bypass (via omental pedicles, anastomosing lymph nodes to veins or direct lymphovenous anastomosis). Complications include recurrent cellulitis and lymphangitis usually caused by *Streptococci*, which respond to penicillin. Lymphangiosarcoma may occur. The tendency is for steady progression of the swelling and recurrent infections.

VASCULAR TRAUMA

This includes penetrating trauma (90%), blunt trauma and iatrogenic trauma. In penetrating trauma, the vessel may be partially or completely transected. High velocity gun shot wounds cause massive tissue loss and extensive vascular damage. With blunt trauma, vessels can be injured directly, e.g. crush injury or indirectly by distraction, e.g. fractures and dislocations. Iatrogenic trauma may occur during surgery, angiography, angioplasty, or while obtaining access to the circulation, e.g. arterial lines and CVP lines. It may also occur with accidental intra-arterial injection, e.g. intravenous drug abusers. Prompt diagnosis and treatment are essential to save life and limb. Complete transection of an artery because of penetrating trauma may stop bleeding, owing to vessel retraction. Partial transection is more serious as the remaining intact wall holds the vessel open, resulting in torrential haemorrhage. Blunt injury usually leads to an intimal tear with a resulting intimal dissection flap, which may compromise the distal circulation. Arteriovenous fistula may occur when an artery and a vein close to each other are injured. Venous injuries are usually due to penetrating trauma. Haemorrhage and/or thrombosis may result.

Symptoms and signs. Mechanism of injury, degree of violence, type of weapon, time of incident. Hypotension. Hypovolaemic shock. Clinical signs can be divided into HARD signs (pulseless cold limb, expanding and/or pulsatile haematoma, palpable thrill or audible bruit and active bleeding) and SOFT signs (history of bleeding from wound, injury close to the course of a major vessel, haematoma, neurological injury). Associated injuries, e.g. nerve injuries, fractures, head injury.

Investigations. There may be no time for investigations, as urgent transfer to theatre may be required.

- Plain radiographs if time permits, e.g. fractures, position of bullets or foreign bodies
- Pulse oximetry can assess oxygen saturation in both limbs – a decrease may indicate injury
- ABPIs – compare injured to uninjured limb – a ratio of <1 in a healthy limb indicates vascular compromise
- Duplex ultrasound
- CT angiogram
- Angiography – this is both diagnostic and therapeutic (placement of covered stents for bleeding and stents for intimal flaps).

Treatment. Principles of treatment include:

- Arrest of haemorrhage
- Management of airway
- Correction of hypovolaemia

- Diagnosis of type and degree of injury
- Repair of vessels
- Management of associated injuries
- Rehabilitation.

Emergency measures. Initial management should be guided by ATLS principles with attention to airway and breathing first. Circulation is addressed with insertion of two large-bore i.v. lines and compression of any external haemorrhage *(tourniquet should not be used)*. Major thoracic penetrating injuries - emergency thoracotomy is occasionally necessary to control bleeding. In exsanguinating penetrating abdominal trauma, it may be necessary to perform a thoracotomy or laparotomy to cross clamp the aorta. Fracture/dislocations with obvious deformity and distal ischaemia need reduction and splinting. If no vascular injuries are obvious (i.e. no hard signs) then any investigations are carried out after the primary survey is completed and the patient is stable.

Principles of surgical management include:

- Fractures should be stabilized before vascular repair. A shunt can be inserted during orthopaedic repairs if necessary (suitable for large and medium sized arteries).
- Simple lacerations may be closed by direct suture.
- Lacerations in smaller arteries can be closed by a vein patch.
- In vessels that are transected, end-to-end anastomosis can be performed. If the ends are far apart, then an interposition graft using either reversed autologous vein or PTFE may be used.
- In complex injuries, bypass procedures may be required after ligation of major arteries. These may need to be extra-anatomic (i.e. running in a different course to the bypassed artery), to provide tissue coverage in major injuries.
- In some cases, the patient may be too unstable for complex vascular reconstruction. In these cases, vessels may be simply ligated (external carotid, subclavian artery, internal iliac artery may be ligated with little sequelae and virtually all veins other than the suprarenal IVC and portal vein can be ligated).
- Packing can be used for venous bleeding but it is unlikely to stop arterial bleeding.
- Fasciotomy should be performed in prolonged ischaemia to prevent compartment syndrome. Rarely, amputation may be required for the unsalvageable limb.

Complications. Thrombosis. Secondary haemorrhage. False aneurysm. AV fistulae. Compartment syndrome. Lymphatic leaks or lymphocele due to damage of lymphatic vessels. Distal vascular insufficiency. Ischaemic muscular contractures.

Procedure

Femoral embolectomy

The stages of a femoral embolectomy are as follows:

- A longitudinal incision is made in the groin over the femoral artery at the mid-inguinal point, i.e. halfway between the anterior superior iliac spine and the pubic symphysis. This is the surface marking of the femoral artery which will not be palpable due to the embolism.
- The incision is extended through the subcutaneous fat to the femoral vessels. The common femoral, superficial femoral and the profunda femoris arteries are dissected free and controlled with vascular slings.
- An arteriotomy is made in the artery directly over the origin of the profunda femoris artery. This may be a transverse incision which is less likely to lead to subsequent stenosis or longitudinal, which is easier to extend if a bypass operation becomes necessary.
- A 5F embolectomy catheter is passed up the common femoral into the iliac vessels. The balloon is inflated and gently withdrawn.
- Once the clot is retrieved, an assistant will need to control the inflow with the vascular sling and a vascular clamp (return of inflow with clot withdrawal will lead to a sudden gush of blood). This is repeated until no further clot is retrieved and the surgeon is happy with the inflow. The common femoral artery is then flushed with heparinized saline and clamped.
- A 4F embolectomy catheter is now passed down the profunda femoris artery and the superficial femoral artery. Once no more clot is retrieved and the surgeon is happy with the degree of back bleeding the vessels are flushed with heparinized saline and clamped.
- The arteriotomy is closed with interrupted 6/0 Prolene sutures.
- Fascia and subcutaneous fat is closed with 3/0 Vicryl and clips are used for skin closure.

CHAPTER 16

Urology

CONGENITAL DISORDERS OF THE URINARY TRACT

KIDNEY AND URETER

Congenital absence of one kidney. Incidence is 1:2500.

Pelvic kidney. Incidence is 1:800. Often associated with reflux or PUJO. Large pelvic kidney may interfere with childbirth.

Horseshoe kidney. Incidence is 1:1000 to 1:1800. The combined kidney lies lower than normal. Renal pelvis rotated anteriorly and the lower pole medially. Often associated with reflux, undescended testes.

Congenital hydronephrosis (PUJO). Aetiology unknown. Lower pole vessel may aggravate but rarely responsible for condition. Failure to thrive, recurrent UTI, mass, hypertension. Often discovered on prenatal USS.

Infantile polycystic disease. Incidence is 1:10 000. Rare, autosomal recessive.

Adult polycystic disease. Incidence is 1:1500. Autosomal dominant, involving both kidneys. Patients usually present aged 30–40 with hypertension, mass, haematuria, renal failure. May be associated with cysts in the liver. Family screening and genetic counselling.

Medullary sponge kidney. Incidence is 1:20 000. Characterized by congenital dilatation or cysts of the distal collecting ducts. May be associated with hypercalciuria, impaired urinary concentration.

Ureteric duplication. Often bilateral. The upper pole ureter lies medial and inferior to the lower pole ureter at the bladder.

Ureterocele. Dilatation of the submucosal portion of the ureter. Filling defect on IVU.

Megaureter. Secondary to either dysplastic (non-obstructed) or obstructed ureter. May be associated with stones, UTI, reflux.

Vesicoureteric reflux. Reflux is the abnormal passage of urine from bladder to the ureter. Primary reflux is due to a defect of the vesicoureteric junction. Usually resolving spontaneously in 70% of cases. Secondary reflux is usually due to outflow obstruction – 20% of children presenting with recurrent UTI have reflux.

Diagnosis. Voiding, micturating cystourethrogram.

Treatment. Consists of antibiotics, regular voiding, ureteric reimplantation.

BLADDER

Ectopia vesica (exstrophy of the bladder). This occurs in 1:20–40 000. It is more common in the male. The anterior wall of the bladder fails to close. The posterior bladder wall, the trigone and posterior urethra are exposed and urine leaks onto the skin. Associated anomalies include wide separation of the pubic symphysis with waddling gait, epispadias, umbilical and inguinal hernias, imperfectly descended testes, and rectal prolapse.

Complications. Ureteric dilatation and pyelonephritis.

Treatment. Involves reimplantation of the ureters into an ileal loop conduit with excision of the bladder and repair of the abdominal wall defect. In some cases, bladder reconstruction may be possible.

Urachal abnormalities. Defects may result from the primitive urachal connections between bladder and umbilicus. If the tract persists, urine may discharge from the umbilicus. An urachal cyst may occur if part of the urachus persists but is closed off above and below. Infection may occur in an urachal cyst. Treatment is by excision.

URETHRA

The urethra may terminate on the ventral aspect of the penis (hypospadias) or on its dorsal aspect (epispadias). Hypospadias may result in difficulty with intercourse. Plastic reconstruction of the urethra may be required. Epispadias is rare and more disabling and difficult to correct than hypospadias. It may be associated with incontinence. Plastic reconstruction or urinary diversions are possible treatments. In the female, the urethra may open on to the anterior vaginal wall.

Urethral valves may occur in the posterior urethra. The condition is rare, occurring with an incidence of 1:5000, 50% of cases occurring under 1 year of age. They cause dilatation of the prostatic urethra, bladder, ureters and pelvis. It is often diagnosed on prenatal USS. Rarely, there may be uraemia with palpable bladder and kidneys at birth. Milder cases present later in childhood with difficulty in voiding, recurrent UTIs and uraemia. Treatment is by transurethral resection of the valves. With early presentation the prognosis is good. With extensive renal damage, dialysis and transplantation may be required.

HAEMATURIA

Haematuria is the passage of red blood cells in the urine. This may vary from a few red cells detected on 'stix' testing to the passage of frank blood. Haematuria may be noted at the beginning of micturition, throughout micturition or at the end of micturition. Care must be taken to avoid menstrual bleeding being mistaken for haematuria. Other causes of red urine include excessive beetroot ingestion, rifampicin, porphyria, haemoglobinuria and myoglobinuria. (For causes of haematuria → Table 16.1.)

Symptoms and signs. Family history, e.g. polycystic kidney. Painless haematuria is suggestive of neoplasia. Loin pain or ureteric colic suggests stone or clot colic associated with tumour. Suprapubic discomfort suggests bladder stone. Terminal bleeding with pain suggests bladder calculus. Urethral bleeding independent of micturition suggests a urethral lesion. Check the drug history. Spontaneous bruising. Palpable kidney. Palpable bladder. Enlarged prostate on examination PR.

Investigations
- Hb, FBC
- ESR
- U&Es

TABLE 16.1 Causes of haematuria	
Kidney	Glomerular disease
	Polycystic kidneys
	Carcinoma
	Stone
	Trauma (including renal biopsy)
	Tuberculosis
	Embolism
	Renal vein thrombosis
	Vascular malformation
Ureter	Stone
	Neoplasm
Bladder	Carcinoma
	Stone
	Trauma
	Inflammatory – cystitis, tuberculosis, bilharzia
Prostate	Benign prostatic hypertrophy
	Neoplasm
Urethra	Trauma
	Stone
	Urethritis
	Neoplasm
General	Anticoagulants
	Thrombocytopenia
	Haemophilia
	Sickle cell disease
	Malaria

- LFTs
- Clotting screen
- Urine microscopy: red cells exclude haemoglobinuria and beetroot ingestion, white cells suggest infection, granular casts suggest nephritis
- Urine cytology
- CXR: secondaries, TB
- KUB
- IVU
- USS
- CT/MRI scan
- Flexible cystoscopy under LA: intravesical lesion, bleeding from prostate
- Ultrasound-guided renal or prostatic biopsy.

Treatment. Appropriate to the underlying condition.

OBSTRUCTIVE UROPATHY

> Hydronephrosis is the distension of the calyces and pelvis of the kidney owing to obstruction to the outflow of urine. It may be bilateral or unilateral. (For causes of hydronephrosis → Table 16.2.)

Symptoms and signs. Loin pain. Upper abdominal pain. Fever. Rigors – if infection. Ureteric colic. Hesitancy, poor stream, frequency, distended bladder with suprapubic discomfort. Uraemia may be presenting complaint. Palpable kidney. Palpable prostate.

Investigations
- Hb, FBC
- ESR
- U&Es
- LFTs
- MSU

TABLE 16.2 Causes of hydronephrosis	
Unilateral	Pelviureteric junction obstruction
	• congenital pelviureteric junction obstruction
	• aberrant renal vessels
	• calculus
	• tumours of the renal pelvis
	Ureteric obstruction
	• calculus
	• ureteric invasion, e.g. cervical, rectal or colonic tumours
	• iatrogenic – damage at surgery
Bilateral	Urethral valves
	Urethral or meatal stenosis
	Prostatic enlargement
	Extensive bladder tumours
	Retroperitoneal fibrosis

Figure 16.1 Intravenous urogram. There is a right-sided hydronephrosis and hydroureter. Note the dilatation of the pelvis with clubbing of the calyces and also dilatation of the ureter down to its entry into the bladder.

- KUB: enlarged renal outline, opaque calculi
- USS: confirms diagnosis and may demonstrate lesion
- IVU (→ Fig. 16.1): early stages show pelvic dilatation with clubbing of the calyces, site of obstruction, function of kidney, trabeculation of bladder, residual urine (if bilateral hydronephrosis and uraemia, no further information would be obtained from an IVU)
- CT scan
- Cystoscopy: cause of bladder outlet obstruction or bladder tumour
- Retrograde pyelogram defines exact site of obstruction.

Treatment. Directed at the underlying cause. With a small ureteric stone the obstruction may be relieved with the passage of the stone. The presence of acute infection or marked renal impairment requires urgent decompression of the urinary tract under antibiotic cover. This may be done by percutaneous nephrostomy, suprapubic cystostomy, ureteric catheter drainage or urethral catheter drainage. A non-functioning kidney, especially if infected, should be removed.

Complications. Infection: pyonephrosis. Stone formation in stagnant urine. Hypertension due to renal ischaemia. Traumatic rupture of a hydronephrotic kidney. Uraemia.

CALCULOUS DISEASE

Urinary calculi are often idiopathic. They also arise secondary to stasis and infection and also in association with metabolic disorders, e.g. cystinuria. Stones may form in the kidney or bladder. Ureteric calculi are in transit from the kidney to bladder. Stones occur in about 1% of the population. The majority is composed of calcium, magnesium ammonium phosphate, or urate.

Types of calculi

Calcium oxalate (75%). 'Mulberry' stones covered with sharp projections. They cause bleeding and are often black owing to altered blood on their surface. Because of their sharp surface they give symptoms when comparatively small. Occur in alkaline urine.

Phosphate (15%). Usually compound of calcium, magnesium and ammonium phosphate. Smooth and dirty white. They may enlarge rapidly and fill the calyces taking on their shape, i.e. staghorn calculus. Occur in strongly alkaline urine.

Urate (5%). Arise in acid urine. Hard, smooth, faceted and light brown in colour.

Cystine (2%). Usually multiple. Arise in acid urine and are of metabolic origin owing to decreased reabsorption of cystine from the renal tubules. White and translucent.

Xanthine and pyruvate stones. Rare. Due to inborn error of metabolism.

About 90% of calculi are radio-opaque. Usually only urates are radiolucent, cystine stones being radio-opaque because of their sulphur content. Precipitating factors include: diet, dehydration, stasis, infection, hyperparathyroidism, idiopathic hypercalciuria, milk-alkali syndrome, hypervitaminosis D, cystinuria, inborn errors of purine metabolism, gout, and chemotherapy (excess uric acid following treatment of leukaemia or polycythaemia).

Symptoms and signs

Renal calculi. May be asymptomatic even with large stone. Loin pain. Haematuria. Dysuria. Signs of uraemia. Colic if stone impacts in pelviureteric junction.

Ureteric calculi. Severe colicky pain radiating from loin to groin. Sweating. Nausea. Vomiting.

Bladder calculi. Dull suprapubic discomfort, terminal haematuria, dysuria, strangury. Patient may have loin tenderness, pyrexia if infection, kidney may be palpable with gross hydronephrosis or pyonephrosis.

Investigations. Emergency for severe renal pain or ureteric colic:

- Urine microscopy
- MSU
- U&Es
- KUB: 90% of calculi are radio-opaque
- CT – non-contrast CT.

Following acute attack or routine for urinary symptoms or incidental finding of stone:

- Hb, FBC
- ESR
- U&Es
- Creatinine
- Calcium
- Phosphate
- Uric acid
- 24-hour urine for calcium, phosphate, oxalate, urate, cystine
- KUB
- IVU
- USS
- Isotope renography to establish functional contribution of each kidney
- Cystoscopy
- Retrograde pyelogram.

Treatment. Acute symptoms – ureteric colic:

- Relieve pain – diclofenac sodium i.m. or p.r.; or pethidine.
- Admit to hospital
- Bed rest
- Intravenous fluids or increased oral fluids
- Collect and sieve all urine to retrieve calculus for analysis
- Check radiographs to assess progress of stone
- Stones <4 mm will usually pass spontaneously; 50% of stones between 4 mm and 6 mm will pass spontaneously. Stones >6 mm usually require removal
- Obstruction and infection require removal of stone
- Stone removal may be carried out by: ureteroscopy and fragmentation of the stone; pushing the stone back into the renal pelvis followed by fragmentation with extracorporeal shock wave lithotriptor.

Routine treatment of established urinary calculus. Removal of renal or bladder calculus by open surgical technique is now rare. Minimal invasive surgery using endoscopic techniques or extracorporeal shockwave lithotripsy is now the treatment of choice.

Percutaneous nephrolithotomy. A nephroscope is inserted into the kidney under radiographic control via a previously dilated track. The stone is then removed by grasping forceps (if small), ultrasonically disintegrated and removed by suction or disrupted into small fragments by electrohydraulic or laser lithotriptors.

Extracorporeal shockwave lithotripsy. This consists of an external energy source focused to provide a high-pressure zone that is directed to fragment the calculus. The calculus is fragmented into small particles, which pass in the urine.

Open surgery. This is used less often. A stone may be removed through the kidney substance (nephrolithotomy), or through the renal pelvis (pyelolithotomy).

Surgery may be needed to correct hydronephrosis associated with a stone. If the kidney is irreparably damaged, nephrectomy is required.

Bladder calculi. Small stones may be removed cystoscopically after crushing with a lithotrite or disintegration using an electrohydraulic lithotriptor. Large stones >5 cm are removed by suprapubic cystostomy.

The stone must be analysed. The underlying cause must be treated if possible, e.g. parathyroidectomy or correction of an obstructive lesion. Attempts should be made to prevent recurrence.

Prevention of recurrence. Up to 50% of patients may have recurrence within 5 years. Prevention involves: (1) high fluid intake, especially in hot weather; (2) reduce milk intake; (3) prompt treatment of urinary tract infections; (4) calcium stones: low-calcium diet, thiazide diuretics, acidify urine; (5) oxalate stones: reduce oxalate intake – exclude rhubarb, spinach, tomatoes, strawberries, tea and chocolate; (6) urate stones: allopurinol, urinary alkalinization.

TUMOURS OF THE RENAL TRACT

KIDNEY

Benign tumours are rare. Adenocarcinoma accounts for 80% of renal tumours. Transitional cell tumours occur in the renal pelvis. Squamous cell carcinomas may occur in the renal pelvis and are associated with squamous metaplasia due to chronic irritation caused by stone or infection.

Renal cell carcinoma

This arises from renal tubular epithelium. Males are affected twice as commonly as females. It usually occurs over the age of 40. There is increased incidence in smokers, coffee drinkers, industrial exposure to cadmium, lead, asbestos, aromatic hydrocarbons; renal cysts in dialysis patients; von Hippel–Lindau disease. Spread is by direct extension into perinephric tissues, by lymphatics to the para-aortic nodes, by the blood, along the renal vein (which may contain tumour), to bone, liver, brain and lung (cannon ball metastases).

Symptoms and signs. The most common presentation of renal cell carcinoma is now an incidental finding on an ultrasound scan performed for unrelated conditions. Haematuria, loin pain, PUO. Palpable mass, anaemia, polycythaemia. Symptoms and signs due to secondaries – hepatomegaly, breathlessness, pathological fractures.

Investigations
- Urinalysis
- Hb, FBC, ESR: anaemia, ESR raised, occasionally polycythaemia
- USS
- CT scan (→ Fig. 16.2) – now standard investigation – diagnosis of primary, lung metastases
- CXR: metastases.

Figure 16.2 Abdominal CT scan. There is a renal cell carcinoma of the right kidney.

Treatment. Nephrectomy. The majority of smaller tumours may be removed by the laparoscopic approach. Occasionally solitary metastases may be treated by surgery. Radiotherapy is palliative for pain due to metastases. Biological modifiers such as interferon, interleukins and tyrosine kinase inhibitors for metastatic disease.

Prognosis. If the tumour is localized to the kidney, nephrectomy offers a 5-year survival of 70%.

RENAL PELVIS AND URETER

These are either transitional cell tumours or squamous cell carcinoma in areas of squamous metaplasia. The tumour may seed down the ureter and involve the bladder.

Symptoms and signs. Haematuria. Infection secondary to hydronephrosis. Ureteric colic due to obstruction or clot.

Investigations
- Urinalysis
- IVU
- Cystoscopy to check for bladder seeding.

Treatment. Nephroureterectomy with excision of a cuff of bladder wall. Chemotherapy – as for bladder cancer.

BLADDER

Some 95% of tumours in the bladder are transitional cell carcinomas but chronic irritation from stones or infection may result in squamous cell metaplasia, giving rise to squamous cell carcinoma. Adenocarcinomas are rare. Aetiological factors include smoking, aromatic hydrocarbons (rubber and dye industry), bladder diverticulae, bilharzia. What were formally regarded as transitional cell papillomas are recognized as well-differentiated transitional cell carcinomas. True transitional cell papillomas are now considered to be extremely rare. Tumours are more frequent in the middle-aged and elderly and occur more frequently in males. Spread occurs by direct invasion into the prostate, urethra, sigmoid colon, rectum or, in the female, to the uterus and vagina. The ureteric orifices may be occluded giving rise to hydronephrosis and renal failure. Lymphatic spread is to the iliac and para-aortic nodes and blood spread occurs late to the liver and lungs.

Symptoms and signs. Painless haematuria. Dysuria, frequency, and urgency. Hydronephrosis. CRF. Pain from pelvic invasion. Examination is usually negative in the early stages. The tumour may be palpable by bimanual examination under anaesthesia.

- T1: Confined to mucosa or submucosa – impalpable
- T2: Superficial muscle involved – localized rubbery thickening
- T3: Deep muscle involved – mobile mass
- T4: Invasion beyond bladder to adjacent structures – fixed mass.

Investigations
- Hb, FBC
- ESR
- U&Es
- Creatinine
- MSU
- Urine cytology
- IVU: filling defects, hydronephrosis
- USS
- EUA to assess tumour spread
- Cystoscopy and biopsy
- CXR
- MRI: for staging of invasive bladder cancer
- Bone scan for metastases.

Treatment of transitional cell carcinoma
- T1: Transurethral resection or cystodiathermy. For multiple small tumours, intravesical chemotherapy with mitomycin or epirubicin. Intravesical BCG therapy is reserved for poorly differentiated superficial bladder cancer or carcinoma *in situ*.
- T2: T2 tumours and above invade the detrusor muscle by definition and should not be managed by transurethral resection alone. A radical cystectomy is the 'Gold Standard' treatment but radiotherapy may be effective in those not fit for surgery.

For T1 tumours there is a 70% chance of recurrence at 5 years and a 10% chance of developing invasive disease. Check cystoscopy should be carried out at regular intervals (6 months to a year) for life.

- T3: This may be treated by radiotherapy, cystectomy or a combination of both. Cystectomy requires urinary diversion by implantation of the ureters into an ileal loop or reconstruction using bowel to fashion a 'neobladder'. The latter can be drained by self-catheterization through a 'continent' stoma, or anastomosed to the urethra to allow normal voiding per urethram.
- T4: Palliative radiotherapy, systemic chemotherapy with cisplatin and gemcitabine may produce remissions.

Prognosis. Early tumours are curable. T1 tumours have an 85% 5-year survival rate, falling to 60% with T2. Approximately 40% of patients with T3 tumours are alive at 5 years. Patients with T4 tumours rarely survive for more than 1 year.

URINARY TRACT INFECTIONS (UTIs)

> These may be divided into those affecting the kidney (pyelonephritis) and those affecting the bladder (cystitis). UTIs are more common in women – the majority of women will have a UTI some time during their life. Risk factors include pregnancy, urinary tract malformations, urinary tract obstruction, calculus, prostatic obstruction, bladder diverticulum, spinal injury, trauma, urinary tract tumour, diabetes mellitus, immunosuppression.

Symptoms and signs
Acute pyelonephritis. This includes loin pain, dysuria, frequency, fever, rigors, cloudy or blood-stained urine. Tender in loin and flank.

Cystitis. Frequency, urgency, dysuria, haematuria, often no fever. Tenderness suprapubically or on examination PR or PV.

Investigations
- Urinalysis
- Microscopy
- Culture
- Hb, FBC
- U&Es
- Creatinine.

May be haematuria and proteinuria. Colony count of >100 000 organisms/mL of a fresh MSU is significant. Microscopy shows pus cells and organisms (usually Gram-negative rods). Common organisms include *Escherichia coli, Proteus, Klebsiella, Pseudomonas*, and faecal *Streptococci*.

Treatment. Drink plenty. Antibiotics – amoxicillin 250 mg t.d.s. or trimethoprim 200 mg b.d. are appropriate initial treatments. Change antibiotic according to organism and sensitivities. Avoid sexual intercourse while infected. If the infection fails to settle on appropriate antibiotics or recurs rapidly after stopping antibiotics, further investigation is required. Two or more UTIs in a female appropriately treated require further investigation. Failure to respond to treatment suggests inappropriate antibiotics, failure to complete the course of antibiotics, resistant organisms, underlying obstruction, calculus, tumour, urinary retention, or specific infection, e.g. TB. Further investigation of recurrent attacks includes ultrasound and cystoscopy.

Sterile pyuria

Pus cells are apparent on microscopy but there is no growth on culture. Causes include inadequately treated UTI, TB, tumour, stone, prostatitis, polycystic kidneys, appendicitis, diverticulitis or analgesic abuse.

Urinary tract tuberculosis

This has shown a decline in the past 30 years but it remains a problem in the Third World and the immigrant population in the UK. Genitourinary tuberculosis is always secondary to TB elsewhere. The urinary tract is involved by haematogenous spread. The kidney is affected most frequently, the lower urinary tract being secondarily infected by descending infection, giving rise to cystitis or infection of the epididymis or seminal vesicles.

Symptoms and signs. The renal lesion is often silent. Repeated UTIs with frequency, dysuria, haematuria. Occasionally dull loin pain. Weight loss, fever, night sweats. Symptoms of uraemia may occur. Epididymitis. Scrotal sinuses.

Investigation
- Hb, FBC
- ESR
- Urinalysis: pus cells, protein, red cells
- MSU: sterile pyuria
- Urine microscopy and ZN staining of early morning specimen of urine may demonstrate acid-fast bacilli
- Culture of tubercle bacilli positive (takes up to 6 weeks)
- CXR: may show primary lesion
- IVU: plain film may show calcification in the renal parenchyma; contrast film may show irregularity of the calyces, obliterated calyces, contractures of ureter or bladder, vesicoureteric reflux
- Cystoscopy: small-capacity bladder with tubercles
- Biopsy.

Treatment. Antituberculous drugs. Surgery may be needed to remove a totally destroyed kidney or to deal with complications, e.g. repair of ureteric stricture or enlargement of small fibrotic bladder (ileocystoplasty, i.e. enlargement of the bladder with a cuff of ileum).

PROSTATE

The three commonest conditions of the prostate are: bladder outflow obstruction due to benign prostatic hypertrophy (over 50s), prostatic cancer (over 65s) and prostatitis in young adults.

BLADDER OUTFLOW OBSTRUCTION

Benign prostatic hypertrophy

This affects most men over the age of 50 but only 10% present with symptoms. The size of the prostate does not correlate with the degree of obstruction. The severity of symptoms depends on the degree of encroachment on the prostatic urethra. Obstruction to outflow occurs and the bladder hypertrophies. Diverticulae of the bladder, urinary infection, hydronephrosis and renal failure may ensue.

Symptoms and signs. The cardinal symptoms are hesitancy (difficulty in starting) and a poor stream. Other symptoms are nocturia, frequency, dribbling, incontinence, acute retention. Haematuria from ruptured dilated bladder neck veins. Palpable bladder occasionally. Smell of stale urine on patient. Enlargement of kidney (hydronephrosis). Examination PR – smooth enlarged prostate, median sulcus, enlarged lateral lobes. Signs of uraemia.

Investigations
- Hb, FBC
- ESR
- U&Es
- Creatinine
- MSU
- USS: assess upper urinary tract (hydronephrosis), bladder, residual urine.

Treatment. Treatment of acute retention (see below). TURP with cystoscopy to check for diverticulae, tumour or stone. The resected prostate should be submitted to histology – unsuspected foci of carcinoma may be present.

Prostatic carcinoma

This is the commonest cancer in men – over 60% of tumours at presentation are localized to the prostate gland. It is rare below the age of 50. Of patients with prostatic cancer in the UK, 25% present with advanced disease, when potentially curative treatment is not possible. Early asymptomatic disease can be detected by prostate-specific antigen (PSA) testing; transrectal ultrasound scanning with guided biopsy. Foci of carcinoma may be found incidentally in specimens resected for bladder outflow obstruction. Spread occurs to adjacent organs, e.g. bladder, urethra and seminal vesicles. Spread to the rectum is rare. Lymphatic spread is to iliac and para-aortic nodes. Blood spread occurs early, especially to the pelvis, spine and skull (osteosclerotic lesions).

Symptoms and signs. Asymptomatic. Incontinence, dysuria, haematuria, hesitancy, dribbling, retention. Bone pain, pathological fractures, sciatica, anaemia, weight loss. Rectal examination may reveal nodule in prostate or hard craggy mass involving whole prostate. The median sulcus between the lobes may be obliterated. Palpable bladder. Tenderness over bones. Hepatomegaly.

Investigations
- Hb, FBC
- ESR

- U&Es
- Creatinine
- PSA: to facilitate early detection and evaluate response to treatment
- Transrectal ultrasound scan and guided biopsy
- CXR: metastases in lungs or ribs
- Bone radiograph: sclerotic deposits in pelvis, spine, or skull
- Bone scan is sensitive indicator of early metastases
- USS: residual urine, upper urinary tract obstruction
- If urinary obstruction, specimens may be obtained at TURP for histology.

Treatment. TURP for obstruction. Treatment for prostatic cancer depends on the staging of the disease. For patients with cancer localized to the prostate gland, the options would include observation with routine monitoring of PSA, external beam radiotherapy, interstitial brachytherapy or radical prostatectomy, which may be carried out as an open procedure, laparoscopically, or robot-assisted. External beam radiotherapy and hormones would conventionally treat locally advanced prostatic cancer. Androgen deprivation therapy for metastatic disease. Subcapsular orchidectomy slows tumour growth. Other techniques of hormonal manipulation include luteinizing hormone releasing hormone (LHRH) agonists, which produce a fall of luteinizing hormone (LH) from the anterior pituitary with consequent reduction of testicular secretion of testosterone, e.g. cyproterone acetate or bicalutamide. Stilboestrol is rarely used nowadays as it causes gynaecomastia, fluid retention and possible thromboembolic complications. Local radiotherapy, especially for bony metastatic pain. Systemic taxane-based chemotherapy for hormone resistant prostatic cancer.

Prognosis. Variable. Dependent on stage at presentation. Patients with clinically localized tumours treated radically may expect a normal life expectancy. Those with metastatic disease at presentation have a median 3-year survival.

Prostatitis

This occurs most commonly in young adults. Acute bacterial prostatitis usually presents as an acute febrile illness. Chronic prostatitis presents with recurrent UTIs. If there is a past history of TB anywhere in the body, suspect tuberculous prostatitis.

Symptoms and signs

Acute bacterial prostatitis. Fever, low back pain, perineal pain, bladder irritation, outflow obstruction. Enlarged tender prostate.

Chronic prostatitis. Symptoms of UTI. Dull perineal ache. Normal or indurated irregular prostate.

Investigations. In acute prostatitis:

- WBC raised
- MSU usually shows growth
- Blood culture may be positive.

In chronic prostatitis:

- Prostatic massage may yield secretions containing white cells and occasionally organisms
- Culture for TB in chronic prostatitis.

Treatment. Acute prostatitis is treated with bed rest, antibiotics (often i.v.) and analgesia. Prostatic abscess or chronic prostatitis may occur as a complication. Chronic prostatitis is treated with long-term antibiotics, e.g. ciprofloxacin for 4–8 weeks. Prostatic massage may be effective. Tuberculous prostatitis is treated with antituberculous therapy.

Urethral strictures

The causes include infection, trauma, foreign bodies, stones, iatrogenic, i.e. postcatheterization or instrumentation, and tumours.

Symptoms and signs. Weak stream, dribbling, acute or chronic retention, UTI.

Investigations
- Flexible cystoscopy under local anaesthetic
- Retrograde or antegrade cystourethrogram.

Treatment. Optical urethrotomy. Intermittent self-dilatation with LoFric catheters. Surgical reconstruction with skin flaps.

URINARY RETENTION

> The retention of urine may be acute, chronic or acute-on-chronic. Patients with acute retention present as surgical emergencies. (For causes of urinary retention → Table 16.3.)

TABLE 16.3 Causes of urinary retention

Local	
Urethral lumen or bladder neck	Urethral valves
	Tumours
	Stones
	Blood clot
	Meatal ulcer or stenosis
Urethral or bladder wall	Urethral trauma
	Urethral stricture
	Urethral tumour
Outside the wall	Prostatic enlargement
	Faecal impaction
	Pelvic tumour
	Pregnant uterus
	Phimosis
General	
Postoperative	
Neurogenic	Spinal cord injuries
	Spinal cord disease, e.g. tabes dorsalis, spinal tumour, multiple sclerosis, diabetic autonomic neuropathy
Drugs	Anticholinergics, antidepressants, alcohol

Symptoms and signs. Previous history of chronic retention. Poor urinary stream, frequency, UTI, urethritis, ureteric colic, haematuria. Backache. Neurological illness. Palpable bladder. Examination PR – prostatic enlargement. Palpate for urethral stone or stricture. Urethral meatus for ulcer. Signs of uraemia. Neurological signs.

Investigations

- Urine microscopy
- MSU
- Hb, FBC
- ESR
- U&Es
- LFTs
- CXR
- USS: to check for upper urinary tract obstruction due to back pressure, bladder tumour, stone
- Cystoscopy: urethral stricture or bladder tumour.

Treatment. Attempt catheterization after giving analgesia. If the catheter will not pass, carry out a suprapubic catheterization.

Postoperative retention may be due to anxiety, embarrassment, supine posture, pain, drugs, fluid overload, previous unrecognized prostatism with minimal symptoms. After urological procedures it may be due to blood clot in the bladder. Before catheterizing a patient in the postoperative period, other attempts should be made to allow the patient to pass urine, e.g. standing up in a warm room relaxed, running tap or bathing in warm water. A short period of intermittent self-catheterization often allows full recovery of bladder function and normal voiding within a few days.

Chronic retention

Chronic retention is painless retention of more than 1000 mL urine.

Symptoms and signs. Overflow incontinence. Uraemia. Painless palpable bladder.

Treatment. Bladder decompression with urethral, suprapubic or intermittent self-catheterization. Watch out for secondary diuresis. Patients often need fluid replacement in the first 48 h after decompression. Videourodynamic assessment of detrusor muscle is important to rule out detrusor failure as a cause. Treatment is that of the cause of bladder outlet obstruction.

TESTES AND EPIDIDYMIS

Imperfectly descended testes

About 5% of full-term babies do not have one or both testes in the scrotum at birth. In the first year of life many descend, leaving only 0.3% undescended at 1 year. When the testes cannot be found in the scrotum it may be because they are:

- retractile
- ectopic
- incompletely descended.

A retractile testis is a normal testis associated with an active cremasteric reflex, the testis being drawn up to the superficial inguinal ring. An ectopic testis is one that has descended to an abnormal site and may be found in the superficial inguinal pouch, the perineum, the femoral triangle or at the root of the penis. An incompletely descended testis lies in the normal course of descent – lying anywhere from the posterior abdominal wall to the top of the scrotum.

Symptoms and signs. The mother may have noticed that the testes are absent from the scrotum. In later life, it may be noticed at a routine medical examination. A retractile testis may be brought down into the scrotum by applying gentle traction with the child relaxed in a warm room. The mother may have noticed that the testes are only present when the child is warm and relaxed, e.g. in the bath. The parents can be reassured that the testes are normal and will eventually take up permanent scrotal residence. An incompletely descended testis cannot be palpated in the inguinal canal because of the tough overlying external oblique aponeurosis. If the testis is palpable easily along the line of the inguinal canal it is almost certainly superficial to the external oblique aponeurosis and therefore ectopic. Absence of both testicles from the scrotum is called cryptorchidism. Some 90% of imperfectly descended testes have an associated inguinal hernia.

Treatment. Retractile testes are normal. Parental reassurance is all that is required. An ectopic or incompletely descended testis must be placed in the scrotum. Treatment of an undescended testis should be carried out as early as possible. The testis is mobilized on the cord, any co-existing hernia repaired and the testis fixed in the scrotum. This is usually done by placing it in a pouch fashioned between the dartos muscle and the skin, i.e. orchidopexy.

Complications of imperfect descent. Defective spermatogenesis with infertility in bilateral cases, risk of torsion, risk of tumour or trauma.

Hydrocele

A hydrocele is a collection of fluid in the tunica vaginalis. A primary or idiopathic hydrocele develops slowly and becomes large and tense. It usually occurs in the over 40 s. A secondary hydrocele tends to be small and lax and occurs secondary to inflammation or tumour of the underlying testes. It tends to occur in the younger age group. Primary hydroceles may be classified as follows:

Vaginal hydrocele. This surrounds the testes in the layers of the tunica vaginalis and does not connect with the peritoneal cavity.

Congenital hydrocele. This is associated with a hernial sac. It connects with the peritoneal cavity.

Infantile hydrocele. This extends from the testes to the deep inguinal ring. It does not connect with the peritoneal cavity.

Hydrocele of the cord. This lies along the cord anywhere from the deep inguinal ring to the upper scrotum. It does not connect with either the peritoneal cavity or the tunica vaginalis. A similar swelling may develop in the female and is known as a hydrocele of the canal of Nuck.

Symptoms and signs. Scrotal swelling. Testes cannot be felt separately. Fluctuant. Transilluminates. Can 'get above it'. Congenital hydrocele in infants may fill during the day and empty while lying down at night. A hydrocele of the cord moves downwards when traction is applied to the testis.

Treatment. A congenital hydrocele may be associated with a hernia. Treatment is by surgical excision of the peritoneal remnant as in herniotomy. An infantile, non-communicating hydrocele usually resolves spontaneously or needle aspiration may be required. A vaginal hydrocele in an adult may be treated by aspiration or by excision. A primary hydrocele in an elderly and unfit patient may be treated by aspiration. This may need to be done every few months. Surgery involves opening the tunica vaginalis longitudinally, emptying the hydrocele, everting the sac after excising the redundant sac and suturing the sac behind the cord – thus obliterating the potential space. Secondary hydroceles require treatment of the underlying condition.

Epididymal cyst

They may be small, large, multiple, unilateral or bilateral. If they contain opalescent milky fluid demonstrated on aspiration, they are called spermatoceles.

Symptoms and signs. Usually occur over 40. Scrotal swelling. Slowly enlarges. Painless. Lie above and slightly behind the testes. Testis can be felt separately. Can 'get above it'. Usually smooth and lobulated. Fluctuant. Transilluminates if contains clear fluid.

Treatment. None unless large – where they may show through the trousers and interfere with walking. Aspiration may help but most cysts are multiloculated. Large cysts require excision, but this will compromise the fertility of that testis. Surgery should be restricted to those who have completed their family.

Varicocele

These are varicosities of the pampiniform plexus. More common on the left side.

Symptoms and signs. Varicose veins in the scrotum on standing. Disappear on lying down. Heavy or dragging sensation in scrotum. The patient must be examined standing or the diagnosis will be missed. The veins in the scrotum are often described as feeling like a 'bag of worms' but feeling like a 'plate of lukewarm spaghetti' is probably a better comparison. Bilateral varicoceles may cause subfertility. The affected testis may be smaller. Sudden onset of a left varicocele which does not disappear on lying down in the older patient may be caused by an obstruction of the left renal vein by a renal carcinoma – USS of the kidney is appropriate.

Treatment. In the asymptomatic patient, no treatment is required – especially if the condition is unilateral. Scrotal support for aching and discomfort. Failure of symptoms to settle with scrotal support or evidence of subfertility are indications for intervention. The majority of varicoceles can be treated by embolization and obliteration under radiological control. If surgery is indicated it is via an inguinal approach, all testicular veins bar one being ligated at the deep inguinal ring.

Infections of the testis and epididymis

Inflammation of the testis and epididymis may be acute or chronic. Acute or chronic orchitis may be due to mumps. Acute epididymo-orchitis may be due to coliform organisms or gonorrhoea. It may follow urethral instrumentation or operations on the prostate. Chronic epididymo-orchitis may follow an acute attack or more commonly is due to TB.

Symptoms and signs. Pain, swelling, redness of the scrotum, often associated with pyrexia. In the young patient, the differentiation from torsion is often impossible and the scrotum should be explored. Enlarged exquisitely tender testis and epididymis.

Investigations
● FBC
● MSU
● TB culture.

Treatment
Acute. Bed rest. Analgesia. Scrotal support. Antibiotic – ciprofloxacin until the results of culture are known. If due to gonorrhoea, treat appropriately. The swelling may take as long as 2 months to resolve.

Chronic. TB – antituberculous drugs. Orchidectomy if improvement does not occur. Long-term antibiotic therapy for non-tuberculous epididymo-orchitis.

Testicular torsion

This is twisting of the testis with interference to the arterial blood supply. The actual torsion is usually of the spermatic cord. It occurs in a congenitally abnormal situation. It is associated with imperfectly descended testis, or high investment of the tunica vaginalis with a horizontal lie of the testis; or when the epididymis and testis are separated by a mesorchium, in which case the twist occurs at the mesorchium.

Untreated, the testis infarcts. The condition is a surgical emergency and to be sure of testicular salvage, untwisting should be carried out within 6 h of symptoms. Incidence is highest between 10 and 20 years.

Symptoms and signs. Sudden onset of severe pain in the scrotum and groin and radiating to the lower abdomen associated with vomiting. May follow strain, lifting, exercise or masturbation. Always examine the testes in a young male with abdominal pain. Examination reveals a swollen, painful, testis drawn up to the groin. Difficult to differentiate from epididymo-orchitis. In the latter, there is usually a fever, leukocytosis and the testis is not drawn up to the groin. Epididymo-orchitis is usually associated with UTI. However, doubt usually exists as to the correct diagnosis, in which case the scrotum must be explored.

Treatment. Explore the testis as soon as possible. Untwist the testis. Establish that it is not irreversibly infarcted and fix it to the scrotum – usually by anchoring it to the scrotal septum. Since the other testis is likely to have an abnormal position, this should be fixed at the same operation. If the testis is infarcted, it should be removed. Leaving behind an infarcted testis may result in the development of sperm autoantibodies with depressed spermatogenesis in the remaining testis.

Testicular trauma

This usually occurs in sports injuries or violence. Trauma may result in bleeding into the layers of the tunica vaginalis resulting in haematocele.

Symptoms and signs. Severe pain, scrotal swelling, bruising, tender enlarged testicle.

Investigations. Scrotal ultrasound – beware of an underlying testicular malignancy.

Treatment. Bed rest. Scrotal support. Surgical exploration may be required to evacuate the haematocele and repair a split in the tunica albuginea. If swelling and irregularity of the testis persists after allowing adequate time for recovery, suspect a testicular tumour and institute appropriate investigations. Unsuspected pre-existing testicular tumours may be unmasked following trauma.

Testicular tumours

This is the commonest malignancy in young men; 90% arise from germ cells and are either seminomas or teratomas. The other 10% are lymphomas, Sertoli cell tumours or Leydig cell tumours. Seminomas occur between 30 and 40 years; teratomas between 20 and 30 years. Imperfectly descended testes have a 20–30 times increased incidence of malignancy.

Symptoms and signs. Painless swelling of the testis. Heaviness in the scrotum. Occasionally painful swelling. Small lax hydrocele. May be history of trauma. Palpable abdominal mass. Spread to para-aortic nodes. Lump in left side of neck – spread to left supraclavicular node. Chest symptoms due to lung metastases.

Investigations
- USS testis
- CXR
- Tumour markers: AFP, βhCG
- CT scan.

Treatment. If there is a reasonable suspicion of tumour, explore the testis through an inguinal incision. Clamp the spermatic cord with a soft clamp to prevent tumour dissemination when the testis is delivered into the wound. Palpate the testis. If obviously malignant, carry out orchidectomy. If not obviously malignant the testis is split ('bi-valve') and examined after packing off the rest of the operative field. If any doubt exists, frozen sections should be carried out. Tumour markers should be repeated after orchidectomy. If they are positive, metastases are likely to be present. CT scan of abdomen and chest are carried out to stage disease. If metastatic disease is present, the following is appropriate treatment.

Seminoma. Very radiosensitive. Radiotherapy to iliac and para-aortic nodes plus chemotherapy as for teratoma. Survival is 90–95% at 5 years.

Teratoma. Combination chemotherapy. Agents used include etoposide, vinblastine, methotrexate, bleomycin, cisplatin, in various combinations of three. Survival is between 60% and 90% at 5 years. Surgery may be used for tumour debulking of retroperitoneal nodes.

PENIS

> The majority of surgical conditions of the penis relate to problems with the foreskin and glans and the need for circumcision. Carcinoma of the penis and Peyronie's disease are rare.

CONDITIONS OF THE FORESKIN

Balanoposthitis
This is inflammation of the glans and foreskin. In children, this may be due to faecal organisms or *Staphylococci*. It may result in phimosis from scarring. Recurrent attacks may occur in adults, associated with poor hygiene. Exclude diabetes, especially if *Candida* is the infecting organism. Treatment is by antibiotics or topical application of antifungal agents. Circumcision may be required.

Phimosis
It is usually congenital. The foreskin is tight and will not retract over the glans. It may be acquired as a result of chronic or acute inflammation of the prepuce. It may be secondary to attempts to retract the foreskin at an early age. It is characterized by ballooning of the foreskin on voiding. In the extreme case, retention of urine with hydroureters and hydronephrosis may occur. However, this is more often due to meatal stenosis, which may be hidden by the phimosis. In adults, phimosis may interfere with sexual intercourse.

Treatment. Circumcision.

Paraphimosis
The foreskin is tight and retracts over the corona glandis and cannot be reduced. It forms a tight constriction around the glans interfering with venous return causing swelling of the glans and foreskin, this further exacerbating the difficulty of reduction. It may occur after masturbation, sexual intercourse, bathing glans or after catheterization when the foreskin is not pulled forwards afterwards (iatrogenic).

Treatment. Apply local anaesthetic jelly. Administer strong analgesic and attempt manual reduction. If the latter is unsuccessful a 'dorsal slit' under local anaesthetic should be carried out. This divides the tight constriction ring and allows the foreskin to reduce. Formal circumcision should be carried out when the oedema has subsided.

Balanitis xerotica obliterans
This is a condition of the foreskin characterized by loss of skin elasticity and fibrosis, resulting in phimosis. Treatment is by circumcision.

Carcinoma of the penis
This is rare. It occurs between 60 and 80 years and is almost unknown in circumcised males. Poor hygiene and accumulation of smegma may be aetiological factors. Histologically, the tumour is a squamous cell carcinoma. The tumour starts

TABLE 16.4 Indications for circumcision
Religious
Phimosis
Paraphimosis
Recurrent balanoposthitis
Diagnosis of underlying penile tumours
Trauma and tumour of foreskin

in the sulcus between the glans and the foreskin. Spread is to the inguinal nodes. Blood spread to the lungs or bone is rare.

Symptoms and signs. Firm ulcerated painless lesion. Offensive bloodstained discharge from under foreskin. Inguinal lymphadenopathy. A red velvety lesion on the glans (erythroplasia of Queyrat) is a premalignant condition.

Treatment. If the urethra is not involved, radiotherapy may be used. If the urethra is involved, amputation of the penis is required. If lymph nodes are involved, block dissection of the groin should be carried out or radiotherapy may be given as a palliative measure.

Circumcision
The indications for circumcision are shown in Table 16.4.

Peyronie's disease
The aetiology is unknown. Ages 40–60 years. Fibrotic plaques occur in the corpora cavernosa. Discomfort, pain and deformity occur on erection. The fibrous plaques are palpable in the shaft of the penis. They may become calcified. Spontaneous resolution may occasionally occur. Treatment is unsatisfactory. Steroids may help but surgical incision of fibrous plaques may be necessary but further deformity may result.

Priapism
This is persistent, painful erection unassociated with sexual desire. Causes include idiopathic, leukaemia, sickle cell disease, disseminated and pelvic malignancy, and patients on haemodialysis.

Treatment
- Aspiration of blood from the corpora cavernosa with a wide-bore needle and irrigation with heparinized saline
- Anastomosis of the great saphenous vein to the engorged corpora cavernosa, thus establishing venous drainage of the corpora.

CHAPTER 17

Orthopaedics

FRACTURES

> A fracture is a complete or partial break in the continuity of a bone. There are several ways of classifying fractures, e.g. according to causation, according to configuration of fracture or according to their relation to surrounding tissues.

Causation

Trauma. The fracture occurs in a normal bone as a result of trauma. The pattern depends upon the direction of the force. Direct force usually results in a transverse fracture. Indirect force, e.g. a twisting injury, usually results in a spiral or oblique fracture. Axial compression results in a comminuted, crush or burst fracture. An avulsion fracture is caused by traction, usually a tendon or ligament tearing off a bony fragment, e.g. patellar fracture with a sudden contraction of quadriceps.

Stress fractures. The bone is fatigued by repetitive stress and resembles the fatigue fractures that occur in metals. This type of fracture occurs in individuals undertaking increased amounts of often unaccustomed exercise, e.g. 'march' metatarsal fractures in soldiers.

Pathological fractures. These occur in bones already compromised by underlying disease. The trauma may be quite minimal. Common underlying causes include osteoporosis and metastases.

Pattern (→ Fig. 17.1)

Transverse fracture. This is caused by direct force.

Spiral or oblique fracture. This is caused by force transmitted from a distance often in a twisting motion.

Crush fracture. This is caused by direct compression in cancellous bone.

Burst fracture. This is caused by strong axial compression of a short bone, e.g. vertebrae.

Avulsion fracture. This is caused by sudden, strong traction by a tendon or ligament avulsing a bony fragment.

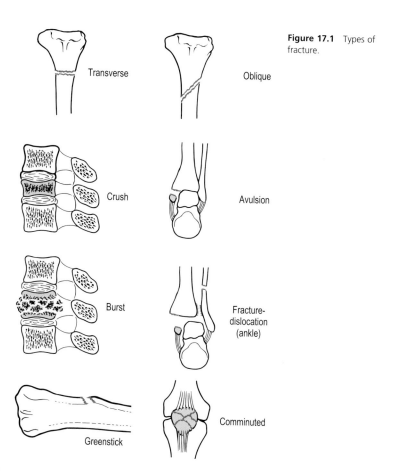

Figure 17.1 Types of fracture.

Fracture–dislocation. This occurs when there is fracture of a bone involved in a joint with complete loss of congruity of the joint surfaces. Partial loss of congruity is a fracture subluxation.

Greenstick fracture. An incomplete paediatric fracture in which the bone buckles and cortical continuity is lost only on one side of the bone.

Comminuted fracture. One in which the bone is broken into more than two fragments.

Relation to surrounding structures

Closed fracture. There is no skin or body cavity wound communicating with the site of fracture.

Open fracture. There is communication between the site of fracture and the skin or body cavity wound, e.g. fractured tibial shaft protruding through the skin.

Intra-articular fracture. The fracture involves an articular surface.

Complicated fracture. There is associated damage to nerves, blood vessels or internal organs.

Symptoms and signs. History to assess mechanism of injury. Pain. Loss of function. Loss of sensation or paralysis. Tenderness. Deformity. Swelling. Crepitus. Abnormal mobility. Discrepancy in length of limbs, associated nerve and vascular injuries. Examine for any associated injuries. Wound associated with open fracture.

Investigations. Radiographs: in two planes at right angles. With long bones include joints at either end. Normal side for comparison. Radiograph – confirms the diagnosis, accurately localizes it, demonstrates the type (e.g. spiral, comminuted, etc.), shows any displacement, shows any pre-existing disease (e.g. pathological fracture through a metastasis), may show foreign body in open fracture, may show associated joint problem. Occasionally a fracture may not be apparent on initial radiograph (e.g. stress fracture, scaphoid fracture) and further radiographs may be required later when callus or late radiolucent line associated with healing is apparent. Further imaging may be required to assess associated damage, e.g. arteriography.

PRINCIPLES OF FRACTURE TREATMENT

First aid

Follow Advanced Trauma Life Support (ATLS) principles (→ Ch. 4). Ensure clear airway. Ensure adequate breathing. Stop bleeding. Splintage to prevent further damage by movement of fragments. If open fracture, cover with Betadine-soaked gauze, administer prophylactic antibiotics and check tetanus status.

Treatment of shock

Considerable blood loss can occur with fractures – 1.5 L can be lost with a femoral shaft fracture. Multiple fractures can lead to considerable blood loss. Ensure adequate treatment of shock with blood or plasma expanders before investigation and treatment.

The fracture itself

1. Reduction, i.e. the restoration of the displaced fragments to their anatomical position
2. Stabilization, i.e. keeping the bony fragments in the reduced position until union occurs
3. Rehabilitation starts as soon as possible after the injury. It is aimed initially at maintaining the function of the uninjured parts and, once the fracture is united, restoring function of the injured parts.

Reduction

Is reduction necessary? Small displacements in extra-articular fractures may be acceptable, although joint surfaces should be anatomically reduced. Initially, reduction is the best form of pain relief. Indications for reduction include functional impairment if not reduced, deformity, interference with blood supply, and interposition of soft tissue between bone ends.

How should it be done? Reduction may be either closed or open.

Closed reduction. This may be by manipulation or traction, the latter being applied via the skin or skeleton. This must be done under anaesthesia, local, regional or general.

Open reduction. This allows accurate alignment of fragments but carries the risk of infection. It is carried out in the following circumstances:

- Reduction cannot be obtained by closed manipulation, e.g. because of soft tissue interposition
- There is inability to maintain reduction – maintenance of reduction requires internal fixation
- Where early mobilization may be appropriate, encouraging rehabilitation and avoiding joint stiffness.

How is reduction held? Some fractures are intrinsically stable and require no additional stabilization. Others require external or internal fixation.

Types of stability

Absolute stability. Fracture fragments are held rigidly together by compression allowing bone healing by remodelling. Little or no external callus forms, e.g. ankle fracture fixation.

Relative stability. Fracture fragments are held approximately opposed without compression. Micromovement occurs at the fracture site and abundant bridging callus forms, e.g. forearm fracture stabilized with a cast.

Methods of stabilizing a fracture

External

Plaster of Paris (or synthetic materials). This may be used for splints, casts or jointed casts. It is usually applied over a layer of wool. Where there is excessive swelling, a slab may be used initially, a full cast being applied at a later date. The cast is radiolucent and the position of the bone should be checked by radiograph after the plaster has been applied. The distal circulation should be observed because a tight plaster may interfere with blood flow. All plasters should be checked 24 h after application. Cast-bracing involves the use of hinged and jointed casts – various segments are connected by specially designed hinges. This allows joint mobility and fracture stability, as well as patient mobility.

Traction. This is used to overcome the powerful pull of muscles, which may cause shortening or angulation. Traction may be fixed, e.g. a Thomas splint for femoral shaft fractures, or sliding (balanced) where the patient's weight is balanced against an applied load. The patient's weight and friction forces counter the applied traction. The patient can move the limb or can move about the bed while traction continues to act in the desired direction. Traction may be applied to the skin via adhesive tape or to bone via pins or wires. Skull traction can be effected by securing a pair of tongs to the skull and applying traction in the longitudinal axis of the neck. Tongs are now used less due to 'halo' traction.

Internal fixation.

Wires. Kirschner (K) wires may be used to internally splint a fracture fragment in two separate planes, e.g. distal radial fracture or used with a figure of 8 tension band wire, e.g. fractures of the olecranon.

Screws. Stainless steel or titanium alloy screws are used. May be used to attach small bony fragment, e.g. fractures of malleoli or to lag two fragments in compression.

Plating. A plate is fastened to both fragments by screws (→ Fig. 17.2). Plates can be designed to compress a fracture, neutralize (support) a fracture compressed by lag screws or bridge a comminuted fracture.

Intramedullary nail. A rod is passed along the medullary cavity of a long bone across the fracture and locked with transverse locking screws. It is used mainly for long bone fractures, e.g. femoral shaft fractures.

External fixation devices. The fragments are transfixed by pins or wires, which are then held in an external fixation device to immobilize the fragments. Difficult, comminuted fractures can be reduced and immobilized by this method. The fracture can be held while surgery for associated injuries, e.g. skin, vascular or nerve, is carried out.

Indications for internal fixation

- Failure to maintain adequate reduction by external methods
- Intra-articular fractures to secure good alignment of joint surfaces and prevent later osteoarthritis
- Need to avoid long periods of immobilization, e.g. elderly patient with fracture of femoral neck
- Patients with multiple injuries where internal fixation may facilitate nursing and patient mobility
- Where damage to other structures, e.g. vessels and nerves, requires stability for good results following repair
- Pathological fractures.

Figure 17.2 A fracture of the radius and ulna fixed with plates and screws. The radial fracture is comminuted.

Open fractures

Principles of management of open fractures include:

- *First aid*: adequate splintage plus coverage with a clean dressing
- *Treatment of shock*: bleeding may be external as well as internal
- *Antibiotic therapy*: as soon as diagnosis is made, large doses of antibiotics are given i.v. (benzylpenicillin 1.2 g 6-hourly and flucloxacillin 1 g 6-hourly)
- *Tetanus prophylaxis*: ± immunoglobulin
- *Photograph wound*
- *Treatment of the wound and fracture:*
  — Clean the wound removing any foreign bodies and all devitalized tissue. A minimum of 6 L of saline washout should be used.
  — Repair any damage to blood vessels.
  — Mark the ends of any nerves that have been severed to facilitate identification for delayed repair.

— Fracture stabilization, usually by external fixation as internal fixation may be associated with increased rates of infection. However, if adequate debridement is carried out, intramedullary nailing may be appropriate, particularly if plastic surgery is required as internal fixation facilitates easier skin cover.
— Clean wounds may be closed primarily.
— Contaminated wounds older than 6 h, or dirty wounds, are further debrided and washed in 48 h.
— Massive wounds may require early free tissue flap coverage.
— If Plaster of Paris is applied a window may be cut in it so the wound can be observed and infection excluded.
— Plastic surgeons should be involved early.

Rehabilitation

The aims should be the restoration of function of the injured part and rehabilitation of the patient as a whole. Specific advice includes: suitable exercises; active use as much as compatible with fracture healing; active exercises; physiotherapy; occupational therapy; advice from social worker; employment advice.

COMPLICATIONS OF FRACTURES

Immediate (at time of fracture)

- Haemorrhage: may be internal or external. Internal haemorrhage can be considerable at the fracture site, i.e. up to 1.5 L with a fractured femoral shaft
- Injury to nerves and vessels
- Injury to underlying structures, e.g. brain damage with skull fractures, splenic rupture with left lower rib fractures, urethral trauma with pelvic fractures.

Early (during the period of initial treatment)

Local

- Gangrene due to vessel damage or tight plaster casts
- Nerve palsies from tight plaster casts, or involved in callus, or iatrogenic injury
- Wound infection or wound dehiscence
- Loss of position
- Pressure sores.

General

DVT. This can occur with fractured neck of femur or generalized immobility in bed. Prophylaxis should be given.

Acute urinary retention. Always exclude the possibility of bladder or urethral injury.

Pneumonia

Fat embolism. This usually complicates fractures of a major long bone at 3–10 days post-injury. Embolization of the pulmonary and systemic microvasculature with lipid globules occurs. The exact source of the fat is controversial. Originally it was thought to be due to fat release from bone marrow adipocytes at the site of the fracture; it is now thought to be more likely to be an abnormal response of fat metabolism to trauma. The main effects are on the brain and lung. The patient may suddenly become drowsy, pyrexial and tachycardic. A petechial rash may appear on the upper trunk. Coma and death may result. With lung involvement the patient develops confusion, breathing difficulties, cyanosis. PO_2 down. Radiograph appearance is similar to ARDS. Renal problems may occur with excretion of lipid droplets. Diagnosis may be confirmed by finding lipid globules in urine or sputum. Treatment is by oxygen therapy, ventilation and renal support. Early operative immobilization of fractured long bones may reduce incidence.

Compartment syndrome. This is elevation of interstitial pressure in a closed fascial compartment that results in microvascular compromised. It may occur with or without arterial injury. Muscle swells and compartment pressure rises. Ischaemia results from pressure on surrounding small arteries. Distal pulses may still be palpable and the diagnosis therefore missed. Awareness of the possibility of the diagnosis is important, particularly when the pain is out of all proportion to the injury. In the lower limb, the posterior compartment (flexors of the ankle), anterior compartment (extensors) or peroneal compartment (evertors) may be involved. The anterior compartment is most commonly involved. Treatment is by prompt fasciotomy, which allows the muscle to expand and relieves the pressure on the vessels.

Crush syndrome. This is due to extensive crushing of muscle or extensive muscle necrosis, e.g. with ischaemia due to arterial injury. Myoglobin is released into the circulation. Myoglobinuria and renal failure may ensue. Oliguria with dark brownish red urine should suggest the diagnosis. Prompt treatment with an osmotic diuretic may prevent renal failure. Removal of all dead muscle, possibly by amputation of the limb, may be required. Dialysis is required for established ARF, which usually recovers.

Late (after the period of initial treatment)

Delayed union. The fracture does not heal in the expected time. Absence of callus and mobility at the fracture site are features.

Non-union. The fracture remains un-united. Non-union may be hypertrophic (due to excessive movement) or atrophic due to poor blood supply, infection or pathological fracture. A pseudarthrosis (false joint) may result. Hypertrophic produces non-bridging callus. Atrophic produces no callus. Treatment is with rigid stabilization, bone grafting, intramedullary bone reaming or pulsed electromagnetic stimulation.

Mal-union. Healing has resulted in a deformed position. This may be because of shortening, mal-rotation, or angulation. Treatment depends on the degree of deformity and the age of the patient. In children considerable remodelling may occur resulting in correction of the deformity. In recent fractures, manipulation, or wedging of the plaster cast, may suffice. In older fractures osteotomy may be required. Deformity may put strain on adjacent joints, resulting in osteoarthritis.

Complex regional pain syndrome (causalgia, reflex sympathetic osteodystrophy, Sudeck's atrophy). The limb becomes painful, swollen and stiff with a reddened, smooth, shiny appearance to the skin. Radiograph shows patchy porosis of the bone. It may be seen after a Colles' fracture, in which case the symptoms affect the hand and wrist. Physiotherapy is required over a prolonged period of weeks or months. The prognosis is usually good.

Avascular necrosis of bone. Part of a bone necroses when its blood supply is interrupted by the fracture. Common sites are:

- The head of the femur is intracapsular where retinacular and intramedullary vessels supplying the femoral head are disrupted.
- The proximal part of the scaphoid bone in fractures across the waist; the blood supply enters from the distal end.

Diagnosis is by radiograph, the avascular fragment being more dense and sclerotic. Early diagnosis may be made by MRI. Osteoarthritis may result.

Myositis ossificans. Calcification with subsequent ossification occurs in a haematoma associated with either stripping of the periosteum and release of osteoblasts into the surrounding muscle and tissue or reactive proliferation in soft tissues causing ectopic calcification. It is most common in injuries around the elbow and those involving quadriceps femoris. Initially treatment involves strict rest, NSAIDs and avoidance of passive movements. When radiographs show that the shadow of calcification has been replaced by a clear outline of ossification, exercise may be reinstituted. Occasionally surgical excision of the ossification is necessary but only when the bone is mature.

Osteoarthritis (OA). This may result from misaligned fractures putting strain on joints, or after intra-articular fractures.

Post-traumatic stress disorder. Compensation neurosis and malingering may occur.

SPINAL TRAUMA

The incidence in the UK of spinal injuries is about 15 per million of the population per year. RTAs account for over 50%, the remainder being due to accidents in the home, industrial accidents, sports injuries and assault. Many patients have associated head, chest and abdominal injuries. The correct management of spinal injuries is essential at every stage to prevent the continuing risk to the spinal cord. Ideal management involves immediate evacuation from the scene of the accident to a centre where care can be supervised by specialists in spinal injuries. A wide spectrum of spinal trauma ranging from minor whiplash injuries to cord transection may occur. All patients complaining of neck/back pain must be thoroughly assessed. All unconscious patients must be assumed to have a spinal injury until proved otherwise.

MANAGEMENT OF SPINAL INJURIES

Scene of the accident

1. Keep the head and neck in neutral position. Avoid any unnecessary movement. Summon help. Do not remove a crash helmet.
2. Medical, paramedical or ambulance personnel. Ensure a clear airway. Apply a collar in suspected cervical injury or a spinal board with an integral head and neck splint prior to extraction from the scene of the accident.
3. Ventilation may be impaired with cervical and upper thoracic injuries. Intubate if necessary with extreme care.
4. Avoid oropharyngeal suction in tetraplegic patients. It may stimulate the vagal reflex, aggravate the pre-existing bradycardia and precipitate cardiac arrest.
5. The casualty who is trapped should be carefully removed and if conscious or intubated placed supine on a stretcher. A 'scoop' stretcher may be fitted together around the casualty on the ground. Unconscious patients who are not intubated are at risk of passive gastric regurgitation and aspiration of vomit if they are nursed on their backs. If intubation is not performed, the patient should be 'log rolled' into a modified lateral position supporting the head in the neutral position. Log rolling should be performed by four people in a coordinated manner ensuring that unnecessary movement does not occur in any part of the spine.
6. Keep the patient warm. Hypothermia may occur owing to paralysis of the sympathetic system.

Initial management at the receiving hospital

1. Follow Advanced Trauma Life Support (ATLS) principles for emergency management.
2. Take a brief history during the primary survey with a more detailed history at the end of the secondary survey.
3. At the start of the secondary survey while removing the spinal board, assess the spine. 'Log roll' for a proper and safe examination of the back. Look for localized bruising and tenderness. Spinal deformity – gibbus or interspinous gap. Assess for other injuries.
4. Full neurological examination to assess the level and the extent of cord damage. Record pin-prick sensation (spinothalamic tracts); fine touch and joint position sense (posterior columns); power of muscle groups according to Medical Research Council Scale (corticospinal tracts); reflexes – limbs, abdominal, anal, and bulbocavernous. Cranial nerves. Priapism indicates a high lesion. A neurological examination should be repeated following the period of potential spinal shock.
5. Radiological investigation: a lateral C-spine radiograph will reveal 85% of cervical spine fractures. However, this is no longer an essential part of the primary ATLS survey, especially if the C-spine is scanned during a trauma CT scan. A CT neck should be requested if the C7/T1 junction is not easily visualized on a lateral radiograph. A C-spine radiograph series comprises an anteroposterior (AP), lateral and odontoid peg view. Unstable fractures

include: fracture-dislocations of the cervical, thoracic and lumbar spine; burst fractures (sometimes); fractures of atlas and axis. CT scan may give clearer view of the damage. MRI shows cord compression and soft tissue damage more clearly.

6. Initial assessment should define two aspects. First, is there a cord injury and is it complete or incomplete (distal sparing easiest to demonstrate as motor activity)? Second, is there a significant spinal injury and is it stable or unstable? Note that these two aspects of the injury can be quite independent (e.g. central cord syndrome after a forced extension injury in a spondylitic patient with no spinal fracture).

WHIPLASH INJURIES

Car struck from behind. Neck extends with sudden acceleration and then flexes forward with sudden deceleration. Usually ligamentous and soft tissue damage only, although there may be pain and paraesthesia in the arms and hands. Radiographs are normal or show mild pre-existing degenerative changes.

Treatment. Rest followed by physiotherapy. Prognosis is variable, some patients recovering while others have prolonged symptoms that may be permanent and require a collar. (In some patients, symptoms settle miraculously after awards of compensation!)

FRACTURES AND DISLOCATIONS OF THE SPINE

Classification by mechanism of injury
- Compression: burst fracture (usually stable)
- Flexion compression: anterior wedge fracture. Possible disruption of posterior ligaments
- Flexion rotation: shearing of all restraining ligaments. Unifacet or bifacet dislocations. These fractures are the commonest cause of neurological damage
- Hyperextension: disruption of the anterior structures. These fractures may cause momentary cord compression leading to 'central cord syndrome'.

Cervical spine fractures and dislocations

Injuries most often occur because of RTAs or sport. A fall on the head with the neck forcibly bent, e.g. flexion and rotation. Subluxation or dislocation occurs with disruption of disc. Forced extension, e.g. a fall on the face or forehead, may occur resulting in cervical spine injury. If a cervical spine injury is suspected the first move should be to safeguard the cord by controlling neck movements. Do not allow the head to flex forward, and do not hyperextend the neck. Keep in a neutral position.

Symptoms and signs. Often associated head injury so patient may be unconscious. Assume cervical spine injury. Conscious patient may have pain, muscle spasm and localized tenderness. Pain may radiate down arms. Look for neurological signs. The patient with damage above C4 is unlikely to survive because of paralysis of all respiratory muscles. Transection above sympathetic outflow causes bradycardia and hypotension.

Investigations

Radiographs

- Lateral to show C1–T1. May need CT scan
- AP through open mouth to show odontoid
- 30° oblique for facet joints (rarely done now because of CT)
- Flexion and extension views to assess stability
- CT scan.

Treatment

Fractures of the atlas. These are usually fractured as a result of vertical compression force breaking the ring into four pieces. Inherently unstable, requiring halo jacket immobilization and fusion if non-union occurs.

C1–C2 subluxation. This is due to failure of the transverse ligament. Treatment is by initial traction in extension then posterior fusion.

Odontoid peg fracture. It is uncommon and easily missed. All but the rare apical avulsion type require traction followed by a halo jacket with posterior fusion for non-union.

Burst fractures. These may be stable, in which case treatment is by halo jacket. If unstable, traction followed by a halo jacket is required. Decompression of the cord and fusion may be necessary.

Anterior wedge fractures. These may be stable (treatment in a collar) or unstable with opening of the posterior elements (halo jacket or posterior fusion).

Facet joint dislocations. They are always unstable. Treatment is by reduction and posterior fusion following MRI to check for sequestrated disc.

Isolated spinous process avulsion. These are stable and require treatment in a collar.

Thoracic spine

Flexion injuries result in crush or wedge fractures, which are usually stable. Such fractures may occur with minimal trauma if the vertebral body is weakened, e.g. osteoporosis or secondary deposits. Fracture-dislocations tend to occur at the thoracolumbar junction and are caused by flexion and rotation injuries, e.g. a fall from a height on to the shoulders or a heavy load falling on the flexed back. If the disc and posterior ligaments are disrupted the injury is unstable. Paraplegia is common in fracture-dislocations.

Symptoms and signs. History of fall from height on shoulder or heavy weight falling on flexed back. Pain over spine. Bruising or abrasions over shoulders. Palpable gap along spinous processus with unstable fracture-dislocations. Associated injuries. Neurological deficit.

Investigations. AP and lateral spine radiographs.

Treatment. Simple flexion injuries with crush or wedge fractures are treated by bed rest and analgesia followed by mobilization when pain allows, occasionally in a plaster or polythene jacket. If trauma is minimal an underlying pathological cause should be sought. Fracture-dislocations may be treated conservatively or operatively. Conservative management includes careful nursing with regular turning on a special spinal bed until core stability returns followed by thoracolumbar support (TLS) orthosis for 3 months. Spontaneous interbody fusion usually occurs. If there is paraplegia, care is as for the paraplegic patient. To offset the problem of long-term bed rest, operative treatment may be undertaken. The fracture may be stabilized by internal fixation.

Lumbar spine

Compression fractures are the most common and may result from a fall from a height on to the heels. With a burst fracture a fragment of bone may be displaced posteriorly and cause damage to the cord or cauda equina syndrome.

Symptoms and signs. History of fall from height on to heels. Pain over lumbar spine. Pain and spasm in paravertebral muscles. Look for associated os calcis fractures or hip injury. Paraplegia.

Investigations. AP and lateral radiograph of lumbar spine (→ Fig. 17.3).

Treatment. Where there is no neurological damage and the fracture is not comminuted, immobilization in a moulded plastic or plaster jacket will suffice until union occurs. Pathological fractures will require fixation.

Figure 17.3 Lateral radiograph of the thoracolumbar spine. There is an anterior wedge fracture of the body of the 1st lumbar vertebra.

Fractures of the transverse processes

The most common are in the lumbar region. It may result from direct violence in a crushing injury or violent muscular contraction. Treatment is symptomatic. There is often severe soft tissue trauma and associated haematoma; prolonged pain may occur. Fractures of L5 transverse process suggestive of pelvic trauma.

Fractures of sacrum and coccyx

This may accompany fractures of the pelvis or occur as isolated fractures due to direct violence. Undisplaced linear fractures are treated symptomatically. Displaced fractures may injure sacral nerves with consequent neurological deficit.

Coccydynia

This causes chronic pain in the coccygeal region. It may follow a fall on the buttocks. The pain interferes with sitting. Treatment is by injection of LA and depot steroid or manipulation under anaesthesia (if fracture-dislocation). If conservative management fails excision of the coccyx may be required.

SPINAL CORD INJURY

Types of spinal cord injury

The extent and level of cord damage is very important in determining recovery and final prognosis. Thoracic cord injuries tend to be complete. Incomplete injuries can be identified by the sparing of some tracts and these injuries tend to show much more recovery. The early picture is obscured by 'spinal shock' where all cord function ceases for 24–48 h.

Anterior cord syndrome. The posterior column still functions (proprioception, vibration sensation).

Central cord syndrome. Relative sparing of motor supply to legs. Sacral sparing (sensation, anal tone).

Brown–Sequard syndrome. Hemitransection of the cord. Preserved contralateral motor function, position, and vibration sense. Preserved ipsilateral pain and temperature sensation.

Mixed syndromes. These are combinations of the above.

Management and complications of cord injury

Respiratory. Impairment of respiratory function is common after injury to the cervical spine. This may relate to partial phrenic nerve palsy, intercostal paralysis, inability to expectorate, and a ventilation-perfusion disorder. Associated chest injuries may be present. Monitor by CXR and ABG. Ventilation and bronchoscopy may be needed.

Cardiovascular. Bradycardia and hypotension may occur owing to damage to sympathetic outflow. Excessive i.v. fluids to attempt to correct hypotension may cause pulmonary oedema. Avoid pharyngeal suction as it may potentiate bradycardia via a vagal reflex and lead to cardiac arrest.

Urinary tract. Insert catheter to avoid overdistension of an atonic bladder. If potential urethral injury (perineal bruising or pelvic fracture) perform retrograde urethrogram. Suprapubic or intermittent self-catheterization may be required later. Stasis in the urinary tract combined with hypercalciuria due to immobilization may lead to repeated UTIs and stone formation. Urinary catheter should be changed frequently.

Gastrointestinal. Paralytic ileus follows a few days after injury. Avoid oral fluids. i.v. fluids and NG suction will be required until bowel sounds return. Beware stress ulceration with perforation. Signs may be lacking. Shoulder tip referred pain may be the only clinical indication.

Hypothermia. Hypothermia may occur owing to paralysis of the sympathetic nervous system. The patient should be kept warm.

Thromboembolism. The incidence of DVT and PE is high. Start subcutaneous low molecular weight heparin 6 h after injury. Continue until the patient is mobile in a wheelchair.

Pressure sores. These form as a result of pressure ischaemia, particularly over bony prominences. Regularly turning in bed every 2 h is essential. The patient's bottom should be lifted off a wheelchair seat every 15 min for a similar reason. Established sores require aggressive treatment with plastic reconstruction if necessary.

LONG-TERM MANAGEMENT OF SPINAL TRAUMA

Nursing care
Good nursing care is essential and should always be in a specialized spinal unit. Objectives include: prevention of secondary complications; facilitation of maximum functional recovery; support for patients and family in adaptation to changed physical status; education of patients and relatives in all aspects of long-term care.

Physiotherapy
This involves care of both the chest and paralysed limbs initially. Later care involves help with strengthening non-paralysed muscles, adaptation to a wheelchair, relearning ability to balance, transfer from wheelchair to bed, toilet, etc. and bracing and gait training.

Occupational therapy
This helps adjustment to a lifetime of disability. Help is given to reach the highest levels of physical and psychological independence at home and at work. Help is provided with the activities of daily living, home alterations, recreation and work.

Social services
This provides help with finance, adaptation of home and employment.

Others

Long-term help with bladder problems, chronic pain, and sexual problems will be required.

PROGNOSIS

It is important to indicate the probable degree of recovery at an early stage to both patients and relatives. Recovery after a complete cord lesion is unlikely. It is, however, difficult to forecast the degree of recovery in an incomplete lesion as improvement may occur after resolution of oedema and contusion. The most encouraging signs are those of incompleteness of paralysis or early return of cord function. Patients with early recovery usually achieve the most recovery. In incomplete lesions improvement may continue for several years. Death in the first days after injury is likely to be due to respiratory failure with high tetraplegia.

The level of cervical transection is crucial to long-term prognosis. Above C4 the patient usually dies of respiratory failure. At C4, patients are able to use their mouth to control a wheelchair. At C5 with special aids they can feed, wash and move their chair. However, they cannot transfer in and out of the chair or dress themselves. At C6 they can drive a special car and dress the upper body but they are unable to transfer themselves from a chair. At C7 their ability is intermediate between that of C6 and C8, the latter being the ability to lead an independent wheelchair life. The other causes of morbidity and mortality include PE, pressure sores and CRF (late).

PELVIC FRACTURES

> The pelvis is a ring of bone and ligaments, which includes the innominate bone, sacrum, sacroiliac joints, and the pubic symphysis. When fractures occur, the ring tends to break in two places. If only one fracture is visible on radiograph the possibility of sacroiliac joint disruption should be considered. Pelvic fractures occur in the younger patient in RTAs. Elderly patients may sustain isolated pubic ramus fractures, which respond to analgesics and mobilization. Mortality for closed pelvic fractures varies between 5% and 15% with a mortality of 50% for open fractures. The pelvis is very vascular and injuries are associated with considerable blood loss. Pelvic visceral and urethral damage may occur.

Symptoms and signs. Fall in the elderly. RTA in young patients (beware of associated injuries). Pelvic pain. Abrasions. Bruising. Shock. Inability to pass urine. Bleeding per urethram. Bleeding PR. Bleeding PV. Perineal bruising. High 'floating' prostate on examination PR.

Investigations
- Pelvic radiograph (anteroposterior and inlet and outlet views)
- CT scan
- IVU
- Urethrogram.

Treatment

Shock. Intensive resuscitation as bleeding may be dramatic (3–4 L). For 'open book' types of fracture, emergency stabilization with an external fixator reduces bleeding. For other fractures, radiological intra-arterial embolization is the best option to slow bleeding.

The fracture itself. Acetabular fractures require accurate reduction and fixation. A CT scan is required to assess for loose bodies and articular congruity. A tertiary referral service should be involved to assess the patient and provide definitive care. A variety of internal fixation methods is available followed by ipsilateral non-weight-bearing for 3 months.

Urethral trauma. Avoid catheterization. If the patient can pass urine and it is clear, all is well. Otherwise, consider suprapubic catheterization or cystotomy. Retrograde urethrogram and IVU may be required.

Complications. Haemorrhage and shock, urethral or bladder injury, rectal injury, paralytic ileus, DVT, damage to hip joint. Late post-traumatic OA may occur in acetabular injuries. Vaginal injury, sciatic nerve injury, mal-union may lead to obstetric difficulties. Sexual dysfunction.

INJURIES TO THE LOWER LIMB

HIP AND THIGH

Traumatic dislocation of the hip

> The majority are posterior and follow impact directed along the femoral shaft when the hip is flexed and adducted, e.g. RTA when the knee strikes the dashboard. Anterior, inferior and central dislocations are rare, the latter being caused by the head of the femur being driven into the acetabulum.

Symptoms and signs. Often other severe injuries. Shock. Thigh is flexed, adducted and internally rotated with posterior dislocations. May be associated injury to femur or patella. Sciatic nerve injury should be assessed prior to reduction.

Investigations
- Good-quality radiograph of hip with lateral film
- Judet views (45° oblique views of hip)
- Radiograph of femur and patella.

Treatment. Reduction under GA with muscle relaxation. If the hip is stable and there is no associated fracture, patient is mobilized with weight-bearing as tolerated. If a bone fragment is displaced from the posterior acetabulum, open reduction and internal fixation of the fragment may be required.

Complications. Associated fractures. Sciatic nerve damage. Avascular necrosis of femoral head. Late OA of hip.

Fractures of the proximal femur

The blood supply to the head of the femur comes from three sources:

- Retinacular vessels in the capsule
- Medullary vessels in the femoral neck
- Via the ligamentum teres.

The main source is via the retinacular vessels and these may be damaged in fractures of the femoral neck. Fractures may be classified as intracapsular (subcapital, transcervical), or extracapsular (basal, intertrochanteric → Fig. 17.4). Extracapsular fractures do not damage the blood supply to the femoral head and therefore there are no risks of avascular necrosis of the femoral head and non-union. They are most common in the elderly, especially females with osteoporotic bones when the traumatic cause is relatively trivial, e.g. a fall in the house. In the young patient they result from major trauma.

Subcapital
Transcervical
Basal

Intertrochanteric

Figure 17.4 Fractures of the femoral neck. The arrowed line separates intracapsular (to the left) and extracapsular (to the right) fracture sites. Intracapsular fractures are associated with avascular necrosis of the femoral head.

Symptoms and signs. Elderly female. Minor trauma. Tripped over carpet. Tripped over pavement. Pain in the hip. Adduction of limb. Shortening and external rotation only if the fracture is displaced. Movements painful. Weight-bearing usually impossible. Beware hypothermia.

Investigations
- Radiographs in two planes (→ Fig. 17.5 AP view)
- Hb
- FBC
- U&Es
- Coagulation screen
- Blood sugar
- CXR
- ECG. In the elderly patient there is the possibility of intercurrent disease.

Complications. These are of the elderly undergoing surgery, e.g. pneumonia, MI, CVA, DVT and PE; 30% of elderly patients are dead within 6 months of the injury. Avascular necrosis of the femoral head. Non-union. Mal-union with varus angulation and shortening.

Figure 17.5 A subcapital fracture of the neck of the femur.

Treatment

General. Pain relief. Bed rest. DVT prophylaxis. Further investigation if pathological fracture suspected (CA, CXR, bone scan, long films to include joints above and below, myeloma screen).

Fracture. Surgery to allow nursing, mobilization, and rehabilitation:

- Intracapsular: undisplaced (fixed with screws); displaced – femoral head replacement, i.e. hemiarthroplasty, e.g. Exeter trauma stem or primary total hip replacement
- Extracapsular: cantilever device, e.g. dynamic hip screw; load sharing device, e.g. cephalomedullary nail, e.g. gamma nail.

Fractures of the femoral shaft

Common in younger people and usually result from severe trauma in RTAs. They may occur at any site and be of variable pattern. Treatment is either conservative (traction – rarely used) or more often operative (internal fixation or external fixator device). There are frequently associated injuries, especially ipsilateral femoral neck fractures.

Symptoms and signs. Severe pain in thigh. Deformity. Shock. Associated injuries. Check head, chest, abdomen, spine. Vascular injury to femoral vessels. Injury to sciatic nerve.

Investigations
- Radiographs in two planes
- Femoral angiography may be required if vascular injury is suspected.

Treatment. Splint leg. Transport to hospital. Pain relief. i.v. fluids. FBC, U&Es. Cross-match (blood loss can be 2–4 units). Check if fracture is open. Give tetanus prophylaxis and antibiotics if open fracture.

Conservative. Skin traction and temporary stabilization in Thomas' splint. *Conservative definitive treatment* – pre-toddler (<3 years) – gallows traction followed by hip spica. Toddler to adult – balanced traction until moves comfortably on bed then hip spica. In adults, skeletal traction with a Steinmann pin and balanced traction applied through the skeletal pin with the knee flexed on a special knee flexion attachment. Fractures heal quickly in children. In adults cast bracing may be used after 6–8 weeks.

Surgical
- Internal fixation: *Open physes* – elastic stable intramedullary nails (ESIN-Nancy nails) aged 5–13. *Closed physes* – achieved by a locked intramedullary nail. This allows accurate reduction and compression and ensures early mobilization of the patient. There is a risk of infection and osteomyelitis. This form of treatment is useful for multiple fractures, pathological fractures and when there is associated vascular injury.
- External fixation: used especially for open fractures where there is soft tissue damage. Pins are inserted above and below the fracture site and reduction and alignment maintained by an external fixator device.

Complications. DVT. PE. Fat embolism. Infection. Shortening. Angulation. Non-union.

FRACTURES AND DISLOCATIONS AROUND THE KNEE

Fractures are usually intra-articular causing haemarthrosis, which should be aspirated to decrease pain. They can be caused by a direct blow (car bumper, car dashboard), vertical compression (fall from a height) or excessive strain (forced abduction at the knee). Associated ligamentous and neurovascular injuries are common. Conservative treatment for these injuries involves a long leg cylinder plaster then a hinged cast brace. This type of treatment is also used after open reduction/internal fixation. The knee joint needs accurate repair of the articular surfaces to reduce the risk of post-traumatic OA.

Supracondylar fractures (→ Fig. 17.6)

These are intra-articular or extra-articular. The distal fragment is pulled backwards by the gastrocnemius. The popliteal artery may be damaged by the distal fragment. Conservative treatment is by skeletal traction via the proximal

Figure 17.6 A supracondylar fracture of the femur. In the lateral view, the distal fragment is tilted backwards and may damage the popliteal artery.

tibia with the knee in about 30° of flexion. Internal fixation is required for all displaced intra-articular fractures (polyaxial/fixed angle locking plates, retrograde intramedullary nails).

Isolated femoral condylar fractures
These are usually displaced so internal fixation is advised with lag screw or headless compression screw.

Tibial plateau fractures
In these fractures, vertical compression forces or strains drive the femoral condyle through the tibial plateau. Fragments of tibial plateau/condyle may be cleaved off, depressed, or both. Both condyles may be damaged. Displaced or depressed fragments should be reduced and internally fixed, often with support from a bone graft and a buttress plate.

Dislocation of the knee
This is an uncommon injury. It is usually associated with damage to the popliteal artery or local nerves. After reduction under anaesthesia any ruptured ligaments should be repaired. Immobilization in plaster then cast brace is required for several months.

INJURIES TO THE EXTENSOR MECHANISM

These involve the following:

- Tear of quadriceps insertion into the patella
- Transverse fracture of patella with separation
- Rupture of the patellar tendon, avulsion of tibial tuberosity.

Forced flexion of the knee against a contracting quadriceps causes the extensor mechanism to give way.

Symptoms and signs. Pain. Knee cannot be fully actively extended against gravity producing extensor lag. Palpable gap and point of maximum tenderness at site of lesion.

Investigations. Radiograph: patella 'high' if patellar tendon ruptured; patella 'low' with upper part tilted forward with quadriceps tear.

Treatment. Operative repair of defect in the extensor mechanism. Immobilization for 4–6 weeks in plaster cylinder with knee in full extension.

FRACTURES AND DISLOCATIONS OF THE PATELLAE

Fractures

An avulsion or transverse fracture is caused by a violent contraction of quadriceps against resistance. A comminuted fracture is caused by direct violence, e.g. a blow from a bat or in an RTA.

Treatment. This depends whether the extensor mechanism is intact and the degree of comminution. If the extensor mechanism is intact and there is no severe comminution, treatment in a plaster cylinder for 3–4 weeks will suffice. Transverse fractures with separation are held with a tension band wire or two longitudinal screws. Mobilization is possible after 3 weeks in a plaster cylinder. If the extensor mechanism is ruptured, surgical repair is required. A long-term complication is OA of the patellofemoral compartment.

Dislocation of the patella

This may be acute or recurrent and occurs laterally.

Acute or traumatic. This results from a blow on the side of the knee. The patella is visibly displaced. The knee remains flexed until the patella is reduced by medial directed pressure. There is usually a tear in the medial capsule or avulsion of the medial side of the patella. May be associated with haemarthrosis. Treatment is by rest in a plaster cylinder followed by quadriceps exercises.

Recurrent. Usually affects adolescent girls. Associated with flattening of lateral condyle, small high-riding patella, or genu valgum. Dislocation occurs spontaneously or with minor trauma. The knee locks in semiflexion. Spontaneous reduction usually occurs. After a single incident, intensive physiotherapy to strengthen vastus medialis. Surgery is indicated in recurrent cases.

FRACTURES OF THE TIBIAL SHAFT

These are common fractures occurring as a result of RTAs, sports injuries, and industrial accidents. They are often open. Oblique and spiral fractures are commonly unstable when reduced. Up to 20% of cases develop non-union.

Treatment. Numerous methods are available depending on fracture.

Stable fractures. Closed reduction under GA is suitable for a transverse fracture. The leg hangs over the end of the operating table, gravity maintaining position of the fragments. The ankle is dorsiflexed to a right angle and a full leg plaster applied with the knee in slight flexion. Positions should be checked with radiographs immediately after plastering and at weekly intervals until no significant risk of displacement.

Unstable fractures. With spiral, oblique or comminuted fractures, a long leg plaster is insufficient. Closed injuries should be fixed with an intramedullary nail. The treatment of severe open injuries is controversial and may be with an Ilizarov frame (fine wire external fixator) or an intramedullary nail at the preference of the surgeon. Either method can be used for open fractures with minimal soft tissue damage.

Open wounds. All open wounds must be explored, irrigated and treated in conjunction with a plastic surgeon if bone is exposed at the base of the wound.

Complications. Delayed union. Non-union. Infection. Stiffness of knee, ankle, foot. Ischaemia of muscles leading to claw toes. Compartment syndrome.

Isolated fractures of the fibula

These are uncommon. They are usually associated with tibial fractures and with direct violence. Beware common peroneal nerve injury in fractures of neck of the fibula. Exclude ankle injury, e.g. diastasis (see below). Treatment is by strapping or below-knee plaster until pain settles.

FRACTURES AROUND THE ANKLE

These are due to indirect forces transmitted from the foot (e.g. twisted ankle). The ligaments and malleoli may be injured in various combinations. Severe force may cause associated dislocation.

Classification (Fig. 17.7)

There are two main classification systems used. The Weber classification is used in everyday practice and describes the X-ray appearance of the fracture. The Lauge–Hansen describes the starting point and deforming force and generally is more useful for research purposes but is actually remarkably similar to the Weber classification. The Weber classification is based on the level of the fracture in

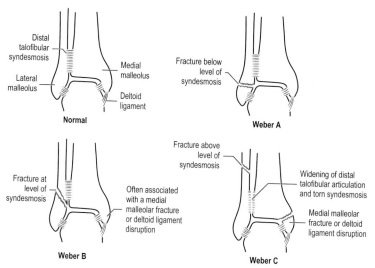

Figure 17.7 Weber classification of ankle injuries.

relationship to the joint syndesmosis of the distal fibular. Three malleoli are described – medial, lateral (distal fibular) and posterior, which is the posterior most distal tip of the tibia.

● Type A fractures are horizontal avulsion fractures found below the syndesmosis. They are stable fractures and are amenable to treatment with closed reduction and a full weight-bearing cast for 6 weeks.

● Type B fracture is a spiral fibular fracture that starts at the level of the syndesmosis. This fracture may be bi-malleolar/tri-malleolar. The importance is the presence of articular congruity in the cast and whether the medial side is tender or not. If non-tender there will be no medial malleolar fracture or disruption of the deltoid medial ligament. Therefore, there will be no possibility of talar shift. This is a stable fracture and may be treated as a type A but with X-ray checks at 1 and 2 weeks. Otherwise, open reduction and internal fixation is required.

● Type C fracture is above the level of the syndesmosis and disrupts and ligamentous attachment between the fibular and the tibia distal to the fracture. These fractures are unstable and require open reduction and internal fixation wit non weight-bearing for 12 weeks.

Axial compression fractures (Plafond fracture)

These are caused by a fall on the foot from a height. The talus is driven into the articular surface of the tibia, which is comminuted. This is a severe injury and is difficult to treat. Massive soft tissue swelling occurs.

Investigations
- AP and lateral films
- Note site of fractures and talus shift or tilt
- CT scan helps delineate fracture anatomy.

Treatment. This is difficult to treat. Initial treatment requires reduction of the ankle joint, immobilization and minimization of swelling with elevation. Consider using a hinged external fixator from tibia to tarsal bones or an Ilizarov external fixator.

Maisonneuve fracture (→ Fig. 17.8)

A twisting injury causes a high fibular fracture with a radiological normal ankle joint. The syndesmosis however is often disrupted along with rupture of the deltoid ligament. There is disruption of the interosseous tibiofibular ligament. Treatment involves syndesmosis screws and non-weight-bearing for 12 weeks.

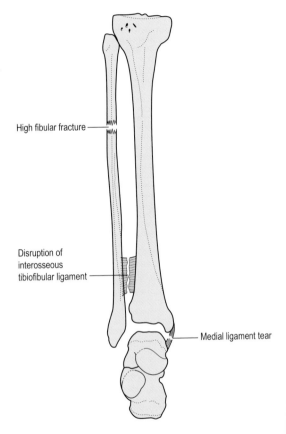

Figure 17.8 Diastasis of the inferior tibiofibular joint with rupture of the interosseous membrane. There is an associated high fibular fracture (Maisonneuve fracture).

High fibular fracture —

Disruption of interosseous tibiofibular ligament —

— Medial ligament tear

FRACTURES AND DISLOCATIONS IN THE FOOT

Os talus

This is rare. The blood supply is from distal to proximal and therefore fractures across the neck may result in avascular necrosis. It is usually caused by forced dorsiflexion. Undisplaced fractures are treated in plaster. The foot should be maintained in plantar flexion following closed reduction of displaced fractures; 8–12 weeks' immobilization is required. Avascular necrosis leads to OA. Displaced fractures require internal fixation after reduction.

Os calcis

This is caused by a fall from height on to the heel. It may be bilateral. Look for fractures elsewhere, especially burst fractures of the spine. Conservative treatment is by bed rest and elevation of the legs to reduce swelling. Operative treatment is offered to non-smokers with fractures of moderate severity. Early subtalar fusion is often beneficial. Ankle exercises are required. Initial non-weight-bearing for 6–8 weeks. Partial weight-bearing on crutches is then permitted. Healing takes up to 10 weeks. Complications include pain, stiffness at the subtalar joint, and local nerve and tendon entrapment.

METATARSAL FRACTURES

Avulsion fracture of the base of the 5th metatarsal is common and is caused by an inversion injury combined with forced plantar flexion, e.g. mis-stepping on a stair. The peroneus brevis tendon avulses the styloid process at the base of the 5th metatarsal. Treatment is in a metatarsal shoe walking plaster for 4–6 weeks. Fracture of the proximal 5th metatarsal is due to direct trauma and may require open reduction and fixation.

Shaft fractures

These occur with crushing injuries and are often multiple. Elevation of the foot followed by mobilization in a below-knee non-weight-bearing plaster for 6 weeks is required. If displacement is gross, manipulation or internal fixation may be required.

Stress fracture ('march' fracture)

This usually affects the second metatarsal neck and is caused by the stress of long hours of walking, e.g. new army recruits. It may not be apparent on an early radiograph but only show on a repeated radiograph when callus is forming. Treatment is a below-knee walking plaster for 6 weeks. In mild cases, rest only is required.

Lisfranc fracture

This is principally a dislocation of some or all of the tarso-metatarsal joints of the foot, particularly the 2nd metatarsal head fitting into the key stone of the cuneiform bones. Clinical suspicion is aroused due to massive swelling and potentially normal X-rays. X-rays should be repeated weight-bearing, anteroposterior, oblique and lateral and the dislocation may be emphasized. CT scan may confirm the diagnosis. Open reduction and internal fixation is required.

FRACTURES OF THE TOES

These are common injuries. Fracture occasionally interferes with circulation, and amputation is required. Otherwise splintage by strapping of the adjacent toe will suffice. Great toe fractures may require fixation.

INJURIES TO THE UPPER LIMB

FRACTURES AND DISLOCATIONS AROUND THE SHOULDER

Dislocation of the sternoclavicular joint

This is uncommon. Usually the medial end of the clavicle dislocates forward and the deformity is obvious. Posterior dislocation is rare and may lead to tracheal compression. Treatment is usually symptomatic. Posterior dislocation requires open reduction to relieve tracheal compression.

Clavicular fracture

This is caused by falls on the outstretched hand or point of the shoulder. The bone usually breaks between the middle and outer third. Fractures of the outer end may be associated with fractures of the coracoid and damage to the coracoclavicular ligament.

Symptoms and signs. Pain in shoulder region. Supports weight of arm with other hand. The proximal portion is drawn upwards by sternomastoid. The distal portion droops owing to the weight of the arm. Tenderness over the site.

Investigations. Radiograph.

Treatment. Support the arm in a triangular sling. With displaced fractures 3 weeks of support is usually sufficient. Rarely, displacement may be sufficient to warrant internal fixation, especially if the skin over the fracture is in danger of necrosis.

Complications. Rare. Occasionally injury to brachial plexus or axillary artery may occur.

Acromioclavicular joint

Subluxation. Seen in rugby players who present with a lump over the joint. Treatment is by rest in a sling until symptoms subside. The lump over the joint often persists.

Dislocation. Complete dislocation occurs only when the coracoclavicular ligament is disrupted. The clavicle is elevated and the point of the shoulder lowered. Tenderness and bruising occur. Radiographs show a gap between coracoid process and clavicle. Treatment is usually conservative with a sling but dependent on percentage displacement, reconstruction may be required.

Scapular fracture

This is usually caused by direct violence. There may be extensive bruising. Treatment is by rest, analgesia, collar and cuff. Mobilize when pain allows. CT if suspicion of glenoid involvement.

Dislocation of the shoulder

The commonest form is anterior (95%), and is caused by a fall on the outstretched hand. In the younger patient the capsule is strong and does not tear. The glenoid labrum and capsule are avulsed from the bone, allowing recurrent dislocations to occur. In the older patient the capsule is torn – this heals after reduction. Recurrent dislocation is less common in the older patient.

Symptoms and signs. Fall on outstretched hand. Pain. Patient supports arm, which is abducted. The normal contour of the shoulder is lost. Check for axillary nerve damage – anaesthesia over skin at insertion of deltoid.

Investigations. Radiograph (→ Fig. 17.9): humeral head not in contact with the glenoid; check for associated fractures of the humeral head and neck.

Treatment. Reduction under GA or intravenous sedation. Two methods are available:

Kocher's method. Flex the elbow to a right angle and apply slow gentle traction in the line of the humerus. Rotate the humerus externally using the forearm as a lever. Adduct the humerus across the trunk. Then internally rotate the humerus. Avoid this method in the elderly owing to risk of iatrogenic fracture.

Figure 17.9 Anterior dislocation of the shoulder joint. The humeral head lies below and medial to the glenoid (arrow).

Hippocratic method. Place the stockinged foot in the axilla and pull downwards on the arm. Use the toes to slip the head back into position. Confirm the position with radiograph. Immobilize the arm in a sling for 3 weeks.

Complications. Early complications include axillary nerve damage and associated fractures. Late complications include stiffness and recurrent dislocation. Complete rotator cuff tear in the elderly.

Recurrent dislocation

This usually follows damage to the glenoid labrum (Bankart lesion) or humeral head (Hill–Sachs lesion) at the time of original dislocation. Dislocation occurs on movement of the arm, especially if raised and externally rotated. Radiograph may reveal a depression on the humeral head (Hill–Sachs lesion).

Treatment. Operative: the operation of choice is Bankart's operation, where the torn glenoid labrum is reattached to the bone. Reconstruction of the anterior labrum is the Gold Standard and should be carried out arthroscopically. Open reconstruction is becoming rarer. Results of surgery are good.

Posterior dislocation is rare. A lateral radiograph is essential for diagnosis.

FRACTURES OF THE HUMERUS

Proximal humerus (→ Fig. 17.10)

This is usually due to indirect violence, i.e. a fall on the shoulder, often in the elderly.

Treatment. Undisplaced fractures are treated with a collar and cuff (for gravitational traction) then physiotherapy. Significantly displaced avulsion of the tuberosities or anatomical neck fractures should be internally fixed with repair of the rotator cuff. Surgical neck fractures are usually treated in a collar and cuff for 3–6 weeks and then physiotherapy.

Complications. Axillary nerve damage. Shoulder stiffness.

Shaft of the humerus

This is caused by a direct blow or a fall on the outstretched hand. The fracture is usually oblique and may be displaced. Check for radial nerve damage (wrist drop and anaesthesia in the first web space on the dorsal aspect especially in midshaft fractures).

Treatment. The weight of the arm effects reduction. A 'U' slab is applied to the upper arm and the wrist supported with a collar and cuff initially. The 'U' slab extends over the shoulder and under the elbow. 'U' slabs are rarely used after the initial 2 weeks when they are replaced with a humeral brace (a thermoplastic moulded splint). Occasionally, open reduction and internal fixation may be required using a plate or an intramedullary nail. Internal fixation is appropriate if the patient requires bed rest for other injuries.

Complications. Radial nerve damage and non-union.

Figure 17.10 A fracture of the neck of the humerus. This shows severe displacement. The axillary nerve is in danger with such a fracture.

FRACTURES AND DISLOCATIONS AROUND THE ELBOW

Supracondylar fracture

This is chiefly a fracture of childhood but may occur in adults. There is a history of a fall on the outstretched hand followed by pain and swelling around the elbow. The lower fragment is usually displaced, rotated and in extension. The brachial artery and median nerve are vulnerable to injury.

Treatment. Reduction under anaesthesia. Longitudinal traction is inserted on the forearm, medial and lateral displacement is corrected along with rotation. Fractures are held with flexion and forearm pronation and stabilized if required with cross K wires (lateral side first) and medial side under direct vision due to the proximity of the ulnar nerve to the medial epicondyle. Check radiograph for position. Check that the radial pulse does not disappear through overflexing the swollen elbow. Admission is necessary to observe the circulation for 24 h. If all is well, the patient is discharged after 24 h, the fracture being immobilized for 4–5 weeks – after which active exercise is commenced.

Problems may occur after this type of treatment. The pulse may not return after manipulation but provided the hand remains pink with good capillary return there is no cause for alarm. Pallor, poor capillary return, excessive pain and inability to bring about full passive extension of the fingers are signs for alarm. Reduce the degree of flexion. If the pulse does not return, extend the arm vertically. If the circulation is not restored, the forearm needs surgical decompression with exploration of the brachial artery.

Complications. This fracture is prone to several complications, particularly in children. Damage to brachial artery. Nerve injury (median). Stiffness. Mal-union causing cubitus varus or gunstock deformity. Epiphyseal damage with later deformity. Myositis ossificans. OA. Volkmann's ischaemic contracture. Chronic regional pain syndrome (Sudeck's atrophy) may occur in adults.

Lateral condyle/epicondyle
Lateral condylar fractures occurring in young children are injuries of the capitellar epiphysis. Displaced lateral condyles should be fixed to prevent valgus deformity and tarda ulnar nerve palsy due to traction. Lateral epicondylar avulsions are very rare and should be fixed if displaced.

Medial condyle/epicondyle
Medial condylar fractures are rare and should be fixed if displaced. Medial epicondylar fractures are more common and are associated with elbow dislocations (50%). They should be fixed if displaced by >0.5–1 cm or fragments need washing out of the joint.

Dislocation of the elbow
It is caused by a fall on the hand with the elbow partly flexed. Dislocation is almost always posterior. Occasionally there are fractures of adjacent bones. Median or ulnar nerve palsy may occur. Damage to the brachial artery is rare.

Treatment. Reduction is usually easy. The elbow is held in slight flexion and then pressure is applied to the olecranon posteriorly until reduction occurs. The elbow is immobilized for 1–3 weeks in a collar and cuff, after which active exercises are encouraged.

Fracture-dislocation of the elbow is a more serious injury involving fractures of the humeral condyles, radial head or olecranon. Manipulative reduction and internal fixation may be necessary. A stiff elbow is the usual outcome. Vascular injury and myositis ossificans may also occur.

FRACTURES OF THE RADIUS AND ULNA

> These are caused by either indirect violence from a fall on the outstretched hand with or without rotation, or direct violence, which usually causes fracture of a single bone.

Fracture of the radial head
This varies from a fine vertical crack to severe comminution. There is localized tenderness over the radial head with minor injury. With comminution the elbow is painful and swollen with restriction of all movement. Minor cracks and undisplaced

fractures may be rested in a collar and cuff sling for 2 weeks. Displaced large fragments may be internally fixed. Comminuted fractures may require excision or replacement of the radial head.

Fracture of the olecranon

This is caused by direct violence as an isolated injury, or as part of a fracture-dislocation of the elbow. Displaced fractures are internally fixed with tension band wires or lag screws.

Fractures of the radial and ulnar shafts

These injuries are common and are often open. They are usually caused by direct violence. An injury to the forearm usually affects the two bones, or one bone plus one radioulnar joint. A displaced fracture of the midshaft of either bone alone can occur if the radial head dislocates with an ulnar fracture (Monteggia's fracture) or the distal radioulnar joint dislocates with a fracture of the radius (Galeazzi fracture). Radiographs of the forearm must therefore include both wrist and elbow joints. Occasionally direct violence fractures only one bone, e.g. the ulnar, as when lifting up the flexed arm to ward off a blow. In children, fractures are of the greenstick type with angulation. In adults the fractures are transverse or oblique.

Treatment

Children. Manipulative reduction is usually successful. Position is maintained in an above-elbow plaster cast from axilla to metacarpal heads with the elbow at a right angle.

Adults. Accurate alignment is essential to allow pronation and supination. Open reduction and plating is usually undertaken followed by 2–4 weeks in plaster.

Fractures of the distal radius

Colles' fracture (→ Fig. 17.11)

This is a dorsally displaced fracture in the elderly 2.5 cm from the wrist joint. It is common in elderly osteoporotic women following a low-energy fall.

Figure 17.11 Colles' fracture. (A) Lateral view. (B) Anteroposterior view.

Distal fragment displaced and tilted backwards

'Dinner fork' deformity of Colles' fracture

(A)

Radial displacement of distal fragment

Avulsion of ulnar styloid

(B)

Figure 17.12 A radiograph of the wrist (lateral view) showing a typical Colles' fracture. There is apex volar angulation, dorsal displacement, and impaction.

Distal radial fracture

A similar fracture is found in younger adults. While there is not the same degree of dorsal cancellous bone collapse as with the osteoporotic Colles' fracture, the high energy nature of the injury often leads to comminution or intra articular extension of the fracture. These are more aggressively treated by surgery due to higher patient demand.

Symptoms and signs. Fall on outstretched hand. Pain. Limitation of wrist movement. 'Dinner fork' deformity. Check for distal neurovascular deficit.

Investigations. Radiograph in two planes (→ Fig. 17.12): distal fragment is displaced dorsally, radially (with pull-off of the ulnar styloid) and supinated; check for intra-articular fracture lines and associated scaphoid fracture.

Treatment. Undisplaced or greenstick fractures require immobilization in a below-elbow plaster for 3–4 weeks. Significant displacement requires manipulation under general or regional anaesthesia (Bier's block). The fracture is disimpacted by traction and increasing the deformity. The distal fragment is levered over the proximal, the wrist flexed, ulnar deviated and pronated. A dorsal plaster slab is applied to hold this position. A check radiograph is taken and the arm supported in a sling. A further radiograph is taken 1 week later to check reduction. Swelling has usually subsided by this time and the plaster is completed and the sling abandoned.

The plaster is removed at 6 weeks and exercises commenced. Operative treatment is required for intra-articular fractures (especially in the young) and failed reduction or failed plaster immobilization.

Complications. Stiffness and oedema of the hand. Mal-union with angulation. This may be associated with pain from subluxation of the inferior radioulnar joint. Median nerve symptoms occur but usually subside spontaneously. Later rupture of the tendon of extensor pollicis longus may occur where it crosses the fracture. Complex regional pain syndrome.

Smith's fracture

This is a fracture of the lower end of the radius with forward (volar) angulation. It is the reverse of a Colles' fracture. Conservative treatment is manipulation using the reverse procedure for Colles' fracture. An above-elbow plaster is applied for 6 weeks with the wrist dorsiflexed and the forearm fully supinated. Operative treatment (volar plating) is often required owing to instability of the fracture in plaster.

Barton's fracture

This is an intra-articular fracture-dislocation of the radiocarpal joints in the coronal plane. Internal fixation is required.

FRACTURES AND DISLOCATIONS OF THE CARPAL BONES

Fracture of the scaphoid

Caused by a fall on the outstretched hand or a blow to the palm of the hand. The blood supply to the bone comes from distal to proximal, and hence there is a risk of avascular necrosis of the proximal fragment. The scaphoid spans both rows of carpal bones hence the high risk of non-union.

Symptoms and signs. Fall on outstretched hand. Painful swollen wrist with tenderness in the anatomical snuffbox and on AP compression of the scaphoid.

Investigations
- Radiograph: scaphoid views
- Bone scan
- MRI.

Treatment. If this fracture is suspected clinically but is not confirmed on radiograph, treat on clinical grounds as a fracture to scaphoid. Re-radiograph in 2 weeks when the fracture may show. A bone scan/MRI may be helpful. The wrist is immobilized in a scaphoid or Colles' cast. The plaster is worn for 6 weeks initially when radiological evidence of union should be apparent. Union may be delayed and a plaster may need to be worn for 3 months.

Complications. Avascular necrosis of the proximal segment. Delayed union and non-union requiring bone grafting and internal fixation. OA of the wrist is a long-term sequel.

Dislocation of the carpus

Commonly missed. Caused by a fall on an extended hand. If the radiograph looks unusual, especially the lateral view, obtain specialist advice. Volar (anterior) dislocation of the lunate is the commonest and may cause acute median nerve compression. Check for associated scaphoid fracture. Closed or open reduction is performed. Methods of immobilization are controversial but application of a plaster ± K wires for 6–8 weeks may be required.

FRACTURES AND DISLOCATIONS OF THE METACARPALS AND PHALANGES

When assessing fractures of the metacarpals or phalanges, beware of rotational displacement. This may not be obvious until the fingers are flexed, when they cross over each other abnormally.

Fractures at the base of the thumb

Extra-articular fractures can usually be treated conservatively by manipulation and plaster casting. Intra-articular fractures of the thumb may produce late OA. Bennett's fracture is oblique and the small fragment is on the ulnar side of the base of the first metacarpal where the deep oblique ligament attaches. Most are treated with closed reduction and K wires under GA, but occasionally open reduction and internal fixation is required. Late OA is rarely seen.

Fractures of the metacarpal bones

These are caused by direct violence or by punching with a closed fist. Very important to identify the 'fight bite' injury where a tooth penetrates the MCP joint. Condition often missed. Requires wash out.

Treatment. Undisplaced fractures are treated in a back slab or by strapping the injured finger to its neighbour. Displaced or multiple fractures require reduction and/or internal fixation. Active movements are encouraged.

Fractures and dislocations of the phalanges

These are often serious injuries and may be associated with tendon and nerve damage.

Treatment. Dislocation can usually be reduced under local anaesthetic. Undisplaced fractures may be treated by strapping the injured finger to its neighbour. Active movements are encouraged. Unstable or displaced fractures may need open reduction and internal fixation with crossed Kirschner wires or miniscrews.

Fractures of the terminal phalanges

These are usually crush injuries and may be open. There may be subungual haematoma that contributes to the pain. The latter can be drained by piercing the nail with a hot wire, giving instant relief. Open fractures are treated with wound toilet, leaving the wound open, tetanus toxoid and broad-spectrum antibiotics. Occasionally, partial amputation of the finger is required.

Mallet finger

This injury is caused by 'stubbing' a finger when it is actively extended. Forced passive flexion leads to avulsion of the extensor tendon from the base of the terminal phalanx often with a flake of bone. Examination reveals a finger in which the distal phalanx is flexed and cannot be actively extended. Treatment is by immobilization of the distal interphalangeal joint in a 'mallet finger' splint, which hyperextends the terminal interphalangeal joint while allowing flexion of the proximal interphalangeal joint. The splint is worn for 6 weeks. Occasionally healing does not occur but the disability is usually slight, although it may be more pronounced and require fusion of the distal interphalangeal joint.

CONDITIONS OF JOINTS

ARTHRITIS

> This is inflammation of a joint. The term is used to describe both inflammatory and degenerative disease.

Osteoarthritis (osteoarthrosis, OA)

This is a term applied to degenerative disease of a joint caused by wear and tear that affects the articular cartilage and subchondral bone. At first, the synovial membrane is normal but later thickening and fibrosis occurs. OA may be primary or secondary. In the former there is no underlying cause. It may arise as a result of senile changes and may affect more than one joint. Secondary OA occurs if there has been previous damage to the joint, e.g. congenital deformity, trauma, infection, avascular necrosis, gout, haemophilia.

Symptoms and signs. Pain. Stiffness. Deformity. Pain increases in severity as the disease progresses. Sleep is often disturbed. Synovial thickening and bony enlargement of joint because of osteophytes. Effusions. Tenderness. Loss of movement. Crepitus. Fixed deformities. Disturbances of gait.

Investigations. Radiographs ($\rightarrow$ Fig. 17.13): narrowing of joint space, subchondral bone sclerosis, subchondral cysts, osteophytes, evidence of other underlying pathology. Symptoms do not necessarily correlate with the severity of radiological changes.

Treatment. Principles of treatment involve pain relief, improvement of mobility and correction of deformity. Management may be conservative or surgical.

Conservative. Analgesia: start with mild analgesia, e.g. paracetamol; NSAIDs are usually required eventually.

- Lose weight
- Walking stick or shoe raise
- Physiotherapy, i.e. heat treatment or short-wave diathermy
- Changing occupation to a lighter job.

Surgical. Disturbance of sleep, severe uncontrolled pain and gross lack of mobility are indications for surgery. The following procedures may be undertaken depending upon the level of symptoms and joint involved:

- Arthroscopy or open debridement: occasionally synovectomy and removal of osteophytes can give temporary relief

Figure 17.13 There is osteoarthritis of the right hip joint. The joint space is diminished and there is sclerosis of the surrounding bone. On the left side, the patient has had an arthroplasty (hip replacement).

- Replacement arthroplasty (→ Fig. 17.13): most joints can be replaced by artificial joints, e.g. hip and knee
- Osteotomy: weight-bearing axis redistributes weight commonly to the lateral side. Pain relief is often dramatic and failure of the procedure is slow
- Excision arthroplasty: for small joints, e.g. small toes
- Arthrodesis: surgical fusion of the joint, relieves pain, e.g. first MTP joint in hallux rigidus.

Rheumatoid arthritis (RA)

Only surgical aspects of management will be dealt with here. (The reader is referred to a textbook of medicine for the details of the symptoms and medical management of this disease.) Surgery is undertaken to improve function, not for cosmetic effect. Procedures include:

- Synovectomy: gives good pain relief. The knees and finger joints are most suitable for this treatment
- Repair or reconstruction of ruptured tendons
- Joint fusion, e.g. painful wrist; atlantoaxial subluxation
- Arthroplasty: the same prostheses and procedures are used as for OA. However, hand deformities are often most trouble in RA and various arthroplasties of the

finger joints are indicated. Flexible silastic implants giving stability whilst allowing movement are the most popular. Infection can be a problem as the patients have often been on long-term steroids.

OTHER CONDITIONS OF JOINTS

Loose bodies

These may occur in any joint but the knee is by far the commonest site. Causes include osteochondritis dissecans (see below), detached osteophytes in OA, osteochondral fractures, torn menisci and synovial chondromatosis, where cartilaginous nodules form in the synovium and may become detached.

Symptoms and signs. Pain and swelling. 'Locking' (an inability to fully extend the knee). Giving way. Occasionally, the loose body may be palpable.

Investigations
● Radiograph
● Arthroscopy.

Treatment. Open or arthroscopic removal.

Osteochondritis dissecans

In this, an area of bone with its overlying articular cartilage becomes necrotic, separates and drops into the joint cavity as a loose body. It is associated with local trauma (50%).

Symptoms and signs. Late childhood or young adults. Commonly affects the knee. Occasionally multiple joints. Knee – usually medial femoral condyle. Pain and swelling. Loose body may cause locking or giving way.

Investigations
● Radiographs
● MRI – high signal or T_2 images deep to the fragment in situ supports diagnosis of loose fragments.

Treatment. In the early stages before separation, rest in a plaster cast or bandage may allow healing. If separation is incomplete, pinning may help revascularization. A loose body needs removal. Drilling the defect may help healing.

Neuropathic joints (Charcot's joints)

A diffuse destructing deformity and dislocation often found in diabetes. A joint which has lost pain and proprioception appreciation is subject to harmful stresses and strains. Destruction of the joint results. The patient usually presents with a painless, deformed joint. Causes include diabetic neuropathy, tabes dorsalis, syringomyelia and leprosy. Vibration sense, position sense and deep pain sensation are absent or reduced. Treatment requires non-weight-bearing immobilization followed by a graduated return to ankle foot orthoses. Arthrodesis and arthroplasty are usually unsuccessful. Supporting appliances may be the most appropriate treatment.

Haemophilia and related disorders

The main orthopaedic problems relate to acute haemarthroses and bleeding into muscles. They may occur spontaneously or as a result of injury, which may be minor. Recurrent bleeding into the same joint results in degenerative changes, capsular fibrosis, contracture and deformity. The knee, elbow and ankle are the joints most frequently affected.

Symptoms and signs. Pain, muscular spasm, swelling over joint. Local tenderness. Bruising. Long-standing cases show deformity of joint. Muscle wasting and synovial thickening. Patients presenting for the first time with a haemarthrosis need detailed haematological investigation.

Treatment. Analgesia, splintage, factor VIII replacement. Large haemarthroses require aspiration under factor VIII cover. The chronically damaged joint is prone to repeated bleeds and a splint (a caliper in case of a knee joint) may be necessary for long-term protection. Synovectomy and soft tissue release for severe contractures.

ARTHROPLASTY

This is surgical refashioning of a joint, the aims being to relieve pain, restore mobility and provide stability. There are basically three types of arthroplasty:

- *Excision*. The joint surfaces are excised. Fibrous tissue forms across the gap. Although considerable pain relief is gained there is residual instability. This method is usually regarded as a temporary measure following failure of a joint replacement where the prosthesis has to be removed and infection allowed to settle before proceeding with a 're-do' joint replacement. It may be a salvage/end stage procedure for pain relief in the elderly, i.e. hip excision (Girdlestone's procedure).
- *Partial or hemiarthroplasty*. This is used where one surface of the joint is in good condition, e.g. a Thompson's prosthesis in fractured neck of femur where the acetabulum is normal. It is rarely suitable for OA.
- *Total* (→ Fig. 17.13). Both articular surfaces are replaced, e.g. Charnley's prosthesis in hip replacement.

Design of joint replacements

- Metal on metal (cobalt – chrome, recently fallen out of favour due to aseptic lymphocyte-dominated vasculitis associated lesion), metal on plastic (high-density polyethylene), ceramic on polythene and ceramic on ceramic
- Fatigue resistant
- Firm bonding to bone, using a cement (polymethyl methacrylate) as grout or osseo-integration to the prosthesis with porous coating or hydroxyapatite coating
- Adequate range of movement
- Stability against dislocation.

Practice of joint replacement

Indications. Pain limiting activity, despite adequate analgesia, and especially pain disturbing sleep.

Preoperative preparation (good practice). DVT prophylaxis. Prophylactic antibiotics. Patient informed of operative procedure. Templating of X-rays. Ultraclean air with unidirectional laminar flow ventilation ('Charnley's tent'), body exhaust suits. Strict aseptic technique. Inclusion of antibiotics in bone cement. Meticulous dissection, positioning of prosthesis, soft tissue reconstruction. Early mobilization.

Complications

Early. As for any major operation, especially bleeding, DVT, PE. Neurovascular injury. Dislocation. Wound infection.

Intermediate. Recurrent dislocation. Heterotopic ossification.

Late. Septic or aseptic loosening (failure of the interface to bone). Implant wear or failure.

CONDITIONS OF MENISCI, LIGAMENTS, TENDONS, CAPSULES AND BURSAE

KNEE

Meniscus tears

This is a common knee injury. The medial is affected more often than the lateral. It occurs in patients whose occupation involves kneeling, crouching, or trauma, e.g. miners, footballers.

Symptoms and signs. Often young male. Twists the knee. Usually knee is flexed and weight is on injured leg. Pain on side of knee where meniscus is torn. Knee may catch, click and 'lock'. Knee swells slowly over 24 h. Settles with resting. Symptoms may then recur with 'recurrent locking'. At time of injury, tenderness, swelling, tender over meniscus, effusion. In the chronic phase – wasted quadriceps, effusion, tenderness over meniscus in joint line. McMurray's test is positive if the tear is posterior. Diagnosis is usually made on classical history and signs.

Investigations
- Plain radiographs normal
- Exclude other conditions, e.g. radio-opaque loose bodies
- MRI scan
- Arthroscopy (for treatment rather than diagnosis).

Treatment

Acute phase. Tears in the periphery of the meniscus can be repaired. Otherwise, minimal meniscal resection. Avoid total meniscectomy because of the high risk of OA.

Chronic phase. Meniscectomy usually by arthroscopic technique followed by course of quadriceps exercises.

Ligamentous damage

Damage to the collateral ligaments and cruciate ligaments occurs frequently in sportsmen. Strains may be associated with an effusion into the joint and tenderness over the affected ligament. In contrast to complete tears the joint remains stable. Strains settle with rest and support followed by graded exercises.

Collateral ligaments

Medial. An abduction strain on the tibia ruptures the medial ligament. Valgus straining with 10° of flexion will demonstrate opening of the joint. If a cruciate ligament is also damaged, the joint will open even in full extension. Clinical diagnosis with confirmation via MRI.

Lateral. Rarely occurs in isolation. Instability is rarer because the biceps femoris tendon helps stabilize the lateral side of the knee.

Cruciate ligament tears

Anterior. Usually caused by non-contact hyperextension or forward movement of the tibia on the femur with the knee flexed. There may be associated meniscal tears or damage to collateral ligaments. Examination reveals an effusion and a positive 'anterior draw sign' – the tibia can be pulled forwards on the femur with the knee flexed. Lachman's test with knee flexed at 20° and tibia drawn forward is more sensitive than 'anterior draw' test. Pivot shift test is most specific.

Posterior. Usually torn by a force drawing the tibia backwards on the femur with the knee flexed. There is almost always other ligamentous injury. Examination reveals 'posterior sag', i.e. the tibia moves backwards on the femur when eliciting the 'posterior draw sign'.

Treatment of ligamentous injuries. Isolated collateral ligament injuries are initially treated in plaster or a brace. Multiple or complex injuries are best treated surgically. Chronic injuries with symptomatic instability benefit from surgery. Acute PCL or posterolateral corner injuries require surgery within 5–12 days. Others may be treated when chronic.

Bursae around the knee

Housemaid's knee (prepatellar bursitis)

Rarely seen now that women do not scrub floors. More often seen in carpet fitters. Leaning forward on the knees brings the prepatellar bursa in contact with the floor. Treatment is by aspiration or excision.

Clergyman's knee (infrapatellar bursitis)

Rarely seen now that clergymen infrequently pray on their knees. After prolonged periods of prayer the clergymen sat back on his heels bringing the infrapatellar bursa in contact with the floor. Treatment is by aspiration or excision.

Semimembranosus bursa

It occurs between the tendon of semimembranosus and deeper structures. Cystic swelling on medial aspect of popliteal fossa. Usually occurs in children and young adults. Most resolve spontaneously. Very rarely excision is required.

Baker's cyst

This is included here for convenience but is not a bursa. It is a cystic lesion of the knee joint most commonly due to a one way valve forming from a meniscal tear in the knee. It presents as a swelling in the popliteal fossa. The cyst usually communicates with the back of the joint through a small defect in the capsule.

Surgery is rarely required unless the cyst becomes tense and very painful. If there is any doubt about the diagnosis MRI should be carried out. The cyst may rupture and cause pain behind the knee and in the calf. It may be difficult to distinguish from a DVT (venography will confirm the diagnosis of DVT). A thrombosed popliteal aneurysm enters into the differential diagnosis of a painful Baker's cyst. Check the other limb (popliteal aneurysms may be bilateral) and the distal circulation.

ANKLE

Sprained ankle

The anterior talofibular ligament is the most common ankle ligament that may be torn during an inversion injury. Pain, swelling and tenderness occur below and in front of the lateral malleolus. Treatment is by analgesia, physiotherapy and occasionally an ankle foot orthosis.

Rupture of the Achilles tendon

This usually occurs during sport, e.g. tennis or due to a missed step. The patient feels 'something give' and feels like 'being kicked in the back of the heel'. Examination usually reveals a gap in the tendon. The calf squeeze test is positive. Conservative treatment is by plaster immobilization in full plantar flexion followed by progressive plasters up to the neutral position. Surgical repair may be necessary in the young, active patient and is followed by immobilization in plaster to reduce the risk of re-rupture. Operative repair is required for re-rupture and delay in diagnosis of >1 week.

Plantar fasciitis

This occurs in late middle age. The pain is under the heel. In the younger patient it may be associated with Reiter's disease. The pain is often worse on standing after a period of rest and improves somewhat with walking. Examination reveals tenderness at the attachment of the plantar fascia to the under surface of os calcis. A lateral radiograph may show an associated calcaneal spur. Treatment is by a soft heel pad, or local injection of steroid and local anaesthetic or both. The condition is self-limiting.

SHOULDER

A variety of conditions may occur in middle life at the shoulder girdle. They probably represent a spectrum of related conditions of low-grade inflammatory or degenerative aetiology. They include conditions variously known as impingement syndrome, rotator cuff tears, frozen shoulder, rupture of the long head of biceps and acromio-clavicular arthritis. Conditions previously known as supraspinatus tendinitis, subacromial bursitis and painful arc syndrome are now grouped together under the title impingement syndrome.

Impingement syndrome

Mechanical impingement of the rotator cuff muscles on the under-surface of the acromion can cause inflammation and pain with overhead activities. The insertion of supraspinatus is a relatively avascular area susceptible to repeated trauma and degeneration. Pain may be felt in the mid-arc of abduction with positive impingement tests – shoulder forward flexed 90° and internal rotation impacts supraspinatus tendon between acromion and greater tuberosity.

Investigations
- Radiographs to exclude arthritis; sclerosis of acromion and tuberosity
- USS – cuff inflammation or tendinosis
- MRI.

Treatment. Modification of activity. NSAIDs. Physiotherapy. Subacromial steroid injection. If symptoms persist arthroscopic subacromial decompression may be required.

Frozen shoulder
Now thought to be due to fibrosis of the capsule of the shoulder joint. Often no predisposing cause is found. There are no adhesions or synovitis. Stiffness and pain predominate with loss of external rotation. May be primary of unknown aetiology or secondary, e.g. trauma. More common in diabetics.

Treatment. Spontaneous resolution usually occurs over 2 years. Manipulation under anaesthetic is often carried out early with good pain relief and improved function. Some patients require open or arthroscopic capsule release.

Rotator cuff tears
Most commonly affects supraspinatus but can involve subscapularis and infraspinatus. Usually occurs in a tendon that is already degenerate. It follows trivial trauma or normal everyday activity. There is a sudden pain in the shoulder and an inability to initiate abduction. If initial abduction can be started passively (e.g. by tilting the body to the side to initiate abduction by gravity) deltoid can continue abduction. Diagnosis may be confirmed by USS, CT or MRI. Surgical treatment may be required for large tears.

Rupture of the long head of biceps
This usually occurs in a previously diseased tendon. There is acute pain, tenderness and 'bunching up' of the muscle in the lower part of the upper arm when the elbow is flexed. There is little residual functional disability.

ELBOW

Tennis elbow
This is chronic inflammation or degeneration of the extensor carpi radialis brevis at its origin on the lateral epicondyle. It affects anyone whose work involves extending and twisting the forearm. In some cases there is no obvious cause. There is pain on the outer side of the elbow radiating down the back of the forearm. It becomes worse on gripping. Tenderness is localized to the lateral epicondyle. Extension of the fingers and wrist against resistance exacerbates the pain. Treatment is by rest and injection of local anaesthetic and hydrocortisone. Surgery is rarely indicated.

Golfer's elbow

This is similar to tennis elbow but affects the medial epicondyle. Pain occurs on hyperextending the fingers and wrist. Treatment is by rest and injection of local anaesthetic and steroid. If the latter treatment is given, remember the close proximity of the ulnar nerve.

Student's elbow (olecranon bursitis)

This occurs owing to prolonged pressure over the olecranon bursa, e.g. a student studying long into the night and resting the head in the hand with the elbow on the table. For obvious reasons, the condition is uncommon in present-day students. Examination reveals a swelling over the olecranon, which may be acutely inflamed. In the acute phase, aspiration (occasionally pus is obtained) and antibiotics are required. NSAIDs are usually given for pain relief. In the chronic phase, straw-coloured fluid is aspirated. Surgical excision may be required.

WRIST

Tenosynovitis

This is inflammation of a tendon sheath. It is caused by the trauma of repetitive movements and affects the tendons of the fingers and thumb, especially dorsally, where they cross the wrist within their synovial sheath. There is localized tenderness and crepitation on movement of digits. Treatment is by rest, local splinting and NSAIDs. A specific form affects the tendon sheaths of abductor pollicis longus and extensor pollicis brevis as they cross the radial styloid (De Quervain's tenosynovitis). Pain occurs at the site and is exacerbated by gripping and by extending the thumb. Forced flexion of the thumb with ulnar deviation of the wrist exacerbates the pain. Treatment in the acute phase involves splints and local injection of hydrocortisone. Chronic cases require surgical division of the tendon sheath.

HAND

Ganglion

A ganglion is a cystic swelling in relation to a joint or tendon sheath. It may represent cystic-myxomatous degeneration of fibrous tissue. It is common on the dorsum of the hand, and also occurs in relation to the wrist and ankle. It is a painless, cystic swelling that is fluctuant and transilluminates, and is filled with a crystal clear gel (some authorities believe it is a protrusion of synovium through an opening in a joint or fibrous sheath and that the fluid is derived from synovial fluid). Treatment is aspiration or surgical excision. The latter should be done under GA or brachial block using a tourniquet as they often extend down inside the underlying joints. Recurrence is less common when treated surgically.

Trigger finger

The fibrous flexor sheath thickens and the lumen narrows. The narrowed area causes friction against the tendon, creating a localized nodule in the tendon. The condition occurs at the level of the metacarpal head or neck. As the nodule passes through the area of stenosis, a click or snap is felt and the digit 'triggers'. Sometimes, the digit frankly locks in flexion and cannot be extended. If the finger is fully flexed the patient may have to extend it passively. A nodule may be palpable at the site of thickening. Spontaneous resolution may occur. Around 70% will respond to steroid injection to the entrance of the tendon sheath. Surgical treatment may by required and is by longitudinal division of the A1 pulley at the opening. Multiple 'triggering' digits should arouse the suspicion of RA.

Dupuytren's contracture

This is a condition of the palmar fascia involving nodules and contractures. Aetiology is unknown but it is associated with family history, diabetes, alcoholism, liver disease and antiepileptic drugs. It may be associated with Peyronie's disease and retroperitoneal fibrosis.

Symptoms and signs. Mainly elderly males but can occur in females. Nodular thickening of the palmar fascia. Contracture of the proximal interphalangeal joint and the metacarpophalangeal joint usually affecting the ring or little finger.

Treatment. If the patient cannot place the hand flat on the table, surgery is required. This involves careful dissection of the palmar fascia, fasciotomy and local fasciectomy. Recurrence may occur. If the deformity is great and involves a single digit, amputation may be appropriate.

MISCELLANEOUS CONDITIONS OF THE LIMBS

UPPER LIMB

Ulnar neuritis

The ulnar nerve lies in a groove behind the medial epicondyle. Pressure or chronic friction may occur in the groove. Cubitus valgus (increased carrying angle) may stretch the nerve. Symptoms include pain in the forearm, paraesthesia in the ulnar one and half fingers and wasting of the small muscles of the hand supplied by the ulnar nerve. EMG studies confirm the diagnosis. Treatment is by decompression or by transposition of the ulnar nerve anterior to the medial epicondyle.

Carpal tunnel syndrome

In this condition the median nerve is compressed in the carpal tunnel. It may be associated with pregnancy, RA, myxoedema, OA, anterior dislocation of the lunate, and arteriovenous fistula at the wrist for dialysis. Middle-aged women are most affected.

Symptoms and signs. Pain, paraesthesia, in the thumb, index and middle fingers. Worse in bed at night. Relieved by hanging arm out of bed. Clumsiness when carrying out fine movements. Wasting of thenar muscles and reduction of sensation in distribution of median nerve in hand occur in advanced cases. No objective findings in early cases. Pressure over the carpal tunnel may reproduce symptoms.

Investigations. Nerve conduction studies may help.

Differential diagnosis. Thoracic outlet syndrome, cervical spondylosis, peripheral neuritis.

Treatment. Mild cases may be treated by splintage at night. Injection of the carpal tunnel with steroid may be appropriate. Carpal tunnel decompression by operative division of the flexor retinaculum. Cases presenting in pregnancy often settle spontaneously after delivery.

LOWER LIMB

Metatarsalgia

This is pain under the metatarsal heads. It is caused by a dropped transverse arch, often in elderly obese ladies. It is tender over the second and third metatarsal heads with callosities. Treatment is with a weight-relieving insole. Morton's metatarsalgia is due to a plantar digital neuroma, probably due to chronic trauma at the confluence of the medial and lateral plantar nerves against the metatarsal transverse ligament. It also affects middle-aged women. Usually it affects the cleft between the third and fourth toes. Treatment is weight-relieving insoles or division of the metatarsal ligament. If symptoms do not settle, wide-toe box shoes and steroid and local anaesthetic infiltration or exploration and excision of neuroma may be necessary. Other causes include stress fracture, plantar warts, inflammatory conditions (e.g. RA), Freiberg's disease.

Hallux valgus

This is common in females. The first metatarsal deviates medially and the great toe laterally creating a bulge often covered with a 'bunion' due to a thickened overlying bursa. The great toe may overlap or under-ride the second toe. It may be a result of wearing unsuitable footwear, especially in adolescence. It is often familial. Metatarsalgia may co-exist.

Treatment. Mild cases require accommodating wide shoe footwear. Surgery is necessary for gross deformity or associated arthritis. If there is no arthritis, realignment operations are appropriate, e.g. Chevron scarf osteotomy or Lapidus procedure should be carried out. Arthrodesis or resection arthroplasty is required if there is secondary OA.

Hallux rigidus

This is OA of the first metatarsophalangeal joint. It is a common condition that occurs in young adults, but the cause is unknown. There is pain on walking, especially 'pushing off', and a stiff, painful, enlarged joint. Radiographs show OA. Treatment in mild cases is by a metatarsal bar in the shoe. Severe cases require arthrodesis.

Hammer toes

This is a toe (usually the second) with a fixed flexion deformity of the proximal interphalangeal joint and compensatory hyperextension of the adjacent joints. Painful overlying corns occur. Treatment is by arthrodesis or excision of the proximal interphalangeal joints with extensor tenotomy.

Mallet toe

This is a toe with flexion deformity of the distal interphalangeal joint with a corn at the tip of the toe or over the joint. Distal interphalangeal joint fusion is indicated.

INFECTION OF BONES AND JOINTS

ACUTE INFECTION OF BONES AND JOINTS

Acute osteomyelitis

This is a disease of growing bones or immunosuppressed or diabetic adults. It is usually due to *Staphylococcus aureus*, and rarely due to *Streptococci, Pneumococci, Haemophilus* or *Salmonella*. The infection usually starts at the vascular metaphysis of a long bone or centre of a short bone. Common sites include the lower end of the femur, upper end of the tibia, humerus, radius, ulna and vertebral bodies. Suppuration occurs and pus under tension causes bone necrosis. Pus breaks out under the periosteum, strips it up, and penetrates through, forming a sinus. Alternatively, the pus can decompress into the joint causing septic arthritis. Necrotic bone is called a 'sequestrum'. New subperiosteal bone forms around the dead bone forming a shell (involucrum).

Symptoms and signs. Young patients. Recent history of infection (e.g. respiratory) or trauma. Pain in limb. Aggravated by movement. Swelling and redness of affected area – usually localized to metaphyseal area. Loss of function. Malaise. Pyrexia. Tenderness and head over site of infection. Oedema. Pus with fluctuation is a late sign. Sympathetic effusion in nearby joint.

Investigations
- WCC ↑
- CRP ↑
- Blood cultures
- Radiographs: negative in early stages. Later, areas of osteoporosis with subperiosteal new bone and later sequestration is seen
- Technetium bone scan
- Indium-labelled WCC scan
- CT scan
- Sinogram.

Treatment. After obtaining blood cultures ± drainage of pus, start antibiotics, e.g. fusidic acid and flucloxacillin i.v. Splint the limb to relieve pain. Prolonged antibiotic therapy up to 6 weeks may be necessary. Resolving temperature and falling CRP are good guides to recovery.

Acute pyogenic arthritis

This is a blood-borne infection, especially in infants. *Staphylococci, Streptococci* and *Gonococci* may be causative organisms. It may arise following osteomyelitis, where the metaphysis is intracapsular, e.g. hip joint. It is a complication of RA in patients on steroids. Occasionally it follows penetrating injuries of joints.

Symptoms and signs. Hot, tender, painful, swollen joint. All movements are painful and there is surrounding muscle spasm. High fever. Rigors.

Investigations
- WCC ↑
- CRP ↑
- Blood culture
- USS
- Joint aspiration with Gram film
- Culture and sensitivity
- Radiographs are of little value in early stages; later, subperiosteal new bone with periarticular porosis.

Differential diagnosis. Osteomyelitis with sympathetic effusion. RA. Reiter's disease. Gout. Rheumatic fever.

Treatment. Washout of joint. Antibiotic. Fusidic acid and flucloxacillin initially and then according to culture. Splintage. Analgesia. Surgical drainage may be necessary.

CHRONIC INFECTIONS OF BONES AND JOINTS

Chronic osteomyelitis

This may follow acute osteomyelitis but is more common following surgery for an open fracture, especially when foreign material is implanted. It may be chronic from the outset, e.g. tuberculosis.

Secondary to acute osteomyelitis

In this condition, the bone becomes sclerotic and thickened. Sequestra are present and involucrum and sinuses may be present.

Symptoms and signs. Flare-ups with pain, swelling, discharging sinus and abscess formation. Spontaneous recovery may occur.

Investigations
- Radiographs: show thickening of bone and cavity formation, sequestra (denser than normal bone) may be present
- CRP ↑
- WCC ↑
- Culture and sensitivity. Drainage if discharge present.

Treatment. Treat acute episodes with appropriate antibiotic. Surgery is indicated if discharge is marked, sequestra or large cavities are present, or attacks of pain and pyrexia are frequent. Open the cavity, allow the wound to granulate, excise sequestra. Rarely, amputation may be necessary.

Complications. Amyloid. Pathological fracture. Squamous carcinoma in a sinus track.

Chronic osteomyelitis may occur secondary to trauma or secondary to insertion of a joint replacement or internal fixation device. Chronic osteomyelitis secondary to trauma is treated as above but fracture stabilization needs an external fixation device. If an internal fixation device or joint replacement is associated with chronic osteomyelitis it must be removed.

Chronic osteomyelitis due to specific chronic infections

This may arise as a result of tuberculosis, syphilis (tertiary) or mycotic infections. Tuberculosis is the most common.

Tuberculosis of bones and joints. This occurs worldwide, especially in under-developed countries. In Europe it is more common in the immigrant population and in the elderly and is on the increase. It is usually blood-borne. The primary site is usually in the lung. Destruction of bone and articular cartilage occurs. The synovial membrane is studded with tubercles, which extend under the articular cartilage, destroying it. Abscess formation occurs, especially in spinal tuberculosis. This may discharge into the psoas sheath and present under the inguinal ligament of the groin as a psoas abscess. Joints are often destroyed and undergo fibrosis or bony ankylosis.

Symptoms and signs. History of TB contact. Infection of bone alone unusual. Usually involves both bone and joint. Malaise, weight loss, night sweats. Local pain, stiffness or limping. Local tenderness, soft tissue swelling, joint effusion. Local muscle atrophy. Discharge of cold abscess with sinus formation. Backache with TB of spine (Pott's disease). Wasting of back muscles, spasm, movement restricted. Localized kyphosis or 'gibbus' due to vertebral collapse. Paraplegia may occur.

Investigations
- WCC ↑ with lymphocytosis
- CRP ↑
- Mantoux test
- Joint aspiration with Ziehl–Nielsen staining and culture
- Biopsy: needle or open
- Sputum and urine culture
- Radiographs show: osteoporosis around joint; erosion of joint surfaces; destruction of bone and intervertebral discs; soft tissue shadows, e.g. psoas abscess
- CXR: initial pulmonary infection.

Treatment. Antituberculous drugs. Rest. Splintage. Traction, e.g. TB hip. Surgery – drainage of abscess, excision of affected bone with grafting, synovectomy, arthrodesis of diseased joints. Spinal tuberculosis is treated initially by immobilization in a spinal support until stability achieved, usually by bony fusion of the vertebral bodies. Drainage of cold abscesses and removal of necrotic bone may be necessary, with surgical fusion of adjacent vertebrae.

BONE TUMOURS

These may be benign or malignant. Secondary tumours are much more common than primary. Secondaries occur from the lung, breast, prostate, thyroid and kidney. Primary malignant tumours are rare but they have a bad prognosis and affect patients in a younger age group. The management of suspected primary bone tumours is a specialist multidisciplinary task and may involve discussion with National Tumour Centres.

Investigations. Diagnosis of primary bone tumours is very difficult. Radiographs show an overlapping spectrum of changes. Various imaging techniques can be used to determine the extent of the lesion. Pulmonary and cerebral metastases should be sought.

Biopsy. Careful surgery reduces dissemination of the tumour and may allow limb-conserving surgery. Histology may be very difficult to interpret.

Treatment. Some combination of surgery (curettage and bone grafting, wide local excision, amputation), and for malignant tumours radiotherapy or chemotherapy. The margin for resection is determined by staging the involvement of adjacent muscles and joints.

BENIGN TUMOURS

Osteoma ('ivory' osteoma)
This is a growth from the surface of bone. It is common on the surface of the vault of the skull. A smooth, non-tender mound, it rarely causes symptoms. If symptomatic, it can be cured by excision.

Osteoid osteoma
It usually occurs in long bones or spine in young males. There is severe continuous boring pain – usually worse at night and with characteristic marked relief by aspirin. It is probably not a true neoplasm. Radiographs show dense sclerosis surrounding a small central lucent nidus (osteoid). Treatment is by radioablation (90% successful), which gives dramatic relief of pain. 50% burn out.

Chondroma
A cartilaginous tumour, common in the phalanges and metacarpals. An enchondroma is a chondroma growing in the centre of a bone. A periosteal chondroma is a chondroma growing on the surface of a bone. Osteochondroma is a cartilage-capped bony outgrowth (commonest bone tumour, malignant potential, especially if >2 cm or multiple). Treatment is indicated only when the swelling is large, when excision should be undertaken. Occasionally multiple enchondromatosis occurs (Ollier's disease) associated with AV malformations (Maffucci's). These have significant future malignant potential.

Fibroma and fibrous dysplasia
This is a spectrum of conditions with failure or partial failure of ossification replaced by fibrous tissue. These are usually asymptomatic and often regress at puberty or after a fracture.

Bone cysts
These are fluid- or blood-filled cavities. They vary from multiloculated cysts containing clear fluid in children and adolescents to large aneurysmal bone cysts that may cause 'bulging out' of one side of a bone. Pathological fractures are common. Treatment is by excision and bone grafting.

MALIGNANT TUMOURS

Primary

Osteosarcoma (osteogenic sarcoma)

This is the most common primary tumour of bone. It occurs under the age of 30 years and is more common in males. It occurs in long bones. In older patients it is usually associated with Paget's disease; in the young it commonly affects the lower end of the femur or upper end of the tibia. It usually affects the metaphysis. Spread is via the bloodstream to the lungs; 10–20% have metastases at presentation.

Symptoms and signs. Bone pain. Swelling. Limp. Cough due to lung metastases. Tumour grows rapidly. Hot, tender swelling on examination.

Investigations

- Radiograph (→ Fig. 17.14): bone destruction, grows out of cortex elevating periosteum with deposition of subperiosteal bone (Codman's triangle), radiating spicules of bone ('sunray' spicules), soft tissue invasion
- ESR ↑
- Alkaline phosphatase ↑
- CT scan: shows invasion of the tumour, lung secondaries
- Biopsy.

Figure 17.14 Osteogenic sarcoma of the lower end of the femur showing 'Codman's triangle' (top arrow) and 'sunray spicules' (bottom two arrows).

Treatment. Classically, amputation was carried out as soon as diagnosis was made. Current treatment involves pre-adjuvant chemotherapy, restaging and then wide excision. If multiple pulmonary metastases at time of presentation, treatment is by chemotherapy alone. Solitary pulmonary metastases may be resected.

Prognosis. The 5-year survival is 60–70%, with pre-adjuvant chemotherapy followed by surgery.

Osteoclastoma (giant cell tumour)

This occurs in young adults, at the ends of long bones. It has a low malignant potential (2%) but is locally recurrent and aggressive. Metastases are uncommon, occur late and are to the lungs.

Symptoms and signs. Pain. Swelling. Pathological fractures.

Investigations
- Radiograph: multilocular cystic lesion expanding the cortex extending into epiphyses
- Biopsy.

Treatment. Excision. Curettage, phenolization and bone grafting or cement leads to 85% recurrence rate.

Ewing's tumour (primitive peripheral neuroectodermal tumour)

It is highly malignant and arises from the marrow. Common sites are the pelvis, knee, femoral diaphysis, proximal humerus. It affects children and young adults and spreads rapidly via the bloodstream to lungs, liver and other bones.

Symptoms and signs. Pain. Tenderness. Swelling. Pyrexia.

Investigations
- WCC ↑
- Radiographs: bone destruction, intense periosteal reaction, soft tissue swelling, 'onion-skin' layers of new bone around lesion
- Biopsy.

Treatment. Aim is wide surgical excision and limb salvage. Chemotherapy and radiotherapy. Amputation may be required for very large lesions.

Prognosis. The 5-year survival rate is approximately 60–70%.

Chondrosarcoma

This is a slow-growing tumour arising from chondroblasts. It occurs between 30 and 50 years and may arise de novo or in a pre-existing osteochondroma (Ollie's or Maffucci's). It occurs in the shoulder/pelvic girdles, knee and spine. Radiographs reveal a diffuse swelling with 'popcorn' calcification. Metastases occur to the lungs. Treatment is by wide excision or amputation. Survival dependent on grade – 50% of patients survive 5 years.

Fibrosarcoma

This is more common in soft tissues (malignant fibrous histiocytoma) and much less aggressive in bone.

Myeloma (plasma cell dyscrasia)

The commonest primary bone malignancy, it arises from marrow plasma cells. It is rare before 50 years. There is very early dissemination with widespread marrow replacement (multiple myelomatosis).

Symptoms and signs. Anaemia. Malaise. Bone pain (backache). Pathological fracture.

Investigations
- ESR (>100)
- Anaemia
- Hypercalcaemia
- Increased gamma globulins
- Urinary Bence–Jones protein
- Bone marrow aspirate
- Radiographs: multiple punched-out lesions.

Treatment. Chemotherapy with radiotherapy for localized pain. Surgery for compression symptoms; prophylactic nailing of long bones.

Secondary

Secondary deposits occur in bone from the lung, thyroid, breast, prostate and kidney.

Symptoms and signs. Bone pain. May be past history of primary tumour or primary may not be apparent. Pathological fracture. Full clinical examination of likely primary sites.

Investigations
- Radiograph individual bone: osteolytic, mixed or osteosclerotic (prostate) lesions
- Bone scan (→ Fig. 17.15)
- Alkaline phosphatase ↑
- PSA ↑
- CA125
- TFTs
- calcium ↑.

Treatment. Severe bone pain at one site may be treated by local radiotherapy or systemic irradiation (thyroid with radio-iodine).

- Pathological fractures are treated by internal fixation and radiotherapy
- Hormonal manipulation. Breast responds to oophorectomy. Prostate responds to hormone manipulation.

BACKACHE

This is an extremely common complaint accounting for about 20% of musculoskeletal triage referrals. Most cases are either traumatic or degenerative but other causes are numerous (→ Table 17.1). The more common causes will be described in this section.

Figure 17.15 A bone scan showing secondary deposits (hot spots) in the bony skeleton, especially in the ribs.

RT ANT LT

Osteoarthritis of the spine

In this condition, disc degeneration causes narrowing of the space between vertebral bodies. The posterior intervertebral facet joints may become osteoarthritic. Osteophytes form and may encroach on nerve roots.

Symptoms and signs. Back pain radiating to buttock or thigh but not beyond. Usually cyclical in nature, associated with overuse or episodes of abnormal movement.

Investigations. Radiographs: disc space narrowing, osteophyte formation.

Treatment. Simple analgesia. NSAIDs. Physiotherapy, heat, exercises, manipulation. Spinal support. Facet joint injections. General advice re: posture, weight loss, lifting, etc. In severe cases, decompression and surgical fusion may be required.

Prolapsed intervertebral disc

This is a common cause of low back pain and sciatica. There is often a history of pain or mild injury, e.g. while lifting. Backache and radicular pain occur. Most disc prolapses are posterior and pass lateral to the posterior longitudinal ligament (paracentral disc) causing compression of the transiting nerve root. Far lateral discs may compress the exiting nerve root also (Fig. 17.16) Central disc prolapses may compress the cord (cord compression) or more commonly, as discs herniated at the level of the cauda equina, cause cauda equina syndrome.

TABLE 17.1 Causes of backache

Congenital	Kyphoscoliosis
	Spina bifida
	Spondylolisthesis

Acquired	
Traumatic	Vertebral fractures
	Ligamentous injury
	Joint strain
	Muscle tears
Infective	Osteomyelitis – acute and chronic, TB
Inflammatory	Ankylosing spondylitis
	Discitis
	Rheumatology disorders
Neoplastic	Primary tumours (rare)
	Metastases (common)
Degenerative	Osteoarthritis
	Intervertebral disc lesions
Metabolic	Osteoporosis
	Osteomalacia
Endocrine	Cushing's disease (osteoporosis)
Idiopathic	Paget's disease
	Scheuermann's disease
Psychogenic	Psychosomatic backache is common
Visceral	Penetrating peptic ulcer
	Carcinoma of the pancreas
	Carcinoma of the rectum
Vascular	Aortic aneurysm
	Acute aortic dissection
Renal	Carcinoma of the kidney
	Renal calculus
	Inflammatory disease
Gynaecological	Uterine tumours
	Pelvic inflammatory disease
	Endometriosis

Symptoms and signs

Back pain. Worse on movement, coughing, straining. May radiate to buttock and thigh without nerve root entrapment. Associated spasm and loss of lordosis. Restricted movements.

Nerve root compression. Most commonly L5 or S1. Dermatomal distribution of pain and anaesthesia. Segmental weakness (L5 – big toe extensor, S1 – foot evertors). Sciatic stretch test (reproduction of radicular leg pain on passive straight leg elevation and foot dorsiflexion). Depressed reflexes, e.g. L3/4 – depressed knee jerk, L5/S1 – depressed ankle jerk.

Cauda equina syndrome. Absolute surgical emergency. Compression of sacral outflow, saddle paraesthesia. Reduced anal sphincter tone. Reduced bladder coordination, painless retention and overflow. Loss of anal reflex. Bilateral leg symptoms.

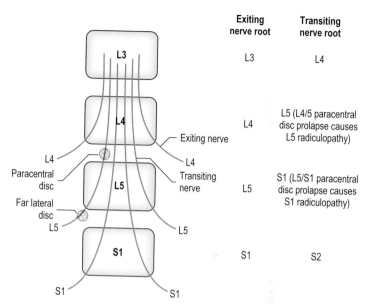

Exiting nerve root | Transiting nerve root

Exiting nerve root	Transiting nerve root
L3	L4
L4	L5 (L4/5 paracentral disc prolapse causes L5 radiculopathy)
L5	S1 (L5/S1 paracentral disc prolapse causes S1 radiculopathy)
S1	S2

Figure 17.16 Prolapsed intervertebral disc. Radiculopathy in relation to transiting and exiting nerve roots. Paracentral disc lesions compress the transiting nerve. Far lateral disc lesions compress the exiting nerve.

Investigations
- Radiograph: often of little help, mild scoliosis, loss of lumbar lordosis, may be loss of disc spacing in chronic cases
- MRI (→ Fig. 17.17).

Treatment. Need correlation of symptoms with MRI.

Conservative. Reassurance. Analgesia. Physiotherapy. Avoid prolonged bed rest. Mobilization.

Surgical. An absolute indication for urgent surgery is bladder paralysis. Muscle weakness is also an indication for urgent surgical assessment. Other indications include failed conservative management for 6 weeks to 3 months: repeated attacks. Operative treatment involves surgical removal of the sequestrated part of the disc. This may be carried out by the open method, i.e. discectomy, partial laminectomy and removal of the disc material pressing on the nerve root, or by microdiscectomy, a minimally invasive technique using a special microscope to view the disc and nerves.

Spondylolisthesis
In this condition, one vertebra slips forward relative to the one below, usually L5 on S1 or less commonly L4 on L5. A classification of spondylolisthesis is shown in Table 17.2.

Figure 17.17 MRI showing a prolapsed intervertebral disc (arrow).

TABLE 17.2 Classification of spondylolisthesis

Type	Classification	Age	Description
I	Congenital (dysplastic)	Child	Congenital dysplasia of superior facet
II	Isthmic (most common defect in pars interarticularis)	5–50	Predisposition leading to elongation/stress fracture of pars interarticularis (L5–S1)
III	Degenerative	Older age	Facet arthrosis leading to subluxation (L4–L5)
IV	Traumatic	Younger age	Acute fractures in posterior elements (other than pars)
V	Pathologic	Any age	Incompetence of posterior elements due to bone disease
VI	Post-surgical	Adult	Excessive resection of neural arches/facets

Symptoms and signs. Chronic backache, worse on standing. May present in late childhood or early adult life. Sciatica. Neurological symptoms in lower limbs. 'Step' palpable in the line of the spinous processes with marked skin creases below the ribs.

Investigations. Radiographs: oblique views show defect in pars interarticularis ('Scottie dog' decapitation sign).

Treatment. Mild slips require conservative treatment with physiotherapy. With severe slips, decompression and spinal fusion are indicated.

Scheuermann's disease (adolescent kyphosis)

The ring epiphyses of the vertebral bodies are affected by osteochondritis. The vertebral bodies grow abnormally and become wedge-shaped. The condition occurs between 12 and 18 years.

Symptoms and signs. Mild backache or no pain at all. A gradual curve or kyphosis develops.

Investigations. Radiographs: wedging of vertebrae and irregularity of vertebral end-plates.

Treatment. Other than postural exercises, treatment is rarely necessary. Occasionally bracing or spinal fusion may be necessary.

Ankylosing spondylitis

This affects young adults, males more commonly than females. It usually starts in the sacroiliac joints and extends to involve the whole spine. Ossification occurs in the ligaments of the spine and intervertebral discs and the spine is converted to a solid column of bone with an increasing kyphosis (bamboo spine). There is an association with HLA-B27.

Symptoms and signs. Young adult males. First sign is often reduced chest expansion. Low back pain, stiffness in the lumbar region. Most marked on rising in the morning and improving with activity initially. Eventually deformity occurs with flexion in the spine and hips and the patient may have difficulty raising the head to look forwards. Iritis and plantar fasciitis may occur.

Investigations
- ESR ↑
- Radiographs: special views of sacroiliac joints, irregularity, sclerosis, fusion. Later changes of ossification in spinal ligaments and discs (bamboo spine).

Treatment. The progress of the disease is rarely influenced. Analgesics. Physiotherapy. Joint replacements may be necessary to deal with deformities. Osteotomy of the spine may be required.

Complications. In the past, this condition was treated with radiotherapy. Leukaemia may develop as a complication of this. Excessive use of analgesia in the past may cause CRF.

Cervical spondylosis

This is a degenerative condition of the cervical spine with narrowing of the intervertebral discs and osteophyte formation of the adjacent vertebral bodies. OA develops in the synovial intervertebral joints. The condition is common in the middle-aged and elderly. It may cause pressure on the nerve roots or the cord itself.

Symptoms and signs. Painful, tender, cervical spine with reduced neck movement. Pain may radiate over the occiput and to the shoulders. When nerve roots are involved pain radiates into the arm and hand. Stiff neck, limited

Figure 17.18 A lateral radiograph of the cervical spine showing cervical spondylosis. There is gross anterior lipping of C5, 6 and 7. There is marked narrowing of the disc spaces.

movement of neck. Diminished reflexes in the arm, dermatomal sensory loss, signs of lower motor neuron weakness. Rarely bladder involvement from cord compression. Rarely spasticity of legs.

Investigations
- AP and lateral radiographs of cervical spine (→ Fig. 17.18): narrowing of disc space, lipping of vertebrae, osteophytes, sclerosis of posterolateral joints with encroachment on foramina
- If neurological symptoms, MRI.

Differential diagnosis. Thoracic outlet syndrome, shoulder disorders, carpal tunnel syndrome, peripheral neuropathy, spinal cord tumour, syringomyelia.

Treatment. Reassurance and symptomatic treatment in mild cases. NSAIDs, collar, short-wave diathermy. Gentle traction. The need for surgery is rare but may be required to decompress the nerve roots or cord.

Cervical disc prolapse
This should be distinguished from cervical spondylosis. It usually occurs in a young adult.

Symptoms and signs
Lateral cervical protrusion. Acute neck pain often with severe pain radiating into the arm or hand with paraesthesia and weakness. Restricted neck movement, spasm

in neck muscles, paraesthesia in dermatomal pattern in arm and hand. Weakness of muscle supplied by affected nerve root. Diminished reflexes.

Midline protrusion. If massive, may cause no root pain but may produce a spastic quadriplegia by interfering with the anterior and lateral columns of the spinal cord. There may also be bladder symptoms. Milder degrees of midline protrusion may cause a spastic gait with reduced fine movements in the hand and associated bladder involvement.

Investigations
- AP and lateral radiographs of cervical spine
- MRI is the investigation of choice
- CT myelography if unsuitable for MRI.

Treatment. In mild cases, analgesia, collar, heat treatment. Acute onset of neurological signs or progressive appearance of neurological signs is an indication for surgery. Surgery involves removal of the disc material by an anterior approach with or without intervertebral fusion.

METABOLIC BONE DISEASE

Osteomalacia and rickets

Vitamin D deficiency causes the failure of osteoid to ossify. Rickets is the childhood form of osteomalacia. In children classical deformities occur, i.e. bowing of the femur and tibia, large head, chest deformity with thickening of the costochondral junctions (rickety rosary), enlarged epiphyses. In adults, bone pain and pathological fractures occur (especially in the elderly with associated osteoporosis). Treatment is with vitamin D and calcium. Orthopaedic correction may be required for severe deformities in children.

Osteoporosis

This is a reduction in bone mass per unit volume. The causes are multifactorial. It is common in postmenopausal women. Pathological fractures are common (hip, wedge fractures of vertebrae, Colles' fracture). Radiograph shows osteopenia, i.e. loss of bone density and cortical widening to increase bending stiffness, when 30–40% of bone mass has been lost. Treatment is difficult but should correct any underlying cause. Calcium and vitamin D should be given if the diet is deficient. Bisphosphonates inhibit bone resorption. HRT helps prevent postmenopausal osteoporosis at the expense of a small risk of endometrial carcinoma.

Hyperparathyroidism (→ Ch. 11)

Pathological fractures may occur.

Paget's disease of bone

This is a difficult disease to categorize but is included here for convenience. The aetiology is unknown. Disorderly bone resorption and replacement leads to softening, increased vascularity, painful enlargement and bowing of bones. It occurs in middle to old age and is more common in males. The skull, vertebrae, pelvis and long bones are affected. Some cases are symptomless, being picked up on routine radiograph (→ Fig. 17.19). Complications include compressive symptoms

Figure 17.19 Paget's disease of bone. The pelvic bones are thickened and patchily sclerotic.

due to skull enlargement (e.g. blindness, deafness, cranial nerve entrapment), paraplegia, pathological fractures, high-output cardiac failure due to vascularity of bone. Osteogenic sarcoma may develop after many years. In mild cases no treatment is required. In severe cases, calcitonin and bisphosphonates may help.

PAEDIATRIC ORTHOPAEDICS

SCOLIOSIS

This is a lateral curvature of the spine in the coronal plane. Untreated, the condition may progress to obvious embarrassing deformities, embarrassment of respiratory function and neurological lesions. Scoliosis may be postural or structural. Postural scoliosis is usually mild and disappears on recumbency. It may be due to a short lower limb, hip deformity, or spasm of the paravertebral muscles, e.g. associated with a prolapsed intervertebral disc. In structural scoliosis, in addition to the lateral curve, the vertebral bodies are also rotated. In the thoracic region this leads to rib asymmetry with flatness on the concave side and a hump on the convex side, which produces the hunchback deformity initially best seen on flexion. Structural scoliosis may be:

- Idiopathic (98%)
- Congenital – failure of segmentation or formation of vertebrae
- Neuromuscular disorders
- Connective tissue disease, e.g. Marfan's Ehlers Danlos
- Trauma
- Infection, e.g. TB
- Tumour.

The management of idiopathic scoliosis is described below.

Adolescent idiopathic scoliosis

This is more common in girls aged 10 onwards. It is usually convex to the right and thoracic curves are most common.

Symptoms and signs. Usually noticed by parents. One shoulder higher than other. Development of rib hump. More obvious on flexion.

Investigations. Radiograph in two planes: used to measure the degree of deformity and to assess progress.

Treatment. Many cases progress. If the scoliosis is minor and not progressing, it can be watched. Curves >30–40° or progressive curves require bracing using a polythene jacket. More severe curves at presentation and those that progress rapidly require surgery. Internal fixation is carried out using various implants to hold the correction until fusion occurs.

CONDITIONS OF THE HIP

Development dysplasia of the hip (DDH)

This describes a wide spectrum of hip abnormalities ranging from mild acetabular dysplasia to complete dislocation of the hip secondary to capsular laxity and mechanical factors. This condition was formerly known as congenital dislocation of the hip (CDH). The incidence is 1.5 : 1000 live births and girls are affected more than boys (85% girls) and the left hip is more commonly affected than the right. There are hereditary factors – an increased risk if one parent has DDH. There is an association with breech delivery and the first born child.

Symptoms and signs. Routine examination in the neonate. Asymmetric groin fold, limited hip abduction in 90° flexion. Hip and knee are flexed to a right angle and the thigh is then abducted. There is a jerk or 'clunk' as the head slips into the joint over the acetabulum (positive Ortolani's test – Ortolani's test relocates a dislocated hip). Barlow's test dislocates the hip with the hip at 90° flexion and in adduction. When reassessed at 3 weeks after the initial test only 1 : 10 of hips will remain unstable. Currently, if risk factors are present or the hip is felt to be unstable, then an USS will be carried out between 2 and 4 weeks post-partum. If the diagnosis is missed at routine testing, the child may present in later life with a limp or a typical waddling Trendelenburg's gait (if the condition is bilateral). Association with torticollis, metatarsus adductus, club foot.

Investigations
- USS <6–8 months old – α-angle – line drawn down lateral edge of ileum and acetabular roof from tri-radiate cartilage (normal >60°)
- Radiographs >10 months old – Shenton's line; positioning of the limb in 45° abduction shows a break in continuity of a line drawn around the margins of the obturator foramen and carried down onto the femoral neck

Treatment. Ideally, all cases should be diagnosed at birth and treatment started immediately. In early infancy, Pavlik harness for 3 months or less. The hip is held in the 'frog' position. Check USS should be carried out to assess acetabular development. If the condition is diagnosed between 6 and 18 months, it is necessary to reduce the hip and maintain reduction until the acetabulum develops enough to hold the femoral head. This may be achieved by hip spica plaster or open reduction. In older children, acetabuloplasty or osteotomies may be required to correct the deformity.

Prognosis. The earlier the treatment the better the result. Delayed diagnosis, especially beyond 18 months, makes it difficult to achieve a good result. OA may develop in later life.

Irritable hip

This usually occurs under the age of 10 years and is more common in boys. The aetiology is unknown and the condition is self-limiting, the diagnosis being one of exclusion of other conditions.

Symptoms and signs. Pain in hip. Limp. Occasionally mild constitutional upset. Mild spasm and restriction of movement.

Investigations
- Radiographs are normal
- CRP
- FBC to exclude sepsis
- USS ± aspiration.

Treatment. Bed rest plus analgesia. Usually settles within 2 weeks.

Differential diagnosis. It is important to distinguish the condition from Perthes' disease, TB and septic arthritis. The patient must be carefully followed up with physical examination and radiographs to exclude other conditions, e.g. developing Perthes.

Perthes' disease

This is a non-inflammatory deformity of the proximal femur secondary to vascular insult leading to osteonecrosis of the proximal femoral epiphysis. It is bilateral in 10%, is commoner in boys and usually occurs between 4–8 years, being maximum around 7–8 years.

Symptoms and signs. Pain in the groin or referred to the knee. Otherwise well. Decreased range of joint movements.

Investigations
- Hip radiographs: early changes include increased joint space and flattening of the epiphyses; later changes show collapse and deformity of the femoral head with new bone formation. Severe deformity of the femoral head risks early arthritis.
- Arthrogram or MRI – assesses congruency throughout the full range of movement.

Treatment. Physiotherapy using muscle strengthening and stretching exercises produces significant improvement in articular range of motion, muscular strength and articular dysfunction. Surgical treatment. Surgery is indicated for children >6 years. Surgery involves various forms of osteotomy. The aim is to produce a congruent joint with maximum contact between immature femoral head and acetabulum.

Prognosis. Prognosis is dependent on age. Less than 6 years of age, outcome is good regardless of treatment. Between 6 and 8 years of age, the results are not always satisfactory with containment of the femoral epiphysis within the confines of the acetabulum. Children older than 8–9 years at an initial onset will have a poor prognosis and may be expected to have a restricted range of movements.

Slipped upper femoral epiphysis

This occurs from ages 10–18 years and boys are more affected than girls. The child may be overweight and may have delayed sexual development in some cases. The capital femoral epiphyses appear slipped downwards and backwards (in actual fact, the neck is the segment displaced); 25% are bilateral, of which 15–30% occur simultaneously.

Symptoms and signs. Pain in hip. Limp. Pain may be referred to knee. Leg lies in external rotation and passive internal rotation is diminished. Classified as stable or unstable depending on whether patient can weight bear.

Investigations. Radiographs: AP and lateral views; both hips should be radiographed. Early slipped upper femoral epiphysis may be identified by Klein's line, i.e. a line drawn along the upper border of the femoral neck should intersect some part of the femoral head on AP X-ray. If not, displacement has occurred.

Treatment. If the patient presents acutely, the head is fixed *in situ* with a single screw to prevent further slipping. Reduction is rarely performed as it increases the risk of avascular necrosis. In the chronic case, pinning should be carried out if feasible, i.e. if the slip is not too great to allow this. Osteotomies may be necessary either as a primary or secondary procedure. Prophylactic fixation of the other side is controversial.

Complications. Avascular necrosis of the femoral head, chondrolysis and osteoarthritis may occur almost exclusively in the unstable group.

CLUB FOOT (TALIPES EQUINOVARUS)

The aetiology of this is unknown but there may be a neurological defect in some cases, and in others intrauterine factors, e.g. pressure or position may be involved. It is more common in boys and may be bilateral. There are three elements of the deformity:

- Equinus – the hind foot is drawn up with a tight Achilles tendon
- Varus – the sole faces inwards
- Adduction of the forefoot – the inner border of the forefoot is concave.

Symptoms and signs. The deformity is as described above. Can be identified by USS *in utero*. Usually picked up at routine postnatal examination. Exclude associated DDH and spina bifida.

Treatment. Commenced at birth. Usually non-surgical (85%). The 'Ponseti regime' corrects the deformity with weekly serial casts for 3 months. Occasionally percutaneous tenotomy of the Achilles tendon is needed. Posteromedial soft tissue release is now rarely carried out, if ever. After serial casts Denis Browne's splint (boots and bars) are used for up to 3 years.

Prognosis. Usually good but relapses may occur. Follow-up for several years is required. Further surgery may be required if relapse occurs.

OSTEOCHONDRITIDES

> A group of conditions in which developing epiphyseal areas, in children and adolescents, are affected. The underlying pathology may be avascular necrosis but trauma and stress injuries have been implicated. Several epiphyses may be involved and there are a number of eponyms in common usage to describe the various conditions: vertebral epiphyseal plates (Scheuermann's disease); femoral capital epiphyses (Perthes' disease); tibial tuberosity (Osgood–Schlatter disease); carpal lunate (Kienböck's disease), os calcis (Sever's disease); tarsal navicular (Köhler's disease); metatarsal heads (Freiberg's disease – usually second metatarsal).

Symptoms and signs. Local pain and muscle spasm.

Investigations. Radiographs: dense and fragmented bone. Progress of the disease is followed by radiograph.

Treatment. These conditions are usually self-limiting. Treatment of the various conditions involves rest, splinting or excision of bone fragments. The three most common of the conditions are Scheuermann's disease, Perthes' disease and Osgood–Schlatter disease. The former two conditions are described elsewhere in the chapter. The latter is described below.

Osteochondritis of the tibial tubercle (Osgood–Schlatter disease)

This is a common condition affecting adolescent boys in which the epiphyses of the tibial tubercle are involved (strictly speaking it is an apophysis). (An apophysis is an insertion of a tendon and does not contribute to longitudinal growth of a bone like an epiphysis.)

Symptoms and signs. Boys 10–14 years. Often related to physical activity, e.g. football. Pain and swelling accurately localized to the tibial tubercle. Examination reveals a tender, swelling. Knee joint is normal.

Investigations. Radiographs: fragmentation of the tubercle.

Treatment. Restriction of physical activity. In severe cases, rest in a plaster cylinder or rarely surgery to remove fragments of bone may be necessary. Most cases settle spontaneously but it may take up to 2 years.

Neurosurgery

HEAD INJURIES

In the UK, head injuries account for annual attendance rates at A&E departments of almost 1 million people. Head injuries account for nine deaths per 100 000 population and in young males, account for 15–20% of all deaths. Some 20% of all patients attending A&E departments with head injuries are admitted, and over 25% of these have alcohol-related head injuries. More than 50% of all patients admitted with head injuries are discharged within 24 h. Head injuries, therefore, cause a considerable workload and bed occupancy. It is therefore necessary to have a protocol to decide which patients need admission and which patients need further investigation.

⚠ **It is recommended that all patients are monitored using the Glasgow Coma Scale after initial resuscitation (→ Table 4.1, in Ch. 4). In all cases, the diagnosis and initial treatment of serious extracranial injuries takes priority over investigations of head injury, or transfer to a neurosurgical unit.**

Criteria for urgent CT scan and consultation with a neurosurgical unit

The presence of one or more of the following:

- Confusion, or other neurological disturbances persisting for more than 2 h, even if there is no skull fracture
- Coma continuing after resuscitation
- Suspected open injury of the vault or the base of the skull
- Depressed fracture of the skull
- Neurological deterioration despite adequate resuscitation
- Penetrating injuries
- Fractured skull in combination with either confusion or other depression of the level of consciousness or focal neurological signs or fits
- CSF leak (usually otorrhoea or rhinorrhoea).

Criteria for hospital admission after recent head injury

The presence of one or more of the following:

- Confusion or any other depression of the level of consciousness at the time of examination
- Skull fracture
- Neurological signs; persistent or worsening headache or vomiting
- Signs suggesting skull base fracture, e.g. haemotympanum, panda eyes, Battle's sign
- Difficulty in assessing the patient, e.g. alcohol, the young, epilepsy
- Other medical conditions, e.g. haemophilia
- The patient's social conditions or lack of responsible adult/relative if discharged.

- Post-traumatic amnesia with *full* recovery is not an indication for admission
- Many patients who appear fully orientated are not. Strict assessment of orientation is necessary prior to discharge
- Patients sent home should be given written instructions about possible complications and appropriate action
- Minor head injury with amnesia or unconsciousness usually causes post-concussion symptoms, which can cause significant morbidity, particularly if not explained to the patient.

Skull radiography after recent head injury

CT scan is the preferred option. A skull radiograph images the skull but provides no information about the brain and therefore is of little use. All patients suffering a significant head injury should have a CT scan, which in most cases will identify any skull fracture.

Simple scalp laceration is not a criterion for skull radiography if the history can exclude a significant impact.

TYPES OF BRAIN INJURY

Primary

This is the damage caused as an immediate result of trauma. It results in contusions, lacerations or diffuse brain damage. Treatment cannot reverse primary brain injury.

Secondary

This develops as a result of complications such as intracranial bleeding, cerebral hypoxia, cerebral oedema and infection. The prevention, recognition and treatment of these secondary complications is the mainstay of treatment of the patient with head injuries.

ASSESSMENT OF HEAD INJURY

Emergency

- **Establish an airway**
- **Ensure adequate breathing**
- **Maintain the circulation**
- **Make a thorough but rapid examination of the patient and exclude significant extracranial injuries**
- **Evaluate the CNS with GCS (→ Table 4.1)**
- **Splint long bone fractures**
- **Assume cervical spine injury until proved otherwise.**

Evaluate CNS injury

Assess the level of consciousness as this is the most significant factor after head injury. Use GCS (→ Table 4.1) and check pupillary reactions. Pupillary changes may indicate brain swelling or compression. Pressure on a cerebral hemisphere causes the third nerve on that side to be stretched over the edge of the tentorium. The resultant paralysis of the nerve allows unopposed action of the dilator pupillae under the control of the sympathetic nervous system and the pupils dilate. There is also loss of light reaction of the pupil on the affected side. If compression continues, the contralateral third nerve is compressed and the opposite pupil also dilates and is fixed to light. Bilateral fixed dilated pupils in a patient with a head injury are a grave prognostic sign and recovery is rare. Pupillary changes are always late signs ('undertaker signs'), and are always preceded by an alteration in conscious level caused by raised intracranial pressure. Direct blows to the eyes can cause dilated pupils in patients without severe brain injury.

Pulse, respiration and blood pressure

As intracranial pressure rises, the pulse slows, the respirations become slow/irregular and eventually of the Cheyne–Stokes type. The BP rises. These are signs of midbrain compression and, properly managed, are avoidable in those with salvageable head injuries.

CNS examination

This may be difficult in the unconscious patient. Observe the pattern of limb movement in response to painful stimuli. Progressive unilateral weakness or focal epilepsy may be helpful localizing signs. Obtain a history from witnesses to the event, e.g. speed of impact, height of fall, state of crash helmet.

Check for CSF rhinorrhoea or otorrhoea

Check for these signs. Periorbital bruising and retromastoid bruising imply basal skull fracture.

Scalp lacerations or depressed fractures

Check these using a gloved finger. If in doubt, perform a CT scan.

Assess amnesia

Post-traumatic amnesia (loss from time of the injury) gives an assessment of the severity of the injury. Retrograde amnesia correlates poorly with the severity of the injury. Post-traumatic amnesia of >1 week signifies severe damage. Patients seen initially may appear fully conscious and orientated. Do not make allowances when assessing. They are often amnesic of events in A&E when asked at a later date.

CT AND MRI BRAIN SCANNING

Computerized tomography (CT) and magnetic resonance imaging (MRI) provide very rapid and highly accurate detail of the brain. CT also provides excellent bone detail and should be performed if a significant brain injury is suspected. Resuscitation must always precede any form of imaging, however sophisticated. MRI is not at present necessary for management of acute head injury but may provide important prognostic data. A cervical spine X-ray or CT scan of the cervical spine is mandatory for all significant head injuries and must include C7/T1.

SKULL FRACTURES

A skull fracture is an indication for hospital admission. Patients with skull fractures are more likely to suffer secondary brain damage. Skull fractures are classified as closed, i.e. the skin over the underlying fracture is intact, or open (compound) where the skin overlying the fracture is broken, or the fracture connects with an air sinus or the external auditory canal.

They may be further classified as follows:

Linear, stellate or comminuted non-depressed. These fractures are serious if they cross major vascular channels, e.g. the groove for the middle meningeal artery.

Depressed fracture. A portion of the vault of the skull is depressed inwards. Surgery may be required to elevate the fracture.

Compound comminuted fractures with damage to the underlying brain. These are treated by removing all bony fragments, debridement and closure. Failure to remove all bony fragments may lead to development of cerebral abscess. They are associated with epilepsy.

Fractures of the base of the skull. They usually involve the anterior or middle cranial fossa. Those affecting the anterior fossa may cause nasal bleeding, periorbital haematoma, subconjunctival haemorrhage, CSF rhinorrhoea and cranial nerve injuries (I–V). Middle cranial fossa fractures involving the petrous temporal bone may cause bleeding from the ear, CSF otorrhoea, bruising over the ear and over the mastoid, and cranial nerve injuries (VII and VIII).

Summary

The emphasis in the management of head injuries is on damage to the underlying structures rather than on any skull fracture *per se*. CT scanning is the investigation of choice for patients with head injury and no patient with a significant head injury should be admitted to a hospital A&E department that does not have immediate 24-hour access to CT scanning.

Management of CSF leakage. It may be difficult to distinguish bleeding from blood mixed with CSF. Place a drop of the blood-stained discharge on a clean white gauze. If CSF is present there will be a spreading yellowish ring around a central stain of blood (halo sign). CSF leakage implies that the dura and arachnoid are torn and therefore there is a potential pathway allowing infection to spread to the meninges and brain. The head of the bed should be elevated 30°. The patient should be advised not to blow their nose. In many cases, the leakage settles spontaneously but all CSF leaks should be referred for a neurosurgical opinion. Where CSF rhinorrhoea occurs do not pass a nasogastric tube. Do not pack the nose or ears.

INTRACRANIAL BLEEDING

> This may be extradural, subdural (acute or chronic) and intracerebral. Subarachnoid haemorrhage commonly follows trauma.

Extradural

This results from bleeding between the bone and the dura. It is most likely to occur when a fracture occurs in the temporal region crossing the middle meningeal artery. It may occasionally occur without a fracture. Usually low-speed injury.

Symptoms and signs. History of head injury (may be relatively minor). Temporary concussion. Recovery ('lucid interval'), then increasing headache, decreased conscious level, coma. There may be no lucid period or the patient may have the signs when admitted unconscious. Falling pulse rate. Rising BP. Reduced and irregular respiration. Dilated ipsilateral pupil. Contralateral hemiparesis or focal fits. May be boggy swelling overlying the site of the fracture as extradural blood may track through the fracture and into the subcutaneous tissues.

Investigations. CT scan. This should *always* be done immediately, before surgery is contemplated.

Treatment. This is a true emergency and requires neurosurgical assistance. If none is immediately available and the patient's condition is critical despite resuscitation, i.v. mannitol should be given and ventilation commenced. A burr hole should be made over the suspected site of clot. Enlarge the hole with bone-nibbling forceps. Gently evacuate the clot. Clip or diathermy the bleeding vessel.

Subdural

Acute

This results from tearing of small bridging veins that bleed into the subdural space and is usually associated with a lacerated brain resulting from high-speed injuries. The haematoma spreads over a large area. The patient usually has marked brain injury at the outset and is comatose but the condition deteriorates further. Can rarely be caused by a ruptured aneurysm, which can cause the patient's collapse and a secondary head injury. The history of the event should distinguish from primary trauma.

Symptoms and signs. Severe head injury. May be rapid deterioration. Signs of raised ICP. Localizing signs. Pupillary inequality.

Investigations. CT scan.

Treatment. Craniotomy. Evacuation of clot. Recovery depends on degree of underlying brain damage.

Chronic
Usually in the elderly. Brain shrinkage makes the bridging veins between cortex and venous sinuses vulnerable. May have only been a trivial and forgotten head injury. It may occur weeks or months after the injury, presenting with neurological signs, headache or coma, confusion or personality change. A brain tumour may be suspected in the differential diagnosis. There may be fluctuating level of consciousness.

Investigations. CT scan.

Treatment. Evacuation of clot via burr holes and short course of dexamethasone. Reaccumulation may occur.

Intracerebral
This occurs as a result of primary brain injury but may expand causing secondary brain damage. It may extend into the ventricles. A discrete haematoma may require craniotomy if the patient's condition deteriorates. Always consider other primary causes for the intracerebral haematoma causing collapse and secondary head injury.

Complications
Meningitis. Organisms enter via compound skull fractures. Prophylactic antibiotics should be used for all compound fractures. Current prophylaxis includes cefuroxime given for a minimum of 1 week. It is not necessary for the drug to cross the blood–brain barrier if given for prophylaxis but it is necessary for it to cross the blood–brain barrier if given for specific treatment of meningitis.

Cerebral hypoxia. This is a major and preventable cause of secondary brain injury. Respiratory failure after head injury may be peripheral or central. Peripheral causes include upper airway obstruction, e.g. tongue; vomit; chest injuries; pneumothorax; pneumonitis; shock lung. Central causes include primary brainstem injury or depressant drugs, e.g. alcohol. Hypertension may also contribute.

MANAGEMENT OF HEAD INJURIES

 Always consider – is this only a head injury or was it caused by something else, e.g. myocardial infarction, fit, intracranial bleed? A good history is vital.

Minor
The most important question is: does the patient need a CT scan and/or admission? The patient should be monitored for 24 h. The majority of complications will occur during this time. If no problems occur after 24 h, the patient can be discharged into

the care of a responsible adult. Patients should be given an information sheet detailing *symptoms and signs* for which they should be on the look-out, with instructions to return to the hospital should any of these symptoms occur. They should be advised about post-concussional symptoms and be referred to a head injury clinic for further management.

Observations during admission

The primary observations are the GCS (→ Table 4.1). In addition pulse, BP, respiratory rate and pupillary size and reaction are monitored. These are carried out by the nursing staff on the ward, the frequency depending on the severity of the symptoms. Hourly observations are usually the norm. Signs of deterioration include falling coma score, falling pulse rate, raised BP, reduced or irregular respirations, dilatation of the pupils, loss of light reflex and asymmetrical pupils. An alteration of conscious level occurs before signs of brainstem compression.

Major

Does the patient need a neurosurgical referral? If the patient deteriorates rapidly and an extradural is suspected, burr holes may be required, but if appropriately diagnosed, it is usually preferable to transfer the patient immediately to a neurosurgical unit. In many patients with head injury, no surgical intervention is warranted. These patients may be in a coma with diffuse cerebral injury and oedema and may require ventilation. Other injuries may be present. Intensive care will be required. The following may be required in management:

- Monitoring of vital signs and neurological status
- Assisted ventilation
- i.v. fluids and nasogastric aspiration
- Avoidance of fluid overload
- Maintain electrolyte balance, avoid hyponatraemia (which exacerbates cerebral oedema)
- Control raised ICP, e.g. i.v. mannitol (osmotic effect reduces cerebral oedema); furosemide; controlled ventilation assists management of cerebral oedema; dexamethasone is not effective in head injuries in the control of cerebral oedema.

Other complications of head injury

Epilepsy

Post-traumatic epilepsy may occur, particularly after prolonged post-traumatic amnesia, depressed fractures and intracerebral haematoma. It is associated with cortical damage and subsequent scarring. Long-term anticonvulsive therapy is usually required. Prophylactic anticonvulsants are given to patients in high-risk categories although efficacy is uncertain.

Post-concussion syndrome

Headache, dizziness, fatigue and poor memory are common after head injury. Loss of ability to concentrate and a labile emotional state are often sequelae. Management includes reassurance and symptomatic treatment. Often strong reassurance is necessary to explain that the condition is usually self-limiting within a few weeks or months. In most patients, symptoms cease within 12 months. Imipramine may be helpful. Strong codeine-based analgesics should be avoided. Failing to recognize and treat the syndrome can cause significant morbidity and psychiatric disturbance (depression). This may be helped by cognitive behavioural therapy.

Brain death

Regrettably, some patients do not recover from head injury and are dependent on life-support systems. The brainstem death criteria were drawn up to allow a way of determining which patients had sustained irreversible brain damage so that they were not kept on life-support systems to no avail and to the distress of relatives and the nursing staff. The diagnosis of brain death depends on the demonstration of permanent and irreversible destruction of brainstem function.

There are prerequisites for the diagnosis of brainstem death:

● The patient must not be medicated with any CNS depressant drugs or neuromuscular blocking agents
● The core temperature must be above 35°C
● There should be no metabolic disturbance
● The cause of the brain damage must be known.

The following tests reflecting brainstem reflexes must then be carried out by two doctors, on two occasions. Both doctors must have been registered for at least 5 years and be of consultant or senior registrar grade. They must be completely independent of any organ transplant team.

● No pupillary response to light – direct or consensual – this reflex involves cranial nerves II and III
● Absent corneal reflex – normally would result in blinking – this reflex involves cranial nerves V and VII
● No motor response in the cranial nerve distribution to stimuli in any somatic area – e.g. supraorbital or nail bed pressure leading to a grimace
● No gag reflex – back of throat is stimulated with a catheter – this reflex tests cranial nerves IX and X
● No cough reflex – no response to bronchial stimulation with a suction catheter – this reflex tests cranial nerves IX and X
● No vestibulo-ocular reflex – head is flexed to 30° and 50 mL of ice cold water is injected over 1 min into each external auditory meatus. There should be no eye movements – this reflex tests cranial nerves III, VI and VIII
● Apnoea test – the patient is pre-oxygenated with 100% O_2 for 10 min. $PaCO_2$ is allowed to rise to 5 kPa (before testing); the patient is disconnected from the ventilator and O_2 insufflated at 6 L per min via a tracheal catheter. $PaCO_2$ is allowed to rise to 6.5 kPa. At this point, there should be *no* respiratory effort.

There is no set time period recommended between the two sets of tests but 6–24 h is usual. Once two sets of brainstem death criteria are satisfied, the decision to discontinue ventilation is made. The official time of death is that of the timing of the first set of tests. The possibility of a patient becoming an organ donor

NEUROSURGERY
HEAD INJURIES ◀ 411

should be discussed sensitively with the next of kin. Many relatives gain some consolation out of the death of their loved ones, knowing that their organs are giving life to others.

MANAGEMENT OF RAISED INTRACRANIAL PRESSURE (ICP)

 Causes Head injury, meningoencephalitis, haemorrhage (extradural, subdural, subarachnoid, intracerebral), tumour, infection, hydrocephalus.

Symptoms and signs. Headache, drowsiness, vomiting, fits, irritability, listlessness, slowing pulse, rising BP. Irregular respiration. As the pressure increases the cerebral hemisphere is pushed through the tentorial hiatus alongside the brainstem. The third nerve is compressed against the edge of the tentorium and the brainstem is compressed by the herniating cerebral hemisphere – symptoms and signs: deepening coma, irregular slow breathing progressing to Cheyne–Stokes respiration and apnoea. Pressure on the third nerve causes ipsilateral and then bilateral pupillary dilatation. Eventually, the patient exhibits the decerebrate posture.

A sixth nerve palsy may be an early false localizing sign. The long intracranial course of this nerve makes it susceptible to stretching.

Investigations
- CT scan
- Cerebral angiography.

Lumbar puncture should *not* be carried out in the presence of raised ICP. If the spinal CSF pressure is reduced by removing CSF, the high ICP may force the brainstem and cerebellar tonsils through the foramen magnum (coning) with fatal results.

Treatment
- Monitor conscious level with GCS (→ Table 4.1)
- Ensure adequate oxygenation
- Avoid fluid overload
- Nurse with head elevated at 15–20° to promote cerebral venous drainage
- Controlled ventilation
- Hyperosmolar agents, e.g. mannitol – osmotic diuretic that reduces oedema in the relatively normal parts of the brain
- Dexamethasone is very valuable in some forms of cerebral oedema, e.g. that associated with cerebral tumours, but not head injury
- ICP monitoring may be helpful in some patients
- Neurosurgical intervention may be required. This must be carried out before signs of midbrain compression become established.

CEREBRAL TUMOURS

> These may be broadly classified as glial and non-glial depending on the cell of origin (→ Table 18.1).

Symptoms and signs
- General, e.g. confusion, dementia, and epilepsy
- Raised ICP, e.g. drowsiness, headache, vomiting
- Focal signs, e.g. weakness, sensory disturbance
- Epilepsy.

Symptoms vary depending upon the site of tumour. A full neurological examination should be carried out. Papilloedema is uncommon (about 15%). Symptoms occur alone or in combination.

Investigations
- MRI
- CT scan
- Angiography
- CXR to exclude primary
- Burr hole
- Biopsy.

Treatment
Medical. Dexamethasone 4 mg q.d.s. if cerebral oedema is present. Avoid overhydration. Consider a diuretic, e.g. furosemide 20 mg b.d.

Surgical. The aim of treatment should be excision with a view to a cure. This is not always possible. If the tumour cannot be completely excised, subtotal removal may be required to decompress the surrounding brain. Postoperative radiotherapy is often given after surgical excision or 'debulking' of the tumour in patients in good clinical condition.

Radiotherapy. For inoperable tumours radiotherapy is used for palliation.

TABLE 18.1 Classification of cerebral tumours	
Primary	
Glial (gliomas)	Astrocytoma
	Medulloblastoma
	Ependymomas
	Oligodendrogliomas
Non-glial	Meningiomas
	Acoustic neuroma
	Pituitary tumours
Secondary	Lung
	Breast
	Kidney
	Melanoma

Chemotherapy. For pineal tumours and medulloblastomas.

Shunting. Ventriculoperitoneal diversion of CSF is required if the tumour blocks CSF flow, causing hydrocephalus.

TYPES OF CEREBRAL TUMOUR

Astrocytoma

The peak incidence of astrocytoma is in early middle age. They vary in malignancy and some are slow growing. All are infiltrative. Most malignant astrocytomas are radio-resistant and survival overall is usually less than 5 years. Surgical cure is usually impossible as they extend into deep structures. In children, the tumour is often well-differentiated and cystic, and occurs in the cerebellum. This type is histologically benign and may often be completely excised with potential cure.

Glioblastoma multiforme

This is the most malignant brain tumour. It is rapidly growing and usually occurs between 40 and 60 years. It is rarely removable surgically and is radio-resistant. Most patients are dead within a year of diagnosis.

Medulloblastoma

This is the commonest glioma of childhood. It occurs in the first decade of life arising in the roof of the fourth ventricle and infiltrates into the cerebellum. It may cause obstructive hydrocephalus. Spread is by the CSF and it may seed on the spinal cord. Radical removal is followed by radiotherapy. Chemotherapy may be required.

Ependymomas

Those arising from the choroid plexus of the ventricles may be totally removable. Those arising from the ventricular walls are difficult to remove. The more malignant forms may seed via the subarachnoid space. Craniospinal irradiation is required and gives good results.

Oligodendrogliomas

These occur in the cerebral hemispheres and are slow growing. Treatment is by tumour debulking and radiotherapy. Most patients are dead within 5 years of diagnosis. Relatively few survive 10 years or more.

Meningiomas

Meningiomas arise from arachnoid cells. They usually occur in females in the 40–60 age group. They compress the cerebral cortex early in their growth and therefore fits may be an early sign. They may rarely cause osteoblastic change in the overlying bone, giving rise to exostosis producing a palpable lump over the vault of the skull. Common sites include parasagittal, along the falx; sphenoid – lesser wing; and olfactory groove. They are usually slow growing and do not invade brain tissue but compress it. Small tumours are usually curable by surgical excision. Even with subtotal excision for large tumours the prognosis is good. They may respond to hormonal therapy.

Acoustic neuroma

This arises from Schwann cells of the nerve sheath of the VIIIth cranial nerve at the internal auditory meatus. As the tumour grows it expands the internal auditory canal and extends into the cerebellopontine angle compressing the pons, cerebellum, and adjacent cranial nerves. It may be a feature of von Recklinghausen's disease.

Symptoms and signs. An acoustic neuroma should always be considered in a patient with unilateral sensorineural deafness, especially with tinnitus. Occurs in those aged 30–60. Facial weakness with unilateral taste loss is a later manifestation. The corneal reflexes are lost relatively early when the trigeminal nerve is stretched by the tumour. Dysphagia, hoarseness and dysarthria may arise owing to involvement of nerves IX, X, XII. Ultimately cerebellar signs and features of raised ICP may occur, but these are now a rare occurrence.

Investigations
- CT
- MRI.

Treatment. Surgical excision. Most can be completely removed with cure. Early diagnosis ensures preservation of facial nerve function and occasionally hearing. Stereotactic radio-surgery may be used, particularly for small tumours <3 cm.

PITUITARY TUMOURS

> These cause symptoms due to their endocrine capacity or due to their effects on the optic chiasma.
> *Secretory tumours* (e.g. prolactinoma) Many tumours contain a mixture of secretory cells. Presentation is influenced by the hormonal production and size of the tumour. These tumours are usually small.
> *Non-secretory tumour* Null cell adenomas – usually grow to a larger size and present because of local effects.

Symptoms and signs. These depend on whether the symptoms are due to the endocrine capacity or local pressure effects. Bitemporal hemianopia results from compression of the optic chiasma. Compression of secretory cells by non-secretory tumours may result in hypopituitarism. Symptoms include reduced libido, infertility, amenorrhoea, myxoedema, depression, loss of sex characteristics and hypoadrenalism. In children, growth arrest may occur. Hormonally active tumours may result in the following:

- Overproduction of growth hormone: before fusion of the epiphyses this will cause gigantism; in adult life, acromegaly results
- Hyperprolactinaemia: this is characterized by amenorrhoea, infertility, galactorrhoea and impotence
- Cushing's disease (→ Ch. 11).

Investigations
- MRI
- CT is contraindicated if MRI available because of radiation of optic chiasma
- Visual field assessment

- Hormonal analysis
- Skull radiograph is never the primary investigation but a pituitary tumour may be discovered incidentally on a skull radiograph (expansion of sella turcica).

Treatment. Surgery or medical therapy in selected cases. Tumour removal may be carried out by the transnasal route. Some pituitary tumours are radio-sensitive and radiotherapy may be used as an adjunct to surgery or rarely as primary therapy in those with large tumours or in poor general health. Radiotherapy may be administered by external beam or stereotactic radio-surgery. Hormonally responsive tumours, e.g. prolactinoma, acromegaly, can be treated with hormonal antagonists.

Craniopharyngioma

This a cystic benign tumour arising in a remnant of Rathke's pouch. It may present in childhood or adult life. Symptoms are those of hypopituitarism due to compression, visual defects or raised ICP. The treatment of choice is radical excision but this may be difficult because of their size.

INTRACRANIAL VASCULAR LESIONS

These include:

- Aneurysms of the circle of Willis at the base of the brain. Most of these are acquired, the remainder being congenital.
- Angiomas that may occur in any part of the CNS. AV malformations may be associated with these.

Aneurysms

The majority are acquired as a consequence of cerebrovascular disease. Most patients are smokers. Mycotic aneurysms are very rare. Some are associated with polycystic kidney disease, Ehlers–Danlos syndrome, coarctation of the aorta and Type III collagen deficiency. Hypertension is a contributory factor.

Symptoms and signs. The classic history is one of sudden severe headache with nausea, vomiting, collapse and often coma. Death may occur within minutes in major bleeds. With less serious bleeding, there may be photophobia, and neck stiffness. Isolated cranial nerve palsy may occur, e.g. third nerve. A sudden onset of headache, particularly accompanied by vomiting, requires further investigation with CT scan in all patients.

Investigations
- CT scan (may miss small bleeds)
- LP (only if the diagnosis is in doubt and the patient is conscious without focal neurological signs); if positive, carry out urgent cerebral angiography.

Treatment. Early consultation with a neurosurgeon. If the patient is conscious with little neurological deficit, angiography is undertaken with a view to endovascular coiling or surgery. Surgery involves an intracranial approach to the aneurysm with clipping of the neck of the aneurysm with a non-magnetic metal clip. Occasionally, angiography fails to show an aneurysm, possibly indicating that thrombosis has taken place in the aneurysm. Such cases may be treated conservatively and often do well. The majority of aneurysms are now coiled. Surgery is reserved for those where coiling is considered inappropriate.

Prognosis. Some 25% of patients die without regaining consciousness; 5% bleed again within 3 weeks of the initial haemorrhage, and in rebleeding, the mortality is high. After 6 weeks, the chances of a rebleed are about 10% per annum, without treatment.

HYDROCEPHALUS

This may be divided into two types:

Non-communicating or obstructive. In this type the CSF cannot escape from the brain through the cerebral aqueduct and ventricular dilatation alone occurs. The aqueduct may be blocked by congenital stenosis, Arnold–Chiari malformation (downward herniation of the fourth ventricle and cerebellar tonsils), infection or tumour.

Communicating. The ventricles communicate with a subarachnoid space and the CSF can escape within the brain but absorption via the arachnoid villae is prevented. This may result from meningitis, intraventricular haemorrhage in premature infants or malignant deposits on the meninges.

Clinically, hydrocephalus may be divided into two groups, congenital and acquired.

Congenital

The commonest causes are stenosis of the aqueduct of Sylvius, stenosis of the foramina of Magendie and Lushka, and Arnold–Chiari malformation.

Symptoms and signs. Developmental delay. Abnormal skull enlargement. Frontal bossing. Prominent scalp veins. 'Setting sun' sign (eyeballs displace downwards). 'Crackpot' sign on percussion of skull. Diffuse transillumination of the skull only if the hydrocephalus is very gross. Bulging fontanelles that fail to close at the appropriate time. Later, there may be epilepsy and profound mental impairment. Associated congenital deformities may occur, especially spina bifida.

Investigations
● USS if fontanelles open
● CT/MRI: ventricular dilatation and may confirm cause.

Treatment. In some infants, natural arrest of the condition occurs. A shunting procedure is usually required to direct the CSF to an absorptive area. In obstructive hydrocephalus, the CSF is shunted from the ventricles into the peritoneal cavity. The shunt incorporates a unidirectional valve set at a specific opening pressure.

Acquired

This usually presents with signs of raised ICP unless it occurs before the age of 3, when the skull may expand as in congenital hydrocephalus. Causes include meningitis, trauma, intrauterine infection, e.g. rubella, syphilis, CMV and cerebral tumours.

Investigations
- USS if fontanelles open
- CT/MRI
- CSF (ventricular tap) to exclude infection.

Treatment. In obstructive hydrocephalus the obstructing tumour or abscess may be removed. Infections, e.g. TB and meningitis, are treated. Ventriculoperitoneal shunting may be required.

SPINAL TUMOURS

Spinal tumours are classified in Table 18.2.

Symptoms and signs. Pain, especially nocturnal. Radiation in dermatomal patterns. Progressive symptoms. Symptoms and signs of cord compression. Sensory changes below lower level of involvement. Motor weakness with spasticity. Bowel or bladder sphincter impairment. Cord compression causes spasticity with increased reflexes and extensor plantar response, together with retention of urine with overflow and constipation. Cauda equina lesions cause a lower motor neuron lesion with flaccidity, diminished reflexes and paralysis of the anal and bladder sphincters with incontinence. Spinal tenderness, especially in the thoracic region, suggests malignant deposits.

Differential diagnosis. Intervertebral disc lesions, especially central disc protrusions. Cord infarction (e.g. vasculitis due to polyarteritis nodosa, syphilis). Syringomyelia. Motor neuron disease. Osteoporosis. Fractures. Extradural abscess. Haematoma. Myelitis. Subacute combined degeneration.

Investigations
- MRI scan is initial investigation
- Spinal radiographs: erosion, vertebral collapse, enlarged intervertebral foramina, calcification in tumour (meningioma)
- CT myelography if MRI not available.

Treatment

Primary tumours. Laminectomy. Surgical intervention is aimed at obtaining tissue diagnosis, removal of tumour and cord decompression. Microsurgery has improved results. Meningiomas and neurofibromas may be completely excised, as may ependymomas.

Metastatic lesions. Radiotherapy and chemotherapy may be helpful in palliation. The prognosis is poor. Surgical biopsy and decompression with stabilization may be required.

TABLE 18.2 Classification of spinal tumours

Extradural	Secondary spinal deposits are most common
	Primary bone tumours, e.g. osteoblastoma and myeloma
Intradural–extramedullary	Meningioma
	Neurofibroma
Intramedullary	Rare and include astrocytomas and ependymomas

SPECIFIC NEURALGIAS

Trigeminal neuralgia

This is a severe lancinating pain in the distribution of, usually, the lower branches of the trigeminal nerve. Exacerbations and remissions may occur. Aetiology is thought to be due to vascular compression of the trigeminal sensory nerve root at the pons but in younger patients, consider inflammatory conditions, e.g. MS.

Symptoms and signs. Severe lancinating pains. Shooting or burning. Exacerbation and remissions. 'Trigger' zones occur on the face, mouth or tongue and patients avoid 'trigger' stimuli, e.g. afraid of eating or shaving.

Investigations. MRI scan for microvascular compression and to exclude tumour and MS.

Treatment. Initially medical. The most effective drugs are carbamazepine and gabapentin. Surgery should be considered in all patients. If fit, microvascular decompression. If the patient is frail, thermocoagulation of ganglion or phenol injection is very helpful. Stereotactic radio-surgery may also be helpful.

Glossopharyngeal neuralgia

This is pain of a similar character to trigeminal neuralgia and is felt deep in the neck at the angle of the jaw and the region of the tonsillar fossa. Diagnosis is confirmed by applying local anaesthetic to the tonsillar fossa, which relieves the pain. Aetiology is thought to be due to vascular compression of the nerve. Surgical treatment involves partial section of the IXth nerve.

Post-herpetic neuralgia

Severe burning pain may persist in the involved segment long after the infection of herpes zoster has settled. Medical treatment should be tried initially. Amitriptyline or carbamazepine may help. TENS may be tried. In severe forms, dorsal route entry zone destruction or dorsal ganglionectomy may be required.

NEUROSURGICAL PROCEDURES FOR PAIN RELIEF

Destructive operations of the nervous system for the treatment of pain should only be used when other simpler measures have been used and failed. These should be undertaken in specialist neurosurgical centres. They are mainly used for relieving the pain of malignant disease.

Cordotomy

The spinal cord tracts that transmit pain to the brain are the anterolateral spinothalamic tracts. If these are divided, the appreciation of pain and temperature is lost on the contralateral side of the body. The procedure can be carried out via a laminectomy but also percutaneously under radiographic control. In the latter procedure, the patient is awake and a radiofrequency current is passed through a needle placed percutaneously in the spinothalamic tract.

Trigeminal thermocoagulation

This is used in the treatment of trigeminal neuralgia in patients who have not responded to medical treatment. Percutaneous radiofrequency rhizotomy of the trigeminal nerve is carried out by introducing a needle into the foramen ovale under radiographic control; 75% of patients get relief at the expense of an area of anaesthesia on the face.

Neurovascular decompression

The aetiology of trigeminal neuralgia is thought to be due to distortion of the nerve by blood vessels. Decompression may be carried out through a small retromastoid craniectomy. No neural tissue is destroyed and therefore there is no anaesthesia. The vessels are separated from the nerve and muscle or silicone sponge interposed; 70–80% gain relief.

Dorsal root entry zone destruction

This may be used for treatment of pain resulting from nerve injury. Suitable conditions include phantom limb pain, post-herpetic neuralgia, and brachial plexus avulsion. Results have been encouraging.

Sacral neurectomy

This may be used for the pain of pelvic cancer. Open laminectomy is carried out. If the sections are limited to the nerve roots below S3, sphincter function is spared.

Procedure

Exploratory burr holes

- Shave and prepare the skull over the temporal region between the ear and the external limit of the orbit on the side of the suspected compression.
- Infiltrate the scalp with local anaesthetic with adrenaline and make a 3 cm incision through the skin and temporal fascia.
- Separate the temporalis muscle and incise the periosteum.
- Control bleeding from the scalp with haemostat supply to the aponeurosis.
- Make the burr hole 2 cm above and behind the orbital process of the frontal bone.
- Use Hudson brace with perforator and once the inner table has been reached, change the perforator for a burr. Use gentle pressure when cutting the inner table of the skull to avoid plunging through into the brain.
- Stop bleeding from diploe with bone wax.
- If extradural haematoma is located it may be necessary to enlarge the opening further with a rongeur.
- Remove clot carefully and wash with saline.
- Control bleeding from middle meningeal artery using cautery or ligature.
- Control venous bleeding with piece of crushed muscle or gelatin sponge.
- If no extradural haematoma is found, incise dura and check for subdural haematoma.
- Meticulous haemostasis.
- Close scalp in two layers.

Plastic surgery and skin

Plastic surgery has evolved from the innovation of techniques concerning the movement and reconstruction of soft tissue defects by the movement of autologous, distant and allogeneic tissue. Knowledge of anatomy, vascularity, wound healing and vessel, nerve and tendon reconstructive techniques are applied. Excision of benign and malignant tumours of the skin and soft tissue (sarcoma) with subsequent reconstruction of resulting defects forms a large part of the workload. Breast reconstruction following partial or total mastectomy defects, soft tissue defects due to trauma and burns and congenital hand, urogenital and craniofacial abnormalities such as cleft lip and palate are also addressed using these techniques. Elective and traumatic hand surgery and reconstruction forms a large subspecialty. Plastic surgeons often work with other specialties to reconstruct defects that cannot close directly, e.g. orthopaedics (open lower limb fractures), general surgeons and gynaecologists (perineal defects), cardiothoracic surgeons (sternal dehiscence and chest wall defects), neurosurgeons (craniofacial defects), and head and neck surgeons (facial reconstruction following tumour excision and trauma, facial palsy correction). The importance of aesthetics in these reconstructions has led to the refinement of cosmetic surgery which forms the minority of the workload. However the recent increased numbers of obese patients undergoing bariatric surgery has increased the volume of referrals for body contouring procedures (abdominoplasty, belt lipectomy, thigh lift, breast reduction/mastopexy, brachioplasty).

THE RECONSTRUCTIVE LADDER

This algorithm is commonly applied when addressing any soft tissue defect. If integrity cannot be restored at the first rung of the ladder, then the second is considered, and so on. The techniques increase in complexity and potential risk as the ladder is ascended. In some circumstances, cosmetic or functional considerations call for the use of the more complex techniques despite the feasibility of simpler manoeuvres.

1. Direct closure
2. Healing by secondary intention
3. Free skin graft
4. Local flap
5. Regional flap
6. Free flap.

PROVIDING SKIN COVER

DIRECT CLOSURE

Following excision of simple skin lesions or debridement of necrotic tissue in small wounds, the edges may approximate without tension and without deforming neighbouring structures such as the eyebrow, nose, lip or eyelid. Direct closure with simple interrupted or continuous suturing techniques is usually the best approach in such circumstances. Eversion of skin edges is essential with the choice of suture and timing of removal related to the anatomical site. Planned excisions are best performed along relaxed skin tension lines to orientate scars into natural skin creases.

HEALING BY SECONDARY INTENTION

Where wounds will not close without tension, small defects with a vascularized bed, rather than exposed bone, tendon or prosthesis can be allowed to heal by secondary intention using appropriate dressings. It is remembered, however, that such wounds will heal slowly with contraction which may distort local structures and limit motion if sited over a joint. Such scars can become hypertrophic and therefore problematic. Good results from secondary intention can be seen after excision of small skin cancers in the inner canthal region and may be the most appropriate choice in lower limb ulcers compromised by venous insufficiency where skin grafts are less likely to survive or a patient is not fit for a surgical procedure.

SKIN GRAFT

A graft tissue is removed completely from one part of the body and inset onto another site. It is separated from its blood supply and therefore depends on being placed on a healthy vascular bed for its revascularization.

Split-skin graft

This consists of the epidermis and upper papillary dermis. This may be shaved with either a freehand knife or a power dermatome. A thin split-skin graft is approximately 0.25 mm thick. The usual donor sites include arms and thigh. The donor site heals by re-epithelialization under semi-occlusive dressings over 10 days, which can be delayed by infection.

Split-skin grafts are used in the resurfacing of burns, and to cover defects after removal of larger skin tumours. The skin graft revascularizes or 'takes' over 3–14 days. Disadvantages include post-graft contracture, lack of resistance to trauma, and absence of normal skin properties, e.g. suppleness, hair growth. The graft can be passed through a 'mesher', which creates multiple holes so that the graft looks like a string vest. Wide meshing allows large areas to be covered, and enables easier contouring and egress of underlying blood. A disadvantage is that the final result also resembles a string vest because the interstices heal by epithelialization alone, as they contain no dermal elements. A 'tie over' pressure dressing can be applied to prevent movement and keep all parts of the graft in contact with the bed or 'quilting' sutures can stitch the graft to the vascular bed.

Full thickness graft (Wolfe graft)

This consists of the epidermis and dermis and therefore includes all skin elements, e.g. hair follicles, sweat glands. Only areas of thin skin can be used as donor sites. Main uses are for facial areas and hands. Usual donor sites include supraclavicular, postauricular, submammary, antecubital and inguinal areas. The donor area requires closure and if this cannot be closed primarily a split-skin graft may be required.

Advantages include the fact that full thickness grafts include all skin elements, are more supple, withstand trauma and undergo the least contraction. Disadvantages include limited donor site area and increased failure of take (compared with split-skin). Successful 'take' depends on the same factors as split-skin grafting. A 'tie over' dressing should be used, often with added 'quilting' sutures.

Factors affecting skin graft take

Skin grafts take over a period of several days. Vascularization commences over the first 2–3 days and is overlapped by a subsequent phase of remodelling and graft maturation lasting several weeks/months. This process is therefore dependent on patient, wound bed and operative factors. The key is good vascularity. If a patient is poorly perfused, for example if peripherally vasoconstricted by noradrenaline administration, is in shock by whatever cause or is a diabetic or peripheral arteriopath, then the graft is less likely to establish. The wound bed needs to be well-debrided and uncontaminated, well vascularized – fat and fascia are less likely to take grafts than muscle, and free from infective organisms especially as *Pseudomonas aeruginosa* and Group A *Streptococcus* species which digest compromised tissue. Operative and dressing technique ensuring meticulous haemostasis prior to insetting the graft prevents a haematoma coming between the graft and the bed, and quilting sutures and/or a firm tie over dressing will help to prevent shear stresses damaging the fragile blood vessels revascularizing the graft. The thicker the graft, the more metabolic demands it has to survive and the longer it takes to revascularize, therefore thin grafts are more likely to take than thick split or full thickness grafts.

FLAPS

A flap is a section of tissue transferred, carrying its own blood supply. They can be defined by their composition, e.g. skin (cutaneous), fasciocutaneous, adipofascial, or muscle with or without skin or bone. They can be local (raised from an area sharing a border with the defect) and move by advancement, rotation or transposition. These can be geometrically designed to rely on the unnamed vasculature from the base of the flap (random pattern → Fig. 19.1) or based on a named or identified vessel – the pedicle, e.g. groin flap, deltopectoral flap or on a vessel perforating from the deeper tissues. These pedicled flaps do not necessarily share a border with the defect (regional), and can be moved into the defect around a pivot point, related to the axis around the pedicle. General indications for flap cover include: avascular areas, e.g. exposed bone or joint surfaces, exposed major blood vessels, irradiated areas or areas to undergo radiotherapy. (For a selection of pedicled flaps, see Figure 19.2.)

Free flaps

The blood supply to the flap is completely divided and the flap transferred to another area of the body where revascularization is affected by microvascular anastomosis. Free flaps may be composed of muscle, fasciocutaneous tissue, bone

Figure 19.1 (A) Some random pattern flap designs used for facial defects and (B) their resultant scars. (a) Bilateral V-Y advancement flaps, move together to complete the primary (excised) defect, without raising eyebrow. The secondary (flap) defects can be closed directly. (b) Rhomboid flap recruits adjacent mobile skin as a transposition flap to cover the primary defect, yet allows direct closure of the secondary defect. (c) Bilobed flap utilizes two transposition flaps recruiting mobile tissue from dorsum of bridge of nose to cover the secondary defect of the transposition flap used to cover the primary defect. (d) Cheek rotation flap utilizes skin laterally via a cheek-lid margin incision extending in the pre-auricular line. (e) Glabellar 'hatchet' flap rotates and advances mobile skin between the brows to cover the primary defect. The secondary defect is closed in a V-Y fashion.

Figure 19.2 Some of the more commonly used pedicled flaps (a–i):

	Name of flap	Composition	Blood supply of flap	Indications
a	Pectoralis major	Muscle ± skin	Thoracoacromial vessels	Head, neck, shoulder defects
b	Rectus abdominis	Muscle ± skin (Vertical skin paddle = VRAM) (Transverse = TRAM)	Deep inferior epigastric vessels or superior epigastric vessels	Perineum, groin, sternum defects TRAM – breast reconstruction
c	Gracilis	Muscle ± skin	Medial circumflex femoral vessels	Groin, perineum, vaginal reconstruction
d	Medial gastrocnemius	Muscle	Medial sural vessels	Knee and upper third leg defects
e	Groin	Fasciocutaneous	Superficial circumflex iliac vessels	Hand, wrist, groin, perineum, abdomen defects
f	Tensor fascia lata (TFL)	Musculocutaneous	Ascending branch lateral circumflex femoral vessels	Groin, lower abdomen, ischium, trochanteric defects
g	Latissimus dorsi	Muscle ± skin	Thoracodorsal vessels	Breast reconstruction, upper arm, thoracic defects
h	Radial forearm	Fasciocutaneous	Radial vessels	Elbow, forearm defects
i	Forehead	Cutaneous	Supratrochlear vessels	Nasal reconstruction

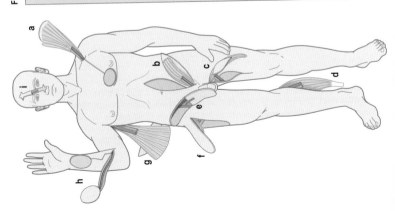

(e.g. fibula, scapula, iliac crest, radius) or a combination of these. Advantages include single-stage reconstruction, a wide choice of donor sites allowing better tailoring and choice of a flap to suit the defect without the constraint of a fixed pedicle and a good success rate (up to 95%). Disadvantages include long operating time and the need for specialized equipment and expertise. (For a selection of free flaps, see Figure 19.3.)

'SURGICAL' SKIN LESIONS: PRINCIPLES OF MANAGEMENT (→ Table 19.1)

- Simple excision for straightforward clinically diagnosed lesions, e.g. skin tags, sebaceous cysts
- Excision biopsy if risk of malignancy, e.g. small pigmented lesions where change may have occurred recently
- Incisional biopsy, e.g. for ulcers which have failed to heal and there is need to exclude malignancy or vasculitis
- Wide excision of adequate margin and depth, e.g. for confirmed malignant lesions
- Radiotherapy for basal cell carcinoma may be an alternative to surgery, especially in sites where skin preservation is important
- Remember that skin lesions may be a manifestation of systemic disease.

COMMON BENIGN LESIONS

EPIDERMIS

Pedunculated papillomas (skin tags)
These small polypoid lesions occur in adults, most frequently on the trunk, neck, axilla and groin. They may catch on clothes and bleed, and are often cosmetically unacceptable. They are removed by excision under local anaesthetic. Small skin tags may be treated by tying a fine ligature around the base, which leads to necrosis.

Warts (verrucae vulgaris)
These are caused by papovavirus, and usually occur in the second decade of life. They are common on fingers, hands and soles of feet (verrucae plantaris). Plantar warts may be very painful. Resolution of warts may occur spontaneously. Treatment may be by curettage, freezing with liquid nitrogen or application of keratolytic agents, e.g. podophyllin.

Seborrhoeic keratoses
These are found in elderly patients, and are often multiple, well-demarcated raised 'stuck on' lesions with varying degrees of pigmentation. It may be difficult to differentiate from malignant melanoma if deeply pigmented. Treatment is to leave alone or treat by surgical excision or curettage.

Figure 19.3 Some of the more commonly used free flaps (a–h):

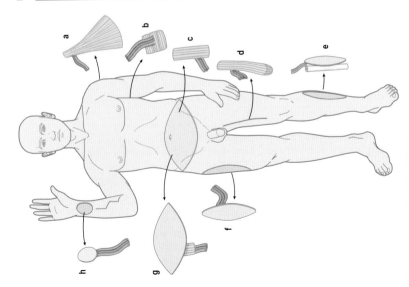

Name	Composition	Blood supply	Indications
a	Latissimus dorsi	Muscle ± Skin	Thoracodorsal or Subscapular vessels	Lower limb, large defects
b	Serratus anterior	Muscle	Thoracodorsal or Subscapular vessels	Lower limb, small defects
c	Rectus abdominis	Muscle	Deep inferior epigastric vessels	Head and neck, tongue, maxilla, skull base, calvarium, lower limb
d	Gracilis	Muscle ± skin	Medial circumflex femoral vessels	Lower limb, mid-sized defects, facial reanimation With skin paddle – breast reconstruction
e	Fibula	Bone ± skin	Peroneal vessels	Bony defects of mandible, lower limb
f	Anterolateral thigh (ALT)	Fasciocutaneous	Descending branch of lateral circumflex femoral vessels	Lower limb, head and neck, general soft tissue defects
g	Transverse rectus abdominis musculocutaneous (TRAM)	Muscle and skin = TRAM flap, Fasciocutaneous based on perforators = DIEP flap	Deep inferior epigastric vessels	Breast reconstruction
h	Radial forearm	Fasciocutaneous ± bone	Radial vessels	Head and neck, floor of mouth, mandible, tongue, larynx, lower limb

TABLE 19.1 'Surgical' skin lesions

Benign	
Epidermis	Pedunculated papilloma, wart, seborrhoeic keratosis, keratoacanthoma
Dermis	Pyogenic granuloma, fibrous histiocytoma, keloid
Appendages	Furuncle, carbuncle, hidradenitis suppurativa, sebaceous cyst, dermoid cyst, pilonidal sinus
Subcutaneous	Lipoma, neurofibroma
Melanotic	Intradermal naevus, blue naevus, compound naevus, spitz naevus, congenital naevus
Vascular	Campbell de Morgan spots, haemangiomas, capillary/venous/arteriovenous/lymphatic malformations, spider naevi, glomus tumours
Premalignant	
Epidermis	Actinic (solar) keratosis, Bowen's disease, erythroplasia of Queyrat (penis)
Malignant	
Epidermis	Basal cell carcinoma, squamous cell carcinoma
Dermis	Kaposi's sarcoma, secondary deposits
Appendages	Sebaceous carcinoma (rare), sweat gland carcinoma (rare)
Subcutaneous	Liposarcoma, neurofibrosarcoma
Melanotic	Malignant melanoma
Vascular	Angiosarcoma (rare)

Keratoacanthoma

This is a nodular lesion with a central crater containing a keratin 'plug'. They progress rapidly in 2 weeks to 2 months. Probably of viral aetiology, they often show spontaneous regression. Occasionally, they are difficult to distinguish from squamous cell carcinomas. Treatment is by excision biopsy or close observation, if the lesion is obviously regressing.

DERMIS

Pyogenic granuloma

This is a dark red nodule of exuberant granulation tissue and polymorphs. There is rapid initial growth, often at the site of trauma. Occasionally, the surface may ulcerate and then must be distinguished from amelanotic melanoma. Treatment is by excision.

Fibrous histiocytoma

This is a well-circumscribed deep reddish-brown tumour. On inspection, it may be mistaken for a malignant melanoma. However, palpation reveals a hard consistency due to the dense fibrous stroma. Treatment is by excision.

Keloid

This involves excessive deposition of collagen beyond and above the wound itself and is covered by normal epithelium. It must be distinguished from a hypertrophic scar in which the wound becomes broad and raised – the latter usually settles within 6 months. Keloid may increase after 6 months. Black Africans and the young are particularly affected. It may follow burns. Treatment is by intralesional injection of steroid, pressure garment therapy, applying silicon-impregnated dressings; or for refractive, problematic lesions, radiotherapy after excision is an option.

SKIN APPENDAGES

Boil (furuncle)

This is an infection in a hair follicle usually caused by *Staphylococcus aureus*. It can occur in any part of the body but is more common in the head, neck, axilla and groins. Diabetes, immunosuppression and general debility are predisposing conditions. Multiple boils (furunculosis) are common in diabetics. Any patient presenting with boils should have the urine tested for sugar.

Usually, they are self-limiting and heal when pus has discharged. Antibiotics should be avoided except in the following situations:

- 'Dangerous' areas of the face, i.e. between the orbit and angle of the mouth where venous drainage is into the cavernous sinus – cavernous sinus thrombosis may occur
- Multiple boils with surrounding cellulitis in diabetics and immunosuppressed patients where septicaemia is a risk.

Carbuncle

An infection which dissects through the dermis and subcutaneous tissues to form connecting channels, some of which open to the surface. There is considerable induration and pus discharges through the sinuses. The back of the neck is a common site. Treatment is with antistaphylococcal antibiotics, e.g. flucloxacillin, with desloughing and adequate drainage of the abscesses if necessary.

Hidradenitis suppurativa

A chronic disease of skin and subcutaneous tissue in apocrine gland-bearing areas, e.g. axilla, groin, perineum and perianal areas. The involved area is indurated, fibrotic and inflamed with sinuses draining pus. *Staph. aureus* is the usual organism grown but occasionally coliforms may be cultured. Treatment is initially by antibiotics. Abscesses are incised and drained. Advanced cases may need wide excision with or without skin grafting. Severe perianal disease may require a diverting colostomy prior to skin grafting.

Sebaceous cysts

These are common on the scalp, face, neck, and back and are soft or firm and spherical. They contain cheesy sebaceous material, which may become infected and discharge. They are attached to the skin and a punctum is usually seen at the point of attachment. Treatment is by excision under local anaesthetic.

Dermoid cysts

These may be congenital or acquired.

Congenital. They are formed in intrauterine life when skin dermatomes fuse and present at birth or a few years after. They are most common in head and neck, e.g. outer end of eyebrow (external angular dermoid). Treatment is by excision. Midline dermoid cysts should be radiologically assessed to exclude intracranial extension.

Acquired. These are implantation dermoids. A piece of skin is forcibly implanted into the dermis as a result of trauma. They are common on fingers. Treatment is by excision.

Pilonidal sinus

This chronic infection in the sinus is caused by penetration of hairs into skin and subcutaneous tissues. Infection leads to pilonidal abscesses. The sinus leads to a cavity filled with hair and granulation tissue. Common sites include posteriorly in the midline over the sacrococcygeal area and natal cleft (usually hirsute males with sedentary occupations); between the fingers in hairdressers; occasionally umbilicus, axilla and nipple. Differential diagnosis includes perianal fistulae, hidradenitis suppurativa, simple boils. Treatment includes:

- Deroofing the track, removing the hairs and packing; the surrounding skin should be shaved until the sinuses have healed
- Injection of the sinuses with methylene blue, followed by wide excision of all tracts until no dye is seen and either packing, primary suture or reconstruction of large defects using local flaps can be carried out under GA
- For pilonidal abscesses, incising, curetting and packing.

DISORDERS OF THE NAILS

Ingrowing toenail (IGTN)

A common condition, it usually appears on the great toe, particularly the lateral side. Caused by a combination of tight shoes and paring the nail downwards into the nail fold rather than cutting it transversely. The sharp edge of nail then grows into the nail fold producing ulceration, infection, and granulation tissue.

Treatment

Non-infected. Give advice on correct cutting of nails, i.e. transversely. Avoid tight, pointed shoes. Tuck a pledget of cotton wool soaked in mild antiseptic under the corner of the nail to lift it out of the soft tissue. Soak feet in warm water regularly.

Infected. With mild infection, it may be possible to adopt the above regimen in addition to the administration of antistaphylococcal antibiotics. If this fails carry out the following:

- Simple nail avulsion with curettage of infected granulation tissue under local anaesthetic. Antistaphylococcal antibiotics should be administered.
- Wedge excision. Lateral or medial nail and nail bed are removed together with granulation tissue and germinal matrix. Liquefied phenol may be applied to the germinal matrix to ensure complete removal.
- Zadik's procedure. This is reserved for recurrent IGTN. The nail is avulsed and the germinal matrix completely excised after raising a skin flap to expose it. To ensure complete removal of the germinal matrix liquefied phenol is applied after protecting the skin. The nails should not re-grow after this procedure.

Complications. Recurrence may occur. This is common after simple avulsion. Spikes of nail may occasionally re-grow after a Zadik's procedure. Infection may occur and it is appropriate to give a course of antistaphylococcal antibiotics prophylactically. Osteomyelitis and septic arthritis may occur after Zadik's procedure.

Onychogryphosis
This is a 'ram's horn' deformity of the toenail. The nail thickens and curls over the end of the toe as it grows. Common in the elderly, it may follow trauma to the nail in the younger patient. It can be treated by either cutting the nail with bone forceps or grinding the nail down. Avulsion is always followed by recurrence. Zadik's operation is curative.

Nail bed lesions
Haematoma. There is a history of trauma, e.g. trapping, or dropping a heavy object on the nail. Very painful. A haematoma is evacuated by piercing the nail with a red-hot paper clip. Small haematomas following trivial injury may closely simulate subungual melanoma. Haematomas grow out with growth of the nail. If there is any doubt, biopsy should be carried out.

Melanoma. Subungual malignant melanoma is not uncommon. The lesion does not grow out with the nail. Biopsy is necessary. If the diagnosis is confirmed, amputation of the digit is required.

Subungual exostosis. This nearly always affects the great toe. It occurs in adolescents and young adults. It lifts the overlying nail and causes deformity. Diagnosis is confirmed by radiograph. Treatment is to remove the nail and excise the underlying bony nodule.

Glomus tumour. See Lesions of vascular origin, below.

SUBCUTANEOUS TISSUES

Lipoma
This is a common, benign tumour of fatty tissue. It is soft, lobulated and pseudofluctuant and the overlying skin appears normal. It is slow growing. Treatment is by excision. Multiple lipomas may occur. These need to be distinguished from neurofibromata by biopsy of at least one lesion. Occasionally, there may be multiple tender lipomas on the trunk (Dercum's disease). Treatment of lipoma is by excision, which is curative. Liposarcomatous change may rarely occur in a benign lipoma.

Neurofibroma
These are benign tumours arising from the connective tissue element of peripheral nerves. They are often multiple and may be asymptomatic, but if closely related to the nerve the patient may get paraesthesia in the distribution of the nerve. Biopsy of one lesion may confirm the diagnosis. If neurofibromata are multiple, congenital and familial, the condition is known as von Recklinghausen's disease. Occasionally malignant change to neurofibrosarcoma occurs.

PREMALIGNANT LESIONS

Actinic (solar) keratoses

These are rough, scaly epidermal lesions on sites of exposure to the sun; 10–20% undergo malignant change. The diagnosis is confirmed by biopsy and then the lesion is excised. Topical chemotherapy with 5-fluorouracil cream has been used in patients with multiple lesions.

Bowen's disease

Intraepidermal squamous cell carcinoma (carcinoma-*in-situ*). A well-defined erythematous plaque with occasional crusting, it occurs in the fourth to sixth decade and may be associated with the presence of internal malignancy. Diagnosis is confirmed by a biopsy. Treatment is by excision, cryotherapy, curettage, topical 5-fluorouracil or photodynamic therapy. Intraepidermal carcinoma may occur on the glans penis and is then called erythroplasia of Queyrat and appears as a reddish-brown velvety plaque.

Leucoplakia

Leucoplakia consists of a thickened white patch on a mucous membrane. It can occur on the vermillion border, oral mucosa and the vulva. It occurs due to chronic irritation. In the mouth, this is usually due to sunlight but can occur due to dentures. Approximately 20% will show dysplasia and may progress to carcinoma. Erythroplasia is a red patch and always represents *in situ* carcinoma.

Lentigo maligna

Also known as Hutchinson's freckle. It occurs on sun-damaged skin in the elderly. It is an irregular flat brown-black lesion. It may increase in size over many years and it consists of an abnormal proliferation of atypical melanocytes in the dermo-epidermal junction. It is essentially malignant melanoma *in situ*. Development of invasion and therefore malignancy is usually heralded by the development of a pigmented nodule within the lesion. Confirmed by incision biopsy, treatment is by excision.

MALIGNANT LESIONS

EPIDERMIS

Basal cell carcinoma (rodent ulcer)

Basal cell carcinoma arises from epithelial cells. It is common in the middle-aged and elderly. Locally invasive; it very rarely metastasizes. Frequently found on skin exposed to sunlight, the commonest area is the face above a line drawn from the angle of the mouth to the lobe of the ear. Other predisposing factors include immunosuppression, radiotherapy, xeroderma pigmentosum and naevus sebaceous.

There are several different types:

- Nodular – most common, starts as a nodule that ulcerates and develops a rolled edge with a pearly appearance and local telangiectasia
- Superficial – presents as red scaly patches

- Morphoeic or sclerosing – forms a flat spreading plaque; it has a fibrous stroma and may cause distortion, i.e. around the eyelids
- Gorlin's syndrome – autosomal dominant condition associated with multiple basal cell carcinomas, dental cysts and a splayed 12th rib; radiotherapy will convert the basal cell carcinoma to a much more aggressive form and is thus contraindicated.

Differential diagnosis includes seborrhoeic keratoses and malignant melanoma. Treatment options include surgical excision (with a 3–5 mm margin) or radiotherapy. Cure rate is high when treated early and adequately. Larger defects may require reconstruction using the principles of the reconstructive ladder.

Squamous cell carcinoma

Squamous cell carcinoma arises from keratinocytes in the epidermis. This may grow rapidly. It metastasizes via lymphatics and rarely via the bloodstream. Exposure to sunlight may be a causative factor. It can also develop in areas of Bowen's disease and erythroplasia of Queyrat. Other causative factors include chemical burns, chronic ulcers (e.g. Marjolin's ulcer, i.e. malignant change in a chronic venous ulcer), irradiation dermatitis.

It starts as a lump, which ulcerates with bleeding and discharge. The edge of the ulcer is characteristically raised and everted. Local lymph nodes may be involved. Differential diagnosis includes keratoacanthoma, basal cell carcinoma, amelanotic malignant melanoma, pyogenic granuloma, traumatized seborrhoeic wart. Diagnosis is confirmed by biopsy. Treatment is by wide excision (with a 4–10 mm margin) or radiotherapy. Block dissection of regional lymph nodes is required if these are affected. Large defects may require reconstruction with skin grafts, local or free flaps as described above.

DERMIS

Kaposi's sarcoma

These are raised purplish nodules. Initially, they are usually single, but gradually multiple nodules occur and may ulcerate. It is the commonest tumour to develop in patients with AIDS; 90% are in male subjects. The solitary nodule should be excised. Local radiotherapy or cytotoxic therapy is useful for multiple lesions.

Metastatic carcinoma

Small, hard, painless, skin nodules may occur. Skin secondaries are commonest with cancer of the breast, lung and bowel. In most patients, the primary will be obvious or will already have been treated. Ulceration of the secondaries may occur. Biopsy confirms the diagnosis. Treatment is given that is appropriate for metastatic disease for that particular tumour, e.g. tamoxifen in carcinoma of the breast.

Others

Malignant change may take place in neurofibromas and lipomas, giving rise to neurofibrosarcoma and liposarcoma. Other soft tissue sarcomas may also arise in this area and are treated by wide excision.

MELANOCYTIC LESIONS

BENIGN LESIONS

Freckle (ephelis)
Related to sun exposure, they consist of an increase in pigment from melanocytes but no increase in the number of melanocytes.

Solar lentigo
Occur in areas of sun-damaged skin, especially on the hands and face. They consist of an increase in the number of melanocytes producing normal amounts of pigment. There is no atypia.

Naevi (→ Fig. 19.4)
A naevus is defined as an increased number of melanocytes in an abnormal position producing normal or increased amounts of melanin. Melanocytes are present

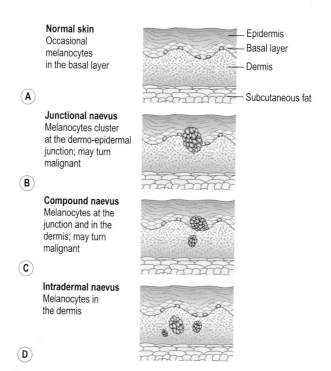

Normal skin
Occasional melanocytes in the basal layer

— Epidermis
— Basal layer
— Dermis

— Subcutaneous fat

(A)

Junctional naevus
Melanocytes cluster at the dermo-epidermal junction; may turn malignant

(B)

Compound naevus
Melanocytes at the junction and in the dermis; may turn malignant

(C)

Intradermal naevus
Melanocytes in the dermis

(D)

Figure 19.4   Pathological varieties of naevus (mole): (A) normal skin, (B) junctional naevus, (C) compound naevus and (D) intradermal naevus.

throughout the dermis and epidermis with similar numbers in all races, which differ in melanin production. At birth, most melanocytes are situated in the basal layer of the epidermis. Over the next few decades, some will migrate to the dermis. Melanocytes within the dermis have no malignant potential as they have lost their ability to divide.

The position of melanocytes can give rise to a number of pigmented lesions:

- Melanocytes in the basal layer form a simple lentigo or *mole*.
- Melanocytes at the dermo-epidermal junction form a *junctional naevus*. These appear as either a macule or papule and are brown, smooth and hairless. They develop at or around puberty and can occur anywhere, including the hands and the soles of the feet. A small percentage may turn malignant but this comprises the vast majority of malignant melanomas.
- Fibroblast migration may draw some melanocytes into the dermis, leaving some at the dermo-epidermal junction. This forms a *compound naevus*. It is clinically indistinguishable from an intradermal naevus. It does, however, have malignant potential.
- As a naevus matures in the late 30s, an *intradermal naevus* is formed, all the melanocytes lying in the dermis. Clinically they appear as a well-defined papule. They are brown or flesh-coloured and often hairy. They have no malignant potential.

Spitz naevus
Benign lesions, usually seen in children and young adults. Clinically they appear as pink, dome-shaped nodules. Histologically, they can be difficult to differentiate from malignant melanomas.

Halo naevus
Benign lesion. Clinically it appears as a lesion surrounded by an area of depigmentation secondary to invasion of lymphocytes. This phenomenon can occur in malignant melanomas and is thus an important differential diagnosis.

Blue naevus
Consists of melanocytes in the dermis. They form lesions with a slate-blue colour. There are two types:

Common. Benign lesion often seen in the head or hands. More common in women and usually seen in women in their 40s.

Cellular. More common in women. More than 50% occur in the sacrococcygeal/buttock area. They are benign but malignant transformation may occur.

Congenital naevi
May be single or multiple. One important variant is the giant pigmented naevus. These lesions are >20 cm in diameter and are flat, pale brown and hairless or lumpy, black and hairy in appearance. Malignant melanoma may develop, usually in the teenage years. Management is usually by excision. This may require extensive plastic surgical reconstruction due to tissue loss.

MALIGNANT MELANOMA

More than 9500 cases of malignant melanoma are diagnosed annually in the UK. They may occur anywhere on the skin or on the retina, oesophageal mucosa or anus. Malignant melanomas can arise in pre-existing naevi or de novo.
  Signs of malignant change in a mole include:

- Change in size, shape or deepening of colour
- Irregular border
- Bleeding or ulceration
- Itching.

Classification

Superficial spreading melanoma. This is the commonest type of melanoma. In males it occurs most commonly on the back; in females most commonly the legs. Prognosis tends to be good, as growth is predominantly radial rather than vertical (this correlates to a reduction in the level of invasion).

Nodular melanoma. Found on the trunk they appear as raised nodules often with ulceration. The growth is almost entirely vertical, thus these tumours have a poor prognosis.

Lentigo maligna melanoma. Arises from lentigo maligna. Occurs in the elderly, i.e. 60–70 years. Tends to have a good prognosis and has low metastatic potential.

Acral lentiginous melanoma. Rare. Occurs on the soles, palms and under nails (subungual).
  Spread of melanoma occurs by local growth and infiltration. Lymphatic spread occurs early. Bloodstream spread occurs in almost any organ, particularly the liver, brain and lung.

Staging

A number of different classifications may be used to stage the level of invasion – this links directly with prognosis. Classifications are as follows:

- Breslow thickness – <1 mm, 1–2 mm, 2–4 mm and >4 mm
- Clarke's level
  - I   Epidermis
  - II Papillary dermis
  - III Junction of papillary and reticular dermis
  - IV Extends to reticular dermis
  - V Subcutaneous tissue
- AJCC (American Joint Committee on Cancer)
  - T1 ≤1.0 mm
  - T2 1.01–2 mm
  - T3 2.01–4 mm
  - T4 >4.0 mm

N1 1 node
N2 2–3 nodes
N3 $\geq$4 or more nodes
M1 Metastatic disease.

Treatment
1. Confirm the diagnosis and depth of invasion. Occasionally a malignant melanoma is clinically obvious but lesions may need to be confirmed by excisional or incisional biopsy.
2. The mainstay of treatment is surgical. Initial excision should be performed with an adequate clearance margin. Following removal of the lesion histology will confirm the diagnosis and allow the measurement of Breslow thickness.
3. After measuring the Breslow thickness, further surgery may be needed. A tumour of <1 mm in thickness requires a 1 cm excision margin. Tumours of greater depth may need a wider margin but margins over 3 cm confer no survival benefit.
4. In patients with involved nodes, a regional lymph node dissection should accompany the removal of the lesion. In patients with no clinical involvement, the management is controversial. As many as 20% of T2/T3 patients may have metastases. Accurate staging is assisted by radiolabelled probe/dye-directed sentinel node biopsy.
5. Chemotherapy is of little value in primary disease. Isolated limb perfusion may be used in local recurrence.
6. Radiotherapy and immunotherapy have been used but are strictly palliative.

Prognosis. Favourable factors include early diagnosis, a depth of penetration of <1 mm, and melanoma in a radial growth phase. Unfavourable factors include lymph node and distant metastases at presentation, increasing depth of penetration, ulceration and presence of vertical growth phase. If the disease is confined to the primary site and has a penetration of <1 mm, then a 5-year survival of 90% may be expected. With lymph node metastases, this is reduced to 30% and with distant metastases, patients rarely survive for 1 year.

LESIONS OF VASCULAR ORIGIN

Campbell de Morgan spots
These are small bright red spots containing capillaries and connective tissue. They are rare before the age of 40 and increase with age. They are of no serious significance. Patients should be reassured and the lesions left alone.

Haemangiomas (strawberry naevi)
Grow rapidly in the first few months of life; are red, soft, compressible fleshy lesions that commonly involute; 50% of haemangiomas have resolved by 5 years of age. Haemangiomas that ulcerate and bleed, obscure vision or hearing or interfere with speech development may require treatment with steroids or excision, otherwise they are treated expectantly during involution.

Capillary malformations (port-wine stains)

These are flush with the skin and occur on the face, lips and buccal mucosa. They can become more thickened during life and are reddish-blue in colour. If the lesion is small, surgical excision may be attempted. Larger lesions are cosmetically distressing. Sclerosing agents and lasers have been used. Advice on the use of cosmetic preparations may be the most appropriate. Lesions in the 5th cranial nerve dermatome (ophthalmic division - VI) may be seen in association with meningeal involvement (Sturge–Weber syndrome), which may cause focal epilepsy. Similar lesions may be seen in the Klippel–Trenaunay syndrome.

Venous malformations, arteriovenous malformations (AVM)

Grow in proportion with the child's growth. High flow lesions (AVM) can progress to high output cardiac failure – treatment is by a combination of radiologically guided sclerotherapy and excision if symptomatic.

Lymphatic malformations

Can be macrocystic (cystic hygroma) or microcystic and localized or involve whole limbs, leading to lymphoedema and limb hypertrophy. Associations with AVM (Parkes–Weber syndrome) and capillary malformations (Klippel–Trenaunay) are recognized. Treatment is usually conservative as lesions often recur after excision.

Glomus tumour

Glomus bodies occur in the subcutaneous tissues of the limbs – especially the fingers, toes and nail bed. They are small arteriovenous communications associated with muscle and nerve (angioneuromyoma). Clinically, they are small, raised, bluish-red lesions. They are painful and exquisitely tender if pressed. Treatment is by surgical excision.

BURNS

A burn is the destruction of tissue due to external stress. Burns may be caused by heat, cold, ultraviolet light, irradiation, electricity, chemicals and friction. In the UK there are about 300 hospital deaths annually from burns, there being approximately 450 000 injuries each year. Domestic burns and scalds, especially in children and the elderly, form a large proportion of the 175 000 patients presenting to A&E units.

CLASSIFICATION OF DEPTH

Superficial

This involves the superficial epidermis only. The underlying germinal layer is intact. It presents with a blanching erythema and pain which resolves over the first 24 h. Analgesia is usually all that is required.

Superficial partial thickness

Damage penetrates to the depth of the superficial dermis. They present with blanching erythema, with blistering and pain. Healing occurs from epithelial elements within the skin appendages (hair follicles, sweat glands, sebaceous glands), taking approximately 3 weeks using appropriate dressings.

Deep dermal

Tissue damage may extend into the remaining dermis, damaging sources of epithelial growth, such as sweat glands and hair follicles. Blistering occurs. The underlying dermis may be non-blanching and white or pink with fixed-staining. There may be some surviving skin appendages, and a second look at 48 h and subsequently, will demonstrate any progression of the depth of the burn and potential for healing without the need for skin grafting. Those that are not anticipated to heal by 3 weeks proceed to skin grafting to prevent wound contracture and hypertrophic scarring.

Full thickness

All layers of the skin are destroyed, presenting with a white, insensate, non-blanching, or brown and leathery appearance or eschar. If left, the wound heals by separation of the eschar and healing by secondary intention with subsequent contraction of fibrous tissue and centripetal growth of the peripheral epithelium. In all but the smallest full thickness burns, skin grafting is required to prevent dense scarring, contractures, and deformity.

MANAGEMENT OF BURNS

First aid

1. Stop the burning process. Dousing with tepid water has both a quenching and analgesic affect. Beware copious cold water irrigation in the young scalded infant, as this may induce hypothermia, and may increase the depth of the burn.
2. If scalding, remove clothes.
3. If a chemical burn, perform copious irrigation with cool water.
4. Remove from smoke. Ensure clear airway.
5. Cover the burn in a clean sheet soaked in cold water, or cling film. Avoid tight circumferential cover, as the wound will swell.
6. Get the patient to hospital.

Assessment of the patient

1. Initial assessment is made using ATLS principles: airway, breathing, circulation, disability and exposure. Do not forget to assess for associated injuries that may be a greater threat to life than the burn itself.
2. Airway – Apply 100% oxygen. Look for signs of inhalation injury, hoarse voice, brassy cough, soot around mouth or nostrils, singed nasal hair, oromucosal oedema and ulceration. Supraglottic thermal burns can swell and obstruct the airway at a frightening pace, and therefore any evidence of airway injury is assessed by a senior anaesthetist for consideration of early endotracheal intubation to protect against later obstruction.
3. Breathing – Inhalation of smoke causes injury to the subglottic airway and systemic toxicity of carbon monoxide, hydrogen cyanide and other toxins may present with an unconscious, confused patient.
4. Ensure an adequate circulation. Obtain i.v. access with two large-bore cannula in burns >15% body surface area (BSA) in adults or 10% in children and resuscitate according to the Parkland formula (see below). If resuscitating, pass a urinary catheter.

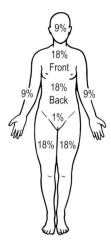

Figure 19.5 The 'rule of 9s'. A guide to estimating the percentage area of a burn.

5. Obtain a history: source of burning, e.g. fire or scald; duration of contact, indoors or outdoors; contact with any toxic gases; first aid given.
6. Assess the site, depth and BSA of the burns. Use the 'rule of nines' to calculate BSA (→ Fig. 19.5) or a Lund and Browder chart. Alternatively, the palm and finger surface of the patient's hand may be used as representing 1% of the BSA. It may be difficult to determine the depth of a burn clinically. Frequently there are areas of partial and full thickness burns. Partial thickness burns may show erythema. Pain is characteristic with normal pin-prick sensation. Full thickness burns are charred, or may be white, grey or leathery. They are usually dry. The surface is pain-free and pin-prick sensation is absent. However, final differentiation between partial and full thickness burns may be dependent on the degree of healing that occurs with time.

Treatment of burns
Patients with burns involving 15% or more of the body surface (10% in children) require resuscitation. Other indications for hospitalization include burns involving the face, hands, eyes, genitalia, and perineum; electrical or chemical burns; smoke inhalation or inhalation of other toxic fumes, suspicion of non-accidental injury. Burns over 20% cause a systemic inflammatory response causing cardiac output suppression, renal impairment, immunosuppression, bowel stasis and a catabolic response.

Full thickness circumferential burns. Around the chest or extremities, these burns threaten ventilation or the vascularity of the limb and require urgent escharotomy along midaxial lines of the extremities, or as a criss-cross on the chest to allow expansion with swelling.

Dressing

Open. The burn is exposed. Blisters are debrided. Wound swabs are taken. Burns are dressed with liquid paraffin. The open method is used for the face.

Closed. The burn is cleansed, covered with silver sulfadiazine cream, paraffin gauze and gauze. The dressings are changed if they become soaked with plasma, or after 48 h. Burns on the hands and fingers are treated with silver sulfadiazine cream and are enclosed in a plastic bag. This allows for encouragement of hand movements.

By 10–14 days, whichever method is used, slough will separate from partial thickness burns leaving an epithelium. This does not occur with full thickness burns, the slough remaining adherent. Removal of the slough reveals granulation tissue, which requires grafting. In some types of burns there is a need for immediate skin grafting. This is particularly the case if the eyelids are involved, where grafting is carried out in order to prevent ectropion and the risk of corneal ulceration. Scarring at certain other sites may cause considerable deformity or disability – these sites include the hands, joint flexures and the face.

Skin grafting of minor burns occurs after 14–21 days when raw areas remained, however major burns are debrided within a few days or hours of injury. If successful, it controls the systemic burn injury, reduces the chances of invasive infection and limits catabolism and heat and water loss. In large burns, the limitation is the availability of autologous skin. In these situations, cadaveric allograft skin or synthetic skin substitutes may be used temporarily, later to be replaced by skin autograft.

General

Pain relief. Frequent small doses of intravenous morphine should be given.

Fluid balance. Hypovolaemic shock occurs from plasma loss. Anaemia occurs owing to destruction of red cells. Intravenous fluids should be given if the burn is >15% (10% in the child). Fluid replacement may be given according to the Parkland formula:

$$\text{Weight (kg)} \times 4\text{mL} \times \text{BSA}\%$$
$$= \text{mL of crystalloid (Ringer's lactate or Hartmann's) over 24h}$$

One half is given over the first 8 h from the time of the burn, the second half over the subsequent 16 h. Children require maintenance fluids with one-half or one-fifth normal saline. Vital signs and urine output should be monitored hourly. The Parkland formula is only a rough guide to the likely fluid needs, and the actual fluid volume given should be related to the clinical response of the patient. Volumes of 5–6 mL/kg per %burns per 24 h have been found to be necessary if inhalation injury co-exists with the cutaneous burn.

Infection. Tetanus cover is mandatory. Regular swabs should be taken. Prophylactic antibiotics are not usually indicated. The usual causes of sepsis are *Staphylococci, Streptococci,* and *Pseudomonas.* Antibiotics should be given on the basis of culture and sensitivity.

Stress ulcers (Curling's ulcer). Prophylactic H_2 receptor antagonists should be given in major burns.

Acute renal failure. This may occur and be due to delayed resuscitation, or myoglobinuria from muscle destruction, particularly in electric burns. Ensure adequate CVP. Treat with mannitol, furosemide, dopamine. Haemodialysis may be required.

Nutrition. Oral feeding via a nasogastric tube is preferred at the earliest opportunity to protect against bacterial translocation, gut stasis and Curling's ulcers.

Multidisciplinary care and follow-up. Burns are managed in a multidisciplinary setting including specialist nurses, dieticians, anaesthetists, occupational therapists, physiotherapists and clinical psychologists. Initial scar care and physiotherapy is key to successful return to function. The long-term management of patients with burns scarring is complex and involves all these disciplines to maintain this function. Secondary revision using a variety of techniques such as skin grafting or local flaps may be necessary and so these patients are often managed over many years in the outpatient setting.

HAND INJURIES

The hand is a sophisticated mechanism from both motor and sensory considerations. Its importance is reflected in the size of its representation in the cerebral cortex. All hand injuries and infections should be referred to a specialist hand surgeon, usually a plastic or orthopaedic surgeon. Often joint management between both is necessary. Expert care is necessary from the outset to preserve or restore function. Careful history and examination are essential. Compensation claims or medicolegal problems may arise later. Accurate notes are essential.

PRINCIPLES OF MANAGEMENT

At place of injury

- Stop any bleeding by direct pressure. Never apply a tourniquet.
- Apply a clean, dry dressing.
- Do not bandage tightly.
- Save any avulsed or severed digit in a clean container. Cool with ice if possible (a bag of frozen peas will suffice). Place the digit in a bag on ice but do not cover in ice, in case the part gets frozen.

At hospital

History

- Age, occupation, dominant hand, any pre-existing anomaly or injury
- The exact details of the injury – how it occurred, when it occurred, where it occurred. Risk of contamination
- Treatment given at the site of accident
- Tetanus prophylaxis status and allergies
- Any drug history or past medical history.

Examination

- Skin loss and viability
- Contamination

- Swelling
- Infection
- Deformity – fractures, ligamentous injuries, flexor and extensor tendon injuries
- Nerve integrity
- Vessel integrity
- Other injuries.

Prophylaxis against infection
Use tetanus prophylaxis; antibiotic.

Surgery
Immediate surgical management of severed digit. Irrigation of wound. Debridement. Repair – bones, tendons, vessels and nerves for reimplantation of digits. Never close incision under tension. Appropriate dressings and splintage – dynamic splints may counteract deformity and assist weakened movements. Splint in the position of function. Elevation to prevent oedema. Physiotherapy.

Delayed primary repair. The patient is transferred to a hand surgical unit. The injury is explored, cleaned and damaged structures repaired as soon as possible. The skin is sutured or the injury covered with a flap of soft tissue and the hand splinted and elevated. Physiotherapy regimes depend on the structures injured.

Secondary reconstructive surgery. This may be required because of extensive soft tissue, nerve, tendon, arterial, or bony injury or loss, gross contamination or infection at the time of original debridement or lack of soft tissue cover, or occult injuries that present late. Structures are reconstructed using bone, tendon or nerve grafts or transfer of neighbouring tendons. Soft tissue cover may require flap reconstruction.

Rehabilitation
This should start as soon as possible. A painful, stiff hand should be avoided. Appropriate early treatment is wasted unless early physiotherapy and occupational therapy are instituted. Career counselling may be appropriate.

HAND INFECTIONS

> The incidence and severity of hand infections have decreased in the past two decades owing to earlier presentation and more appropriate treatment with antibiotics. The gross infections of the palmar spaces seen in the pre-antibiotic era are rare today. However, they should be recognized and treated appropriately to avoid long-term or permanent disability to the hand. Care should be taken with hand infections in patients with already compromising conditions, e.g. steroids, immunosuppressive therapy, diabetes, rheumatoid arthritis and other collagen diseases, and patients with poor peripheral circulation, e.g. Raynaud's phenomenon.

Paronychia (Whitlow)
In this condition, pus accumulates between the cuticle (eponychium) and the nail matrix. The pus tracks round the nail margin or under the nail. The causative

organism is usually *Staph. aureus.* In chronic cases, *Candida* may be responsible. In the acute case, spontaneous rupture may occur. If it is treated early, antibiotics and rest may suffice. Often surgical drainage is required. Incision is through the nail fold. Removal of the base of the nail may be necessary if pus is trapped beneath it. Chronic paronychia requires swabs and scrapings. If fungus is located, long-term oral antifungal agents may be used or the nail may be avulsed followed by application of a topical antifungal agent as the nail re-grows.

Pulp space infection (felon)

The origin of the infection is usually a minor penetrating injury. Pressure builds up in the pulp space with oedema and suppuration, and the terminal branches of the digital vessel may thrombose owing to pressure from the pus. Necrosis and osteomyelitis of the terminal phalanx may result. Treatment is by surgical drainage via a longitudinal incision over the point of maximum tenderness. Antistaphylococcal antibiotics should be given.

Suppurative tenosynovitis

This is most common in the flexors of the fingers. Organisms reach the tendon sheath either from a direct puncture wound or by extension from an undrained pulp space infection. An exudate, which becomes purulent, forms in the sheath and, if untreated, may discharge and infect the palmar spaces.

Symptoms and signs. Following minor injury, there is rapid onset of pain and swelling. The finger is held semiflexed and attempts at extension cause severe pain. Eventually a red, hot exquisitely tender finger results.

Treatment. In early stages, i.v. antistaphylococcal antibiotics, rest and elevation may suffice. If there is no improvement in 24 h or pus is present at presentation, the tendon sheath should be opened proximally and distally, a fine catheter passed down the sheath and irrigation with antibiotic solution carried out. Rest, elevation and systemic antibiotics should be given. Active exercises should be undertaken as pain subsides.

Deep palmar space infection

This is rare and may arise as a result of penetrating trauma, infection of a callosity, or as a complication of suppurative tenosynovitis. The infection occurs in the space deep to the flexor tendons but superficial to the interossei. The deep palmar space is divided into two by a septum attached to the third metacarpal. The space medial to the septum is the midpalmar space, the space lateral is the thenar space.

Symptoms and signs. Oedema of the dorsum of the hand. The skin is looser here and the swelling initially forms on the dorsum of the hand, although the infection is on the palm. Ballooning of the palm or thenar eminence. Acute throbbing pain. Fingers held flexed. Attempts at extension painful. Pain on pressure over affected space. Fever. Malaise.

Treatment. Incision and drainage. The midpalmar space is drained by an incision in the web space between the 4th and 5th or 3rd and 4th metacarpal heads. The thenar space is opened by an incision posteriorly in the web space between the thumb and index finger. Rest. Elevation. Antistaphylococcal antibiotics.

Bites

Human or animal bites to the hand are serious. Most human 'bites' are the result of teeth and knuckles coming into contact in a fight. They frequently become infected, always with oral commensals, predominately anaerobic bacteria. Dog bites are common, and usually cause more extensive injury than human bites.

Symptoms and signs. Obvious with dog bites. Check for teeth marks on the hand, particularly the knuckle area after fights. Oedema, cellulitis, and frank suppuration may be apparent with delayed presentation.

Treatment. Antibiotic and tetanus prophylaxis. Explore all wounds where the skin is breached. Remove foreign bodies or tooth fragments. Take swabs for bacteriology. With extensive dog bites, excise any ragged areas of skin. Avoid primary closure in infected wounds. Elevate the hand postoperatively. If nerves or tendons are damaged in an infected wound, delayed repair is more appropriate.

COSMETIC (AESTHETIC) SURGERY

In assessing a patient for cosmetic surgery, the surgeon must assess the effect that the 'abnormality' is having on the patient and whether or not surgery will be truly beneficial. In many cases, the patient wants a surgical improvement on nature or control of the natural ageing process. The patient must understand that while surgery may alter the appearance, it rarely alters the person. In some cases, a formal psychological assessment may be appropriate prior to surgery. The decision to operate on prominent ears in a child who is the subject of taunts at school is easy, while to alter the facial appearance of a young woman simply because she does not like the way she looks, is more difficult.

The following are some indications for cosmetic surgery.

RECONSTRUCTIVE BREAST SURGERY

Augmentation mammaplasty

Indications

Small breasts (developmental or involutional after pregnancies); breast asymmetry with hypoplasia of one breast.

Treatment. By silicone implant with textured silicone envelopes containing silicone gel. Implants may be placed in the plane between the breast and the underlying pectoralis major muscle or under pectoralis major via a submammary approach.

Complications. Infection. Haematoma. Development of a firm capsule around the prosthesis may lead to distortion of the breast and discomfort. Silicone gel may leak out of the implant. There is no evidence that silicone prostheses increase the incidence of carcinoma.

Reduction mammaplasty

Indications

Abnormally large breasts may cause backache, neck ache, intertrigo. Interfere with active sports. Taunts and sexual harassment.

Treatment. Several techniques are described. All involve removal of breast tissue and skin with transposition of the ptotic nipple and areola to a higher level. Care must be taken to preserve the blood supply to the nipple. In very large breasts a free nipple graft may be required. The satisfaction rate among patients is high.

Complications. Haematoma, infection, nipple or fat necrosis.

Reconstruction following mastectomy

This may be carried out at the same time as mastectomy or several months later. If the soft tissue is adequate, the breast can be reconstructed with a silicone implant. A tissue expander may be necessary to form a space to insert a prosthesis later. If there has been extensive surgery or irradiation, reconstruction importing vascularized tissue is required. A pedicled latissimus dorsi musculocutaneous flap is most commonly used to cover an implant, but free and pedicled flaps from the abdomen, based on the rectus abdominis muscle, or from the buttock or thigh can also be used. Reconstruction of the nipple and areola may be carried out at the time of reconstruction or at a later stage.

Gynaecomastia

Treatment is by liposuction and/or excision of breast tissue to restore the normal breast contour, preserving the nipple. A circumareolar incision is used when possible.

OTHER TYPES OF SURGERY

Rhinoplasty

This is correction of congenital or acquired nasal defects. It may be carried out for cosmetic or functional reasons (breathing difficulties). Controlled nasal bone fracture is combined with excision or augmentation of varying amounts of bone and cartilage. The operation can be carried out totally through intranasal incisions (closed rhinoplasty). Alternatively, a columella incision can be made extending along the inferior edges of both lower lateral (alar) cartilages, then the skin is raised off the dorsum of the nose to access the bony and cartilaginous framework of the tip and dorsum for augmentation, reduction or realignment procedures (open rhinoplasty).

Prominent ears

A child with prominent ears may be taunted at school. The operation should be carried out at about 7 years as the ear cartilage has undergone 85% of its growth by this time. This can be done using sutures placed posteriorly to draw the ear back, or moulding the underlying the cartilage through anterior scoring to recreate a deficient antihelical fold.

Blepharoplasty

This is used to treat excess upper and lower eyelid skin and herniating fat and through upper and/or lower lid skin incisions. Removal of too much skin from the lower eyelid may result in ectropion (out-turned lower eyelid) with a watery eye that is difficult to correct.

Face lift

This is used to treat the 'ageing face'. There are various techniques commonly employed that excise excess skin of the face and neck and excise or tighten the underlying fascial suspension – the subcutaneous musculoaponeurotic system (SMAS). Excess skin is excised at hair-bearing areas, thus hiding the suture line. The skin of the face and neck are tightened, smoothing out wrinkles and giving a more youthful appearance. Complications include haematoma, skin necrosis, infection and damage to branches of the facial nerve and great auricular nerve. The large majority of these operations are carried out in the private sector.

Abdominoplasty

This is excision of redundant abdominal skin and fat. It is indicated in patients who have undergone massive weight loss and in women who have had repeated pregnancies where there are redundant skin folds and a lax anterior abdominal wall. For some minor or moderate degrees of tissue laxity a limited transverse lower abdominal excision may be sufficient (combined with umbilical transposition). When the operation is carried out after bariatric surgery or after massive weight loss a 'fleur-de-lys' excision pattern is used leaving an inverted T-shaped scar, or the excision is continued around the back (belt lipectomy).

Liposuction

This is carried out for the removal of localized deposits of fat, e.g. hips, thighs, buttocks. It is not indicated for generalized obesity and is therefore not a weight-reduction procedure. Cannulae are inserted through remote stab incisions and the subcutaneous fat removed through a series of tunnels using suction. Complications are rare, the chief problem being uneven removal of fat. Temporary numbness and bruising may occur. Occasionally, when large amounts of fat are removed significant fluid replacement is required to prevent hypovolaemia.

Filler injections

These are used for correcting minor irregularities of skin contour, e.g. static wrinkles on the face. A variety of filler materials are available, biological and synthetic, and include autologous fat and dermis, hyaluronic acid, poly-L-lactic acid, and bovine collagen.

TISSUE EXPANSION

The principle involves localized stretching of the skin using an inflatable silicone implant, which is surgically implanted underneath normal skin, adjacent to the tissue that is to be excised. Over the ensuing weeks, the implant is inflated through a remote valve by injecting normal saline. Once sufficient skin expansion has been produced, the silicone expander is removed, the lesion excised and the defect is repaired with the excess skin produced by the expander. Basically, a skin flap has been created at an adjacent site to the defect, which allows repair of the defect. The time required to inflate the balloon in order to produce more skin may take 4 weeks to 6 months and depends on the site, amount of skin required and the age of the patient. The patient has to attend hospital at least twice weekly to have the expander further inflated. Complications include haematoma, infection and extrusion of the device through the skin. They may be used, for example:

- to replace hair-bearing scalp where there has been extensive hair loss from trauma, adjacent hair-bearing skin being expanded to replace the defect
- to allow expansion of skin following mastectomy prior to insertion of a permanent prosthesis.

CLEFT LIP AND PALATE

Cleft lip occurs in 1:750 live births. Cleft palate occurs in 1:2000 live births. In half the affected children, cleft lip and cleft palate occur together. Cleft lip may be complete or incomplete and it may occur unilaterally (70%) or bilaterally (25%) or, rarely, in the midline. A unilateral cleft lip usually occurs on the left. Clefts of the palate may be unilateral and usually affect the soft palate and posterior third of the hard palate. They may be complete, incomplete or submucous. Bilateral clefts usually affect the soft and hard palate.

Symptoms and signs. Cleft lip is obvious at birth. Cleft palate is discovered on routine inspection soon after birth or may be discovered when difficulties occur with feeding. Beware missing a submucous cleft in which the palate initially appears intact. Late presentation may occur with speech and hearing difficulties.

Treatment. The problem and its treatment must be explained to the parents. Cleft care is coordinated via a network of specialist centres, and paediatricians refer to a cleft care nurse who sees the patient and their parents urgently. Isolated cleft lip babies can normally breast- and bottle-feed successfully. In cleft palate, feeding may be a problem. Sucking may be difficult, making breast-feeding and bottle-feeding a problem. Swallowing is normal. Feeds may be delivered to the back of the tongue via a spoon or pipette or using a bottle with a specialized teat. Feeding in the upright position prevents regurgitation.

The aims of surgery are to achieve an intact lip, alveolus and palate and to permit normal speech and dentition, and to address the associated nasal deformity. The timing of operations on cleft lip and palate remains controversial. Although some surgeons are now carrying out neonatal lip repair, the majority would undertake primary lip repair from 10 weeks. The methods of lip repair are numerous, but the principles involve realignment and repair of the orbicularis oris muscle, supplementing the deficient medial mucosa and philtrum with skin and mucosal tissues from the lateral side. Operation on cleft palate should be undertaken before the child starts to articulate sounds. This is normally around 9–12 months. The aims of treatment of cleft palate are:

- To close the cleft, thus separating nasal and oral cavities
- To ensure adequate length of the soft palate, allowing separation of the nasopharynx and oropharynx on phonation.

Various relaxing or plastic procedures may be necessary to achieve this.

Prognosis. Surgery for cleft lip and cleft palate is confined to some 10 centres nationally. A good cosmetic result is normally achieved in closing cleft lip. With cleft palate, satisfactory speech is achieved in about 80% of cases; however 20% may require a pharyngoplasty due to velopharyngeal incompetence (abnormal nasal escape during speech, nasal regurgitation of fluids). All children need speech therapy. Occasionally, secondary procedures may be required such as secondary alveolar bone grafting at 9–11 years and corrective rhinoplasty around the age of 16 years. The Cleft Lip & Palate Association (www.clapa.com) is available for advice and support.

Paediatric surgery

This chapter will cover some of the paediatric surgical emergencies that arise in the newborn and also the more common paediatric surgical problems presenting at outpatient departments and common paediatric surgical emergencies.

ALIMENTARY TRACT EMERGENCIES IN THE NEWBORN

Oesophageal atresia
The commonest type is a blind-ended, upper oesophagus associated with a tracheo-oesophageal fistula involving the lower oesophagus ($\rightarrow$ Fig. 20.1). Oesophageal atresia may occur alone or with a tracheo-oesophageal fistula. The incidence is approximately 1:3000 births. There may be co-existing anomalies of the heart, kidneys and intestines.

Symptoms and signs. Association with maternal polyhydramnios. Dribbling of saliva, inability to swallow feeds, production of frothy mucus, choking, cyanotic attacks, aspiration pneumonia.

Investigations
- Pass an orogastric tube – it will arrest at the obstruction
- CXR including neck to see the position of tube at obstruction: cardiac anomalies, aspiration pneumonia
- AXR: gas in stomach and intestine will indicate the presence of a tracheo-oesophageal fistula.

Treatment. Rehydration. Treat any chest infection. Keep upper oesophageal pouch empty by continuous aspiration. Urgent surgical ligation of tracheo-oesophageal fistula and correction of atresia by primary end-to-end anastomosis of the oesophagus.

Prognosis. There is a 90% survival in regional paediatric surgical centres in the UK.

Duodenal atresia
This occurs in 1:6000 births. The common bile duct may open proximal or distal to an atresia. There is an association with Down's syndrome and congenital heart disease.

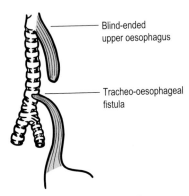

Blind-ended
upper oesophagus

Tracheo-oesophageal
fistula

Figure 20.1 The commonest form of oesophageal atresia.

Symptoms and signs. Associated with maternal polyhydramnios. Vomiting in first few hours of life usually bile-stained.

Investigations
- Antenatal diagnosis is possible with USS
- AXR shows 'double bubble' sign, i.e. gas bubble and fluid level on each side of upper abdomen owing to gas in stomach and proximal duodenum (→ Fig. 20.2).

Treatment. Rehydration. Urgent surgery. Duodenoduodenostomy, i.e. a side-to-side anastomosis between proximal and distal duodenal segments.

Prognosis. Mortality depends on associated abnormalities and is high with Down's syndrome and cardiac anomalies.

Small bowel atresia
The incidence is 1:20 000 births in the UK. It is somewhat more common in other parts of the world. It may occur at any level and may be multiple.

Signs and symptoms. Bilious vomiting. Abdominal distension. Visible peristalsis.

Investigations. AXR: distended bowel with fluid levels.

Treatment. Rehydration. Urgent surgery. Resection of areas of atresia or stenosis with end-to-end anastomosis.

Malrotation (volvulus neonatorum)
In the first trimester, the midgut herniates outside the abdominal cavity but returns at the end of the 3rd month, rotating as it does so. Several rotational abnormalities may result. Obstruction may consequently result from a variety of causes from peritoneal bands to volvulus of the midgut. Failure of normal rotation invariably occurs in patients with exomphalos and diaphragmatic hernia.

Symptoms and signs. Bile-stained vomiting and abdominal distension. The symptoms are similar initially to duodenal atresia. However, volvulus will lead to venous and subsequently arterial obstruction, gut infarction and consequent potential short bowel syndrome.

Figure 20.2   Duodenal atresia. AXR with 'double bubble' gas sign and no gas pattern beyond the duodenum.

Investigations
- USS to identify mesenteric vein/artery relations – the position of the vein and artery in relation to one another changes with rotation
- Contrast meal: abnormally placed duodenojejunal junction
- Contrast enema: may show abnormally placed caecum but the latter may also be normal in position.

Treatment. Emergency laparotomy. Untwist the volvulus. Tease out mesenteric base to prevent recurrence. Excise any gangrenous bowel.

Meconium ileus
This occurs in 15% of patients with cystic fibrosis. Meconium becomes inspissated in the terminal ileum with soft meconium above associated with distended proximal small bowel.

Symptoms and signs. Infant born with distended abdomen. Bilious vomiting. Meconium is not passed and the rectum is empty.

Investigations
- AXR: dilated loops of bowel

- Gastrografin enema will show an empty colon and may relieve the obstruction by refluxing into the terminal ileum and 'loosening' the meconium
- Prenatal diagnosis may be made with USS.

Treatment. Some 50% may have associated atresia, perforation, or volvulus and then laparotomy is required. The terminal ileum is opened and the inspissated meconium washed out. A temporary ileostomy may be required.

Complications. Meconium peritonitis. May occur *in utero* or postnatally. The chemical peritonitis resulting is treated by peritoneal lavage and repair of the perforation. The mortality rate is 10%.

Anorectal abnormalities

These occur with an incidence of 1:5000 births. Management depends on accurate definition of the abnormality.

Symptoms and signs. Infant fails to pass meconium. Rectal inspection reveals imperforate anus or other abnormality. There may be associated abnormalities of the GU system.

Investigations
- Tape a metal marker over the anus (or if absent, anal dimple)
- Place infant in knee–elbow position for 2 min and take a lateral shoot-through pelvic radiograph
- Assess the distance between the gas shadow and metal marker.

Treatment. Low lesions can be treated by a simple anoplasty. Higher lesions should be managed with a sigmoid loop colostomy, allowing further evaluation prior to a more complicated reconstructive procedure.

Necrotizing enterocolitis

This is an ischaemic disorder of the intestine of the newborn. The aetiology of the disease is unknown but bacterial infection, hypoxia and umbilical artery cannulation have been implicated. It is more common in premature infants and 'epidemics' have occurred on neonatal intensive therapy units, suggesting an infective aetiology.

Symptoms and signs. Diarrhoea, blood, mucus per rectum. Abdominal distension and bilious vomiting.

Investigations
- AXR shows distension of bowel with fluid levels
- Later, a diagnostic radiological sign is intramural gas indicative of bowel wall necrosis
- Free gas confirms intestinal perforation.

Treatment. This is initially non-operative unless perforation occurs. Resuscitation includes i.v. fluids and NG suction together with intravenous broad-spectrum antibiotics. Laparotomy is required if there is evidence of perforation or failure of patient to improve on medical treatment. Gangrenous bowel is excised with a temporary ileostomy or colostomy.

Prognosis. The mortality rate is high in severe cases. Stricture may develop in healing bowel and present later.

Diaphragmatic hernia

This occurs with an incidence of 1:4000 births. A hernia may occur through the foramen of Bochdalek, i.e. a defect in the pleuroperitoneal canal; through the foramen of Morgagni, between the xiphoid and costal margin; through a deficiency in the central tendon; or through a congenitally large oesophageal hiatus. Herniae through the foramen of Bochdalek are most common. Normal development of the ipsilateral lung is impaired and that of the contralateral lung may also be impaired.

Symptoms and signs. May be diagnosed by prenatal USS. Presents with respiratory distress at birth. Apex beat displaced. Bowel sounds in chest. Scaphoid abdomen if the hernia is large and most of the bowel is in the chest.

Investigations
- CXR
- AXR: mediastinal shift, abdominal viscera in thorax; lack of intestinal gas pattern in abdomen (→ Fig. 20.3).

Treatment. Urgent respiratory assistance and maintenance of circulation. When ventilation is adequate and the patient is haemodynamically stable, closure of the defect is undertaken. May require prosthetic patch.

Figure 20.3 CXR of a neonate with a left diaphragmatic hernia. Note the hypoplastic lungs, mediastinal shift to the right, and gas in abdominal viscera in the left chest.

Prognosis. Mortality is high, especially with large defects, and is due to consequences of pulmonary hypoplasia.

Hirschsprung's disease

This occurs in 1:5000 births. There is a defect in the parasympathetic ganglia in the submucosal and myenteric plexus of the bowel wall. The aganglionic segment is present for a varying distance upwards from the anus and always involves the rectum. Rarely it affects the whole colon and even more rarely, the small bowel. The peristaltic waves stop at the affected segment and the proximal bowel becomes dilated and hypertrophied. The aganglionic segment remains contracted. It is more common in males than females.

Symptoms and signs. Delayed passage of meconium in the newborn period. However, presentation may be delayed, especially with short segment involvement, when it presents in infants and older children with constipation and abdominal distension. Digital rectal examination may demonstrate an empty rectum, which feels 'tight' on the examining finger.

Investigations
● AXR: dilated loops of bowel with fluid levels
● Barium enema will demonstrate the level of obstruction
● Rectal biopsy shows absence of ganglion cells.

Treatment
1. If the baby is healthy, and only rectosigmoid Hirschsprung's is suspected, it may be managed by regular rectal washouts to clear the bowel and early operation at 4–6 weeks, avoiding a colostomy if possible.
2. If the baby is ill and if a longer segment Hirschsprung's is suspected, then management is as follows:
   — Initial defunctioning colostomy (normal innervation of the segment of bowel used for the colostomy should be confirmed by frozen section)
   — Resection of the affected segment between 3 and 6 months of age and pull-through of the ganglionic bowel to the rectum
   — The defunctioning colostomy is closed 3–4 weeks later.

ABDOMINAL WALL DEFECTS

These occur with an incidence of 1:6000 births. There are two types, gastroschisis and exomphalos. Aetiology is unknown.

Gastroschisis

In this condition, there is a defect in the abdominal wall immediately adjacent to the umbilicus but the abdominal wall itself is completely formed. Coils of gut have no protective covering and are thick, oedematous and matted together. The diagnosis is obvious at birth.

Treatment. Primary closure of the defect may be possible after decompressing the gut and returning it to the peritoneal cavity. However, it may be necessary to cover the defect temporarily with a silastic sheet. Staged repair requires daily reduction of bowel into the peritoneal cavity, after which the defect may be repaired. It may be weeks or months before normal GI motility is restored – long-term TPN may be required.

Exomphalos

In this condition, the opening is at the umbilicus. The umbilical cord coverings continue into a sac, which covers the visceral protrusion. Chromosomal abnormalities, heart defects and also genitourinary malformations frequently occur, e.g. ectopia vesica and cloacal abnormalities. The condition is obvious at birth.

Treatment. This is by either primary closure or staged repair with larger defects using a silastic sheet.

ALIMENTARY TRACT PROBLEMS IN OLDER INFANTS AND CHILDREN

Congenital hypertrophic pyloric stenosis

The aetiology of this condition is unknown. Progressive hypertrophy of the circular muscle of the pylorus occurs. The condition affects boys more than girls, being four times more common in boys, and occurs with an incidence of 1:4000 births. The first-born male child is most commonly affected. There is a familial tendency, especially on the maternal side.

Symptoms and signs. The infant thrives for the first 3–4 weeks of life and then presents with projectile vomiting after feeds. The vomit is rarely bile-stained. The infant is usually hungry and eager for further food after vomiting. Wasting is rare nowadays but weight loss and dehydration are presenting features.

Diagnosis. This is clinical. A test feed is carried out. The abdomen is inspected for visible peristalsis passing from left to right across the epigastrium. Palpation is carried out during feeding for the classical 'lump', which is felt deep to the right rectus muscle in the RUQ. The 'lump' has the size and shape of an olive. Never sit facing the infant during this examination. You may experience the full impact of the projectile vomit.

Treatment. Ramstedt's operation (pyloromyotomy). This is an elective operation and should be carried out only after correction of any dehydration and metabolic alkalosis. The stomach is emptied via an NG tube and saline lavage. The pylorus is exposed either through an upper, right transverse abdominal incision or a periumbilical incision. It is then incised longitudinally along its anterosuperior border. The incision is deepened by blunt dissection until the mucosa pouts out.

Complications. Postoperative recovery is rapid. There should be no mortality. Morbidity relates to accidental mucosal perforation, which, if unrecognized at the time of surgery, will lead to peritonitis.

Intussusception

This is the invagination of a portion of intestine into its lumen. It is commoner in children than adults. The peak incidence is between 6 and 9 months, although it may occur any time between 3 months and 2 years and occasionally in those younger and older than this age range. Most cases are ileocolic but ileo-ileal and ileo-ileocolic may occur. In most cases, the aetiology is unknown but hypertrophied Peyer's patches, polyps, Meckel's diverticulum or intramural haematomas (Henoch–Schönlein purpura) may be contributory. An intussusception is composed of three parts:

- The entering inner tube
- The returning or middle tube
- The sheath or outer tube.

The outer tube is called the intussuscipiens: the inner and middle tubes are called the intussusceptum (→ Fig. 20.4).

Symptoms and signs. An otherwise healthy child presents with colicky abdominal pain and vomiting. The child often screams, draws up its knees to its chest, and goes pale with an attack of colic. In between bouts of pain, the child appears normal. A first stool passed after onset of the pain may be normal but 30% of subsequent stools contain blood and mucus, the so-called 'redcurrant jelly stool'. Palpation of the abdomen reveals a palpable sausage-shaped mass in the line of the colon. An empty RIF may be apparent on palpation as the swelling moves into the upper abdomen with peristalsis. PR examination may reveal blood or mucus. Occasionally, the apex of the intussusception may be palpable per rectum.

Investigations
- AXR may show typical gas distribution and may show small bowel obstruction
- USS or contrast enema (→ Fig. 20.5)
- Adequate resuscitation with i.v. fluids.

Treatment. At an early stage, the intussusception may be reduced by the pressure of either an air or fluid enema under ultrasound control. Operation is required in patients with peritonitis, radiological signs of perforation, or failure of hydrostatic reduction. At operation, the intussusceptum is reduced by gentle retrograde reduction, squeezing the apex out of its containing bowel. Traction should not be applied to the proximal bowel. If the bowel cannot be reduced or is gangrenous, resection is required.

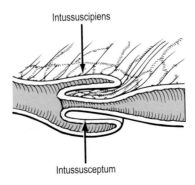

Intussuscipiens

Intussusceptum

Figure 20.4 An intussusception.

Figure 20.5 Barium enema showing the typical appearance of an ileocolic intussusception. The ileum (arrow) has progressed as far as the proximal transverse colon.

Prognosis. Recurrence occurs in 1–2%. Mortality is very low if treatment occurs in the first 24 h but increases if resection is required.

Obstructed inguinal hernia

This is a common cause of surgical admission in boys under the age of 2 years. It may also occur in girls when bowel or ovary may become irreducible. It is associated with a patent processus vaginalis. There is a high incidence in premature babies. The condition is often bilateral.

Symptoms and signs. Mother usually notices a tense lump in the groin of her crying child. Examination reveals an irreducible lump, which may extend into the scrotum.

Treatment. If the lump is not red or tender, analgesia and sedation may be given and a gentle attempt made to reduce the hernia when the child is well sedated. If the hernia does not reduce, surgical repair should be undertaken. If infarcted bowel is found, this must be resected. If the hernia does reduce, surgery should be delayed for 24–48 h to allow oedema to resolve. It is prudent to electively repair inguinal herniae in young children as soon as they are discovered.

Acute appendicitis

This is dealt with more fully in Chapter 14. Certain points, however, are relevant to appendicitis in children. The condition is rare under the age of 6 months. The stool is liquid and the appendiceal lumen relatively wide. Therefore, acute obstructive appendicitis is rare. It does, however, occur and may present with diarrhoea and vomiting and consequently be mistaken for gastroenteritis. Careful and repeated examination is therefore essential.

Mesenteric adenitis

This is enlargement of mesenteric lymph nodes caused by an adenovirus infection. *Yersinia enterocolitica* has also been implicated. It affects young children and adolescents. Usually there is a preceding history of URTI, with sore throat and cervical lymphadenitis. Essentially, mesenteric adenitis is inflammation of Peyer's patches with secondary mesenteric lymphadenitis. The fever is usually higher than that of appendicitis, usually 38–39°C. The abdominal pain is more diffuse and examination reveals shifting tenderness rather than sharply localized tenderness in the RIF. Headache and mild photophobia may occur. These never occur in appendicitis. The WCC is usually raised but there is a relative lymphocytosis rather than neutrophil leukocytosis as seen in acute appendicitis. Treatment is symptomatic. If there is doubt over the diagnosis, appendicectomy is advisable.

Constipation

This is a common problem in children. The child is usually afebrile and relatively well, despite the abdominal pain.

Urinary tract infections (UTIs)

There is abdominal pain and high pyrexia associated with dysuria, frequency and cloudy urine. Right pyelonephritis or cystitis may be mistaken for appendicitis. An FBC reveals neutrophil leukocytosis. An MSU and microscopy reveal cells and organisms. Beware the presence of cells alone. Pelvic appendicitis may irritate the bladder, producing frequency and pyuria but organisms will be absent on microscopy. Beware the presence of organisms *alone* as it may be due to contamination from the foreskin or vulva. Treatment of UTI is with appropriate antibiotics. Further investigation is with USS.

Lower lobar pneumonia

In this condition, pain may be referred via the thoracic nerves to the lower abdomen. Right lower lobar pneumonia may refer pain to the RIF and be mistaken for acute appendicitis. It is important to observe the breathing pattern and auscultate the chest. Anteroposterior and lateral CXR will confirm diagnosis.

Testicular torsion (→ Ch. 16)

> ⚠️ **This may radiate to the iliac fossa. The child may be embarrassed to draw attention to scrotal symptoms. Always examine the scrotum in a child with abdominal pain.**

Crohn's disease

Acute regional ileitis may occur in children.

Gynaecological problems

Remember pregnancy may occur in very young girls. Onset of periods may be associated with acute lower abdominal pain. Torsion of ovarian cyst or ovarian dermoid may occur.

INFANTS WITH JAUNDICE

Neonates often develop physiological jaundice starting about 2 days after birth and lasting up to 2 weeks. Persistent jaundice beyond the first 3 weeks of life requires investigation. The two most common surgical causes are biliary atresia and choledochal cysts.

Biliary atresia

This occurs with an incidence of 1: 25 000 live births. The aetiology is unknown. It appears to develop after birth.

Symptoms and signs. Presents from 4 weeks to 4 months. Usually a healthy child with jaundice. Jaundice may be intermittent. Pale stools. Dark urine. Later hepatosplenomegaly, ascites. Without treatment, death from liver failure occurs within 2 years.

Investigations
- LFTs
- USS: dilated ducts, absent gallbladder
- Liver biopsy: bile duct proliferation with hepatocellular necrosis
- Isotope scan demonstrates absence of bile drainage
- Diagnostic laparotomy with operative cholangiography – if a normal duct system is demonstrated, hepatitis should be suspected as a diagnosis
- α_1-Antitrypsin deficiency and cystic fibrosis must also be excluded.

Treatment. If an extrahepatic duct can be found a Roux loop of jejunum is anastomosed to it – this is called correctable biliary atresia. If an extrahepatic duct cannot be found (incorrectable biliary atresia), a hepatoportal enterostomy (Kasai procedure) is carried out. A patent duct is exposed in the porta hepatis and a Roux loop anastomosed to it. Intrahepatic biliary atresia (total absence of intrahepatic ducts) requires liver transplantation.

Prognosis. Good with correctable form. Incorrectable extrahepatic and intrahepatic forms have a poor prognosis but this may be improved with a more widespread use of liver transplantation.

Choledochal cyst

Cystic dilatation of the bile ducts is usually extrahepatic involving the common bile duct. The aetiology is unknown.

Symptoms and signs. It occurs between 3 months and adult life. More common in females. Pain, jaundice, abdominal mass.

Investigations
- LFTs
- USS
- ERCP.

Treatment. Excision of CBD with Roux choledochojejunostomy. Severe forms with involvement of the intrahepatic ducts require liver transplantation. Residual CBD can develop malignancy.

ABDOMINAL MASSES IN CHILDHOOD

An abdominal mass is an uncommon reason for surgical referral in children. (For causes → Table 20.1.)

Symptoms and signs. In addition to the mass, failure to thrive, nausea, vomiting, weight loss, abdominal pain, constipation, diarrhoea. Anaemia. Jaundice. Uraemia. UTI symptoms. Spontaneous bruising.

Investigations
- Hb
- FBC

TABLE 20.1 Abdominal masses in childhood	
Gastrointestinal system	Pylorus (congenital pyloric stenosis)
	Crohn's disease
	Constipation (faecal masses)
	Intussusception
Hepato-pancreatico-biliary system	
Liver	Biliary atresia
	Portal hypertension
	Metastases
	Hepatitis
	Hepatoblastoma
Bile duct	Choledochal cyst
Pancreas	Pseudocyst (traumatic)
Genitourinary system	Hydronephrosis
	Nephroblastoma (Wilms')
	Bladder (urethral valves)
	Ovarian tumour or cyst
Other	Neuroblastoma
	Lymphoma
	Splenomegaly
	Retroperitoneal sarcoma
	Teratoma
	Other rare malignancies, e.g. primitive neuroectodermal tumour, rhabdomyosarcoma

- ESR
- U&Es
- LFTs
- Urinalysis: 24-hour urine (VMA in neuroblastoma)
- α-Fetoprotein (tumour marker for teratoma and hepatoblastoma)
- AXR
- CXR (metastases)
- USS: solid-v-cystic lesions
- CT scan: solid-v-cystic spread
- Bone scan, bone marrow aspirate
- Biopsy.

Treatment. This is of the underlying cause.

ABDOMINAL MALIGNANCIES IN CHILDHOOD

The commonest are neuroblastoma and nephroblastoma (Wilms' tumour). Neuroblastoma is the commonest extracerebral malignant solid tumour in children. Wilms' tumour accounts for about 10% of all the childhood tumours.

Abdominal neuroblastoma

This is a highly malignant tumour arising from the neural crest. The commonest site is the adrenal gland. It occurs in children under the age of 5; 70% occur under 1 year. Metastases occur early.

Symptoms and signs. Abdominal mass. Failure to thrive. Anorexia, nausea, vomiting, diarrhoea. Metastases occur to liver, orbit, skull, long bones, spinal canal. Fever. Abdominal mass has a hard irregular surface and tendency to cross midline.

Investigations
- AXR: calcification
- USS: solid lesion
- CT with contrast: size, site and metastases, and demonstrates displaced kidney
- 24-hour urine VMA and HVA grossly elevated.

Treatment. Localized tumours are excised. Unresectable primary and metastases require combination chemotherapy. Irradiation may be necessary. In neonates, tumour regression may be permanent. The older the child the worse the prognosis.

Nephroblastoma (Wilms' tumour)

This is an embryonic tumour of the kidney. The majority occur in the first 3 years of life. Less than 5% are bilateral. Metastases occur to the liver, lungs and regional nodes.

Signs and symptoms. Abdominal mass. Pain. Haematuria. Weight loss. Pyrexia. May be associated with abnormalities of the GU tract. Aniridia.

Figure 20.6 An abdominal CT scan of a child with an abdominal mass. There is an extensive nephroblastoma (Wilms' tumour) of the right kidney.

Investigations
- USS: solid tumour
- CT (→ Fig. 20.6): size, site, metastases.

Treatment. Surgical excision. Chemotherapy with or without radiotherapy depending on the stage; 80–90% chance of cure. If the condition is bilateral dialysis will be required unless partial nephrectomy is possible. If there is no evidence of recurrence after 2 years, renal transplantation is indicated.

RECTAL BLEEDING IN CHILDREN

This is not an uncommon problem. Causes include fissure-in-ano, rectal polyps, rectal prolapse, Meckel's diverticulum, intussusception and blood dyscrasia.

Fissure-in-ano
Constipation causes a split in the mucosa of the anal canal. It is usually painful on defaecation. A vicious circle occurs with worsening constipation owing to fear of defaecation. There is blood on the stool and toilet paper. The fissure is often in the midline, usually posteriorly. Treatment involves explanation of the condition to the parent. Lactulose helps to relieve constipation, and LA is applied locally before and after defaecation. Most cases settle on this regimen. Persistent fissures require exclusion of Crohn's disease and TB.

Polyps

In addition to bleeding, they may prolapse on their stalk if they are low enough in the rectum. Occasionally they may twist and auto-amputate and are passed PR. Occasionally they may precipitate intussusception. Treatment is by excision. If they are in the rectum, this may be done under GA using a proctoscope, the stalk being cut with diathermy. Higher polyps can be snared at colonoscopy.

Rectal prolapse

This usually occurs around 2 years. Most cases settle spontaneously. Straining at stool precipitates the condition initially, which may then occur every time the child defaecates. There may be an underlying abnormality, e.g. spina bifida, previous anoplasty for imperforate anus or cystic fibrosis. Prolapse may involve the mucosa only or may involve the full thickness of the rectum.

Symptoms and signs. Usually prolapse occurs with defaecation and returns spontaneously. The prolapsed mucosa may ulcerate and bleed.

Treatment. May settle spontaneously with toilet training and laxatives to relieve constipation. Persistent mucosal prolapse may be treated by submucosal injection of phenol in almond oil. Rarely rectopexy may be required.

Meckel's diverticulum

This is a remnant of the vitellointestinal duct which was attached to the umbilicus and is found on the antimesenteric border of the terminal ileum about 60 cm from the ileocaecal valve in an adult and proportionately nearer in a child. Rarely, this may bleed if it contains gastric mucosa, which produces acid and ulcerates the adjacent small bowel mucosa. This may cause either bright red or dark red bleeding, depending upon the degree of haemorrhage. Abdominal pain is usually absent. The presence of gastric mucosa in a Meckel's diverticulum may be demonstrated by a technetium scan. Treatment is by excision.

Intussusception

In this condition, rectal bleeding may occur and is classically the appearance of a redcurrant jelly stool associated with attacks of abdominal pain.

General investigation of child with rectal bleeding

Full history and examination. Often the cause is obvious and no further investigation is required.

- Hb
- FBC
- Clotting screen
- Examination under anaesthesia including PR, proctoscopy, sigmoidoscopy and colonoscopy under GA
- Barium enema
- Technetium scan.

Treatment. This is of the underlying condition.

CHRONIC AND RECURRENT ABDOMINAL PAIN

A common problem in children of school age, and many are referred to general surgery clinics. In many cases, the pain has a non-organic basis. Organic causes include chronic constipation, Crohn's disease, UTIs, hydronephrosis, peptic ulceration and, rarely, gallstones (may be associated with haemolytic anaemia). If the child has had previous abdominal surgery, adhesions may be responsible. It is the author's opinion that chronic and recurrent abdominal pain in children should initially be referred to a paediatrician and subsequently referred to a surgeon if necessary. The reader is referred to a textbook of paediatrics for further discussion of this topic.

NECK LUMPS IN CHILDREN

The general management of lumps in the neck is dealt with in Chapter 8. However, lumps in the neck are common in children, the most common cause being due to reactive lymphadenitis secondary to tonsillitis. The other causes of lumps in the neck in children are shown in Table 20.2.

Symptoms and signs. Child may otherwise be well. Malaise. Pyrexia. Lethargy. Weight loss. Bruising. Bleeding. Rash. Cough. Signs of URTI, tonsillitis, inflamed tympanic membrane. Examine head and neck thoroughly for sites of primary lesion (infective or neoplastic). Check for lymphadenopathy elsewhere. Check for hepatosplenomegaly.

Investigations
- Hb
- FBC
- ESR
- U&Es

TABLE 20.2 Lumps in the neck in childhood	
Anterior triangle	Lymph nodes: • primary infection, e.g. atypical mycobacterium, TB, toxoplasmosis • secondary infection, e.g. lymphadenitis • primary tumours, e.g. Hodgkin's, leukaemia • secondary tumour – rare Thyroglossal cyst Dermoid cyst Goitre Submandibular gland Branchial arch remnant
Posterior triangle	Lymph nodes Cystic hygroma (lymphangioma) Sternomastoid tumour Parotid swelling

- LFTs
- TFTs (goitre)
- Paul–Bunnell
- Toxoplasmosis screen
- Mantoux
- CXR
- USS of lump
- CT: lump, spread.

Treatment. This is of the underlying disorder.

Organ and tissue transplantation

Transplantation has developed from an experimental procedure over 50 years ago, to an established therapeutic option for most types of end-stage organ failure. For kidney, heart and liver transplantation, a 1-year graft survival in excess of 85% can be expected.

CLASSIFICATION

This depends on the relationship between donor and recipient.

Autograft. Tissue is transferred from one area of the body to another in the same individual, e.g. skin grafts.

Isografts. Tissue is transferred between genetically identical individuals (e.g. monozygotic twins).

Allografts. Tissue is transferred between genetically dissimilar individuals of the same species (e.g. deceased donor renal transplants).

Xenografts. Tissue is transferred between species. The only clinically applicable xenografts at the present time are temporary porcine skin grafts in human burns victims.

ORGAN AND TISSUE DONORS

Organs and tissues may be obtained from:

- deceased donors – donation after brain death (DBD; heart beating donors) or donation after cardiac death (DCD; non-heart beating donors)
- living donors.

DECEASED DONORS

Donation after brain death (DBD)

General criteria (→ Table 21.1)

As the organ shortage became more severe, it was realized that ideal requirements for selection of organ donors were not feasible. Selection criteria for solid organ donors have therefore recently been relaxed. Organs that long ago would not have been considered for transplantation, are currently being used, bringing in a new class of organ donor termed the 'expanded criteria donor; ECD' formerly known as 'marginal' donor. ECD is any brain-dead donor aged >60 years or a donor aged >50 with two of the following conditions: a history of hypertension; a terminal serum creatinine level >150 µmol/L, or death resulting from a cerebrovascular accident. Selection of liver and heart and heart/lung donors depends on size match with the recipient. Also, no attempt is made to match other than on blood group compatibility with these organs. HLA typing and cross-matching are not currently undertaken.

Obtaining permission for deceased organ donation

1. A potential donor should be identified by the consultant in charge of the patient.
2. Contact may be made with a transplant team prior to establishment of brainstem death to assess if the donor is suitable for organ donation.
3. The first set of brainstem death criteria are carried out. If they are satisfied, the question of organ donation may be raised with the relatives. Consent should not be obtained until two sets of brainstem death criteria have been obtained.

TABLE 21.1 General criteria for deceased donors

Brainstem dead with intact circulation

Cause of death:
- cerebral trauma
- cerebral haemorrhage
- suicide
- primary cerebral tumour (histologically proven)
- cardiac arrest with brain death

Exclusions:

Absolute
- HIV infection
- Creutzfeldt–Jakob disease (CJD) – plus any patient who has received a dura mater graft or human pituitary growth hormone

Relative
- chronic renal disease
- metastasizing malignancy
- severe hypertension
- Hepatitis B and C infection (can be considered in recipients who are HBV- or HCV-positive)
- i.v. drug abuse
- age >75 years
- prolonged renal warm ischaemia
- oliguric renal failure
- death from sepsis or viral infection

4. If the relatives wish to know more about what is involved in transplantation, the Transplant Coordinators will speak to them and explain the details.
5. Blood is taken for tissue typing, blood group, HIV and hepatitis B and C screening.
6. Confidentiality must always be maintained.
7. Bereavement counselling and follow-up support should be arranged for the family; the Transplant Coordinators can also help with this.

Donation after cardiac death (DCD)

This type of organ donation applies to renal transplantation and liver transplantation only but tissues such as heart valves, corneas, bone, etc. can also be removed from this type of donor. The distinction between a DBD and DCD donor lies in the mode of death. DBD donors usually die from an intracranial catastrophe (→ Table 21.1), the mode of death being classified as 'brainstem death'. In DCD donors, the patient dies from a cardiorespiratory arrest, their death being classified as a 'cardiac death'. After death, kidneys are viable for around 30 min (maximum of 45 min in young donors).

There are four types of DCD donors (Maastricht criteria). They may be classified as *controlled* (cardiac arrest is anticipated and gives time for organization of necessary resources; category III) or *uncontrolled* (donor dies without warning, thus the ischaemic time is longer as resources are not readily available; categories I, II and IV). The groups of DCD donors are classified as follows:

I. Dead on arrival at hospital
II. Unsuccessful resuscitation
III. Awaiting cardiac arrest
IV. Cardiac arrest in brainstem dead patient.

Brainstem death

This is covered in Chapter 18, as this is the province of doctors independent of the transplant team.

LIVING DONORS

> This type of organ donation relates chiefly to renal transplantation, although it is now possible to transplant segments of pancreas, segments of liver and lobes of lung from living donors. At the present time, more than 30% of transplants in the UK are carried out from living donors owing to the shortage of deceased donors. Living donation, like deceased donation, is regulated by the Human Tissue Authority under the Human Tissue Act 2004.

Organ donation and transplantation is governed by the Human Tissue Act 2004, which supercedes the Human Organ Transplant Act 1989. The Human Tissue Authority (HTA) was established in 2005 to implement the provisions of the Act, which came into force in 2006.

Categories of living donation established under the Act are:

1. Directed (i.e. the organ is directed to a known recipient)
   — genetically related (formerly living related)

— emotionally related (living unrelated)
— paired.
2. Non-directed (i.e. the organ is for a recipient whose identity is unknown as with deceased donation)
— domino
— altruistic.

Directed

Genetically and emotionally related

This is donation to a known person, i.e. brother to sister, parent to child, husband to wife or between friends. Under the Human Tissue Act, the approval process is the same for directed genetically and directed emotionally related organ donation. Both will be dealt with by a local independent assessor who is trained and accredited by the HTA and who will assess all donor/recipient pairs, and where the requirements have been met, will give approval for the transplant to proceed.

Paired donation

This relates to circumstances where a close relation, friend or partner is fit and able to donate but is not well-matched to the potential recipient. That couple can be matched to another couple in a similar situation so that both people in need of a transplant receive a well-matched organ, i.e. Mrs A wants to give Mr A a kidney. Mrs B wants to give Mr B a kidney. Mrs A does not match Mr A. Mrs B does not match Mr B but Mrs B matches Mr A and Mrs A matches Mr B. In these circumstances, Mrs B gives a kidney to Mr A, while Mrs A gives a kidney to Mr B. Hopefully, everyone lives happily ever after!

Non-directed

Domino

This is when a normal organ is removed as part of a patient's treatment. It may then be suitable for transplantation into another person. For a patient requiring a lung transplant, e.g. a cystic fibrosis sufferer, it is technically easier to transplant the heart and lungs as a unit, removing the recipient's normal heart. This can then be offered for a recipient in heart failure in the same way as a heart from a deceased donor.

Altruistic

This is when a person offers to donate an organ to anyone who might benefit, i.e. a complete stranger. Before such organ transplants are undertaken, it is essential that all medical, surgical and psychiatric assessments necessary to ensure fitness to donate have been completed. The independent assessor must be satisfied that all procedures have been fully complied with before any application for a non-directed altruistic donation is sent to the HTA panel for approval.

Independent assessors

Independent assessors are trained persons, i.e. medical consultants or someone of equivalent registered professional status, independent of the transplant team. They are trained to approve all living organ donations, both directed and non-directed. The role of the independent assessor is to act on behalf of the HTA in an altruistic capacity and in order to satisfy the requirements of the Human Tissue Act. The independent assessor must be satisfied that:

- A registered medical practitioner has given the donor an explanation of the nature of the medical procedure and risks involved
- The donor understands the nature of the medical procedure and the risks and consents to removal of the organ in question
- The donor's consent to the removal of the organ in question was not obtained by coercion or the offer of an inappropriate inducement
- The donor understands that he or she is entitled to withdraw consent at any time and understands the consequences of withdrawal for the recipient
- The donor–recipient relationship is as stated
- There were no difficulties in communicating with the donor and/or recipient and if so how these were overcome
- Any interpreter used should have no personal involvement with either party to the transplant.

Work-up for a living donor

For a genetically related donor, there are three potential histocompatibility matches:

- 'Perfect match' (2 haplotype match): all antigens match. There is a 25% chance of this occurring
- 'Half match' (1 haplotype mismatch): half the antigens match. There is a 50% chance of this occurring
- 'No match': no antigens match. There is a 25% chance of this occurring. In the past it was rare to use such a donor but it is now clear that the results from a 'no-matched' live related donor are almost as good as those from a well-matched deceased donor.

The following sequence is undertaken:

- Identify a potential donor
- Take blood for blood group, tissue typing and cross match to identify compatibility
- Give full explanation of procedure and risks
- Urinalysis: exclude proteinuria, haematuria, infection
- FBC, ESR, U&Es, creatinine, LFTs, glucose
- Infection screen: HBV, HCV, HIV, HTLV (counselling required prior to HIV testing)
- Creatinine clearance, GFR via ^{51}Cr-EDTA
- CXR
- ECG.

If all of the above are satisfactory, the patient undergoes an angiography (usually CT angiography and urography) to assess the renal vasculature and to check for any abnormality in the excretory system. It is ideal that at least one kidney should have a single artery to anastomose to the recipient's artery (either end-to-end) to the recipient's internal iliac artery (or end-to-side) to the recipient's external iliac artery.

Although kidneys with multiple arteries can be used in deceased donor transplantation as they can be removed with a Carrel patch of aorta, clearly this is not the case with a living donor. However, with living donors it is possible to use kidneys with multiple arteries, e.g. two equal sized arteries may be anastomosed in a double-barrelled fashion before being anastomosed to the recipient's arteries; or a small polar artery may be anastomosed to the side of the main renal artery.

If angiography and urography are normal, the donor recipient pair will be referred to the independent assessor who will send a report to the clinician responsible for the donor and a copy to the HTA indicating that the transplant may go ahead.

Living donor nephrectomy

This may be carried out by an open technique either via a loin incision excising part of the 12th rib or transperitoneally by a subcostal incision. More living donor nephrectomies are being carried out via a laparoscopic technique, the kidney being removed through a small 6–10 cm suprapubic incision. Laparoscopic donor nephrectomy (LDN) has resulted in less pain, shorter hospitalization, a reduced duration of convalescence and better cosmesis, compared with the open flank approach. LDN is done through transperitoneal or retroperitoneal approach, which can be either total or hand-assisted.

Complications of living donor nephrectomy

These include: mortality (1:3000); bleeding; infection; DVT; pulmonary embolus; chest infection; pneumothorax; urinary tract infection, persistent wound pain and incisional hernia. The donor should be warned that if subsequently they develop trauma to, or a tumour in, their one remaining kidney, they may require nephrectomy and dialysis themselves.

Tissue matching

ABO compatibility

In the past, ABO compatibility has been essential. However, currently, ABO-incompatible transplants are being carried out with good success (see below.)

Histocompatibility matching

Human leukocyte antigens (HLA) are encoded on the short arm of chromosome 6; these code for the antigens involved in transplant rejection. Class I molecules consist of HLA-A, B, and C; Class II molecules consist of HLA-DP, DQ and DR. HLA-A, B and DR are generally considered the most important, a perfect match at the DR locus being associated with improved graft survival in deceased donor renal transplants. Each locus is highly variable and thus gives rise to numerous combinations. The HLA matching of patients is expressed as the HLA 'mismatch' – this describes how well matched the kidney is.

Some examples of HLA matching are given below:

a. A6, A3	B27, B15	DR3, DR15 Donor
A2, A3	**B7, B8**	**DR3, DR12 Recipient**
b. A1, A24	B8, B44	DR4, DR15 Donor
A1, A3	**B27, B15**	**DR4, DR15 Recipient**

In example (a) the recipient is a 1-2-1 mismatch. In example (b) the recipient is a 1-2-0 mismatch.

Cytotoxic cross-match
It must be negative. The recipient's blood is tested for cytotoxic antibodies against antigens on donor T lymphocytes using either complement-dependent lymphocytotoxicity or flow cytometric crossmatch techniques. If such antibodies are present, they would attach to and destroy the transplanted kidney, and therefore the donor is unacceptable.

ABO-incompatible living donor kidney transplantation
The presence of anti-A/B blood group antibodies has been considered a contraindication to transplantation for the risk of hyperacute rejection. Currently, kidney transplants between ABO-incompatible donor and recipients are carried out by removing the antibodies pre-transplantation, by either immunoabsorption or plasmapheresis until a low level of antibody (1:8) is reached. The patient then receives rituximab (anti-CD20 monoclonal antibody against B cells) or intravenous immunoglobulin. Induction with anti-thymocyte globulin or basiliximab in combination with tacrolimus, mycophenolate mofetil and prednisolone followed by maintenance with last three drugs has produced a 1-year graft survival of over 95%. Frequent monitoring of antibody levels, low threshold for biopsy and aggressive treatment for antibody-mediated rejection is needed for good outcome. Similar strategy is adopted for renal transplantation in highly sensitized recipients in the presence of positive cross-match.

ORGAN PRESERVATION

> Organs are perfused with a balanced salt solution, e.g. hyperosmolar citrate or University of Wisconsin solution at 4°C, and are stored surrounded by the same solution in sterile bags, which in turn are surrounded by crushed ice. Kidneys may also be preserved by hypothermic pulsatile perfusion on a machine. This is ideal for kidneys taken from DCD donors.

Warm ischaemic time. This is the time from cessation of circulation until perfusion with cold preservative. In DBD donors, this time is theoretically zero.

Cold ischaemic time. This is the time from perfusion with ice-cold preservative until circulation is re-established in the recipient. Table 21.2 shows appropriate times for warm and cold ischaemic time for different organs.

SITING OF THE TRANSPLANT

Orthotopic. The organ is situated in the place where the diseased organ had been, e.g. heart and liver transplantation.

Heterotopic. The new organ is placed in a different site from the native organ, e.g. renal transplantation – the kidney is placed in the iliac fossa.

TABLE 21.2 Warm and cold ischaemic times

Organ	Warm	Cold
Kidney	30 min	Up to 48 h
Heart	0	Up to 4 h
Heart/lung	0	Up to 4 h
Lung	0	Up to 4 h
Liver	0	Up to 18 h
Small bowel	0	As soon as possible
Pancreas	0	Up to 12 h

REJECTION

There are four types of rejection.

Hyperacute. This occurs with ABO incompatibility or preformed cytotoxic antibodies. It occurs on the operating table and in the case of the kidney it is seen to be flaccid, cyanotic and eventually thromboses. Nephrectomy is required, often at the time of transplantation or within 24 h.

Accelerated acute rejection. Rapid onset within a few days after transplantation. It results from prior sensitization to HLA antigens. Injury to the kidney results from antibody-mediated responses.

Acute rejection. This is the most common form of rejection and occurs within 3 months of transplantation. Two distinct types are seen:

Cellular. >90% of cases of acute rejection. Damage is predominantly cell-mediated and is easily reversed by appropriate treatment (see below).

Vascular. 5–10% of acute rejection episodes are due to antibodies directed against graft endothelial cells. This type of acute rejection tends to be more severe and less responsive to treatment.

Chronic allograft nephropathy (chronic rejection). This is the commonest cause of late graft loss. The process is not fully understood and it is thought to be due to a number of immune and non-immune factors. Clinical manifestations include proteinuria, hypertension and progressive deterioration of renal function. Histology shows interstitial fibrosis, tubular atrophy, glomerulosclerosis and obliterative arteriolopathy. Management includes use of least nephrotoxic immunosuppressive drugs, control of hypertension and proteinuria with ACE and ARB-inhibitors.

IMMUNOSUPPRESSION

All transplant patients require immunosuppression for life. Large doses are given in the perioperative period but these are gradually scaled down to maintenance dose over a few months post-transplant. Drugs used include corticosteroids, antiproliferative drugs, e.g.

azathioprine and mycophenolate mofetil (MMF), calcineurin inhibitors (CNIs), e.g. ciclosporin and tacrolimus, and mTOR inhibitor, e.g. sirolimus and everolimus. Rejection episodes are treated with pulsed doses of methylprednisolone, polyclonal (ALG or ATG) or monoclonal (OKT3 and rituximab) antibodies. Polyclonal or monoclonal (basiliximab and daclizumab) antibodies are being used routinely as induction agents in combination with other agents. The immunosuppressive agents are tailored to the individual recipient based on the degree of HLA-mismatches, sensitization and graft function. The most commonly used regimen includes basiliximab, tacrolimus, MMF and prednisolone combination

Corticosteroids

Prednisolone is usually used in combination with CNI and antiproliferative agents. It has multiple anti-inflammatory effects as well as immunosuppressive effects, the latter mainly the result in inhibition of cytokine (IL-1 and TNF-α) production and non-specific effects on cell-mediated and humoral immunity. A high dose of prednisolone is given during transplantation (500 mg i.v., followed by 0.3 mg/kg body weight/day), which is gradually decreased to 5 mg/day over a 6-month period and continued long term. Several early steroid withdrawal or sparing regimens have shown to avoid the side-effects of steroid therapy without compromising the graft outcomes. Pulsed doses of methylprednisolone are an effective treatment for acute rejection episodes. The side-effects of corticosteroid include cushingoid features, hypertension, peptic ulceration, poor wound healing, acne, easy bruising, osteoporosis, myopathy, cataracts, stunted growth, pancreatitis, avascular necrosis of bone, hyperglycaemia and diabetes.

Antiproliferative drugs

These include azathioprine, which was the first widely used immunosuppressive drug, and the newer drug, mycophenolate mofetil (MMF). Azathioprine is metabolized to 6-mercaptopurine by the liver and this in turn inhibits DNA and RNA synthesis by interfering with purine metabolism. In so doing, it inhibits proliferation of lymphocytes in response to antigenic stimulation and impairs antibody response. Side-effects include nausea and vomiting, rashes, agranulocytosis, leukopenia, hepatic dysfunction, malignancy (especially skin malignancies and lymphoid tumours). MMF has a greater effect than azathioprine in preventing rejection, the active compound being mycophenolic acid. It blocks the proliferation of T and B cells by the reversible inhibition of the enzyme inosine monophosphate dehydrogenase (IMPDH). This enzyme is involved in the synthesis of guanosine nucleotides, which are required for DNA and RNA synthesis; lymphocytes are preferentially affected as other cells have salvage pathways. In addition, MMF has been shown to prevent smooth muscle proliferation that might have additional benefit in preventing chronic allograft nephropathy. The main side-effects of MMF include haematological effects (anaemia and leukopaenia) and gastrointestinal effects, particularly abdominal pain, diarrhoea and, in some cases, gastrointestinal haemorrhage. The GI side-effects are managed by reducing the dosage of MMF, increasing the frequency of administration (four times instead of twice daily), or by switching to the newer product, mycophenolate sodium.

Calcineurin inhibitors

These include ciclosporin and tacrolimus. Ciclosporin is a fungal metabolite that inhibits the enzyme calcineurin, thereby preventing the dephosphorylation and translocation of the nuclear factor of activated T-cells (NF-AT), which is essential for interleukin-2 (IL-2) gene transcription within the nucleus. This prevents IL-2 production, which is essential for the proliferation and clonal expansion of cytotoxic T lymphocytes . It has considerably improved the results of organ transplantation since its introduction in 1983. The dose is titrated to trough level in the blood. Side-effects include nephrotoxicity, hypertension, hirsutism, tremor, gingival hyperplasia, hepatotoxicity, hyperlipidaemia and gout. Tacrolimus is 100 times more potent than ciclosporin and has a similar mechanism of action to ciclosporin. Tacrolimus is proven to be more effective in reducing the incidence of acute rejection and prolonging the graft survival, compared to ciclosporin. This has led to a wider use of tacrolimus in solid organ transplantation. The side-effects of tacrolimus are similar to those of ciclosporin except that there is a lower incidence of hirsutism and gingival hyperplasia with tacrolimus, but is more neurotoxic and diabetogenic compared to ciclosporin. The incidence of BK polyoma virus has increased with the use of tacrolimus.

mTOR inhibitors

Sirolimus and everolimus are potent immunosuppressive agents that impair T cell proliferation by inhibiting the mammalian Target of Rapamycin (mTOR) and thereby IL-2 gene transcription. This results in cell cycle arrest in late G1 phase. They also inhibit proliferation of smooth muscle cells, fibroblasts and tumour cells *in vitro* and in animal tumour models. Sirolimus, in combination with ciclosporin, has reduced acute rejection rate significantly and has proven useful in the management of chronic allograft nephropathy. Side-effects include electrolyte abnormalities, thrombocytopaenia, hypercholesterolaemia and hypertriglyceridaemia, wound dehiscence and lymphocele.

Polyclonal antibodies

Polyclonal antibodies are produced by immunizing horses or rabbits with human lymphoid tissue/thymocytes. The resulting immune sera are then harvested. Two types are used:

- Antilymphocyte globulin (ALG)
- Antithymocyte globulin (ATG).

They can be used for induction of immunosuppression and the treatment of rejection. Severe depletion of both T and B lymphocytes occurs following their administration through complement mediated and antibody-dependent cellular cytotoxicity. Complications include anaphylaxis and a high incidence of viral infection, particularly CMV.

Monoclonal antibodies

Monoclonal antibodies in clinical use are:

- Anti-CD3 (cluster of differentiation-3) antibodies – OKT-3
- Anti-IL-2 receptor (IL-2R) antibodies – basiliximab and daclizumab
- Anti-CD20 antibody – rituximab.

OKT-3 is directed against the CD3 antigen of T lymphocytes, binding leading to a reduction in the number of CD3 +ve T lymphocytes in the circulation. It can be used for induction immunosuppression and in the treatment of steroid-resistant acute rejection. Release of cytokine following lympholysis results in fever, hypotension, pulmonary oedema and fatal myocardial depression. Administration of antihistamines, steroid and antipyretic is needed to ameliorate these manifestations. There is a higher incidence of herpes virus reactivation, opportunistic infections (cytomegalovirus and fungi), and Epstein–Barr-associated lymphoproliferative disorders and B cell lymphomas.

Anti-IL-2R antibodies bind to the IL-2 receptor and thus inhibit IL-2 mediated responses. They are given preoperatively in combination with ciclosporin and prednisolone in high-risk sensitized patients in an attempt to decrease acute rejection. They are not used in the treatment of acute rejection. Side-effects have not been reported.

Anti-CD20 monoclonal antibody is used in transplants involving ABO incompatibility. It is also used as induction therapy in highly sensitized patients prior to kidney transplantation and as rescue agent to treat antibody-mediated rejection.

SPECIFIC ORGANS

KIDNEY TRANSPLANT

Recipient
Almost any kidney disease is suitable for transplantation. Some diseases may recur in the transplant kidney, e.g. mesangio-capillary glomerulonephritis, focal segmental glomerulosclerosis and IgA nephropathy. If malignancy was the cause of renal failure, e.g. bilateral nephrectomy for Wilms' tumour or renal carcinoma, a period of time should be allowed for recurrence to occur. If it does not occur within that time period, then the patient is reassessed for transplantation.

Donor
HLA typing is essential. Cross-match should be negative. Kidneys can be safely kept for 36 h, and occasionally up to 48 h.

Operation. This is heterotopic, the kidney being placed extraperitoneally in either the RIF or the LIF. The renal vein is anastomosed to the external iliac vein. The renal artery is anastomosed either end-to-end to the internal iliac artery or end-to-side to the external iliac artery. The ureter is anastomosed to the dome of the bladder. Some 80% of kidneys from BDB donors function immediately; 20% show delayed function due to ATN and require dialysis until the kidney begins to function. Kidneys DCD donors show a delayed function rate of around 70%.

Diagnosis of rejection
- Clinical: general malaise, fever (rare), increased weight, decreased urine output
- Laboratory: increased serum creatinine, decreased creatinine clearance
- Radioisotope scan: MAG3 scan shows reduced perfusion
- Biopsy: core biopsy with a Tru-cut needle. This is the Gold Standard.

Complications

Early

- Vascular – bleeding, renal artery thrombosis, renal vein thrombosis
- Urological – ureteric leak and ureteric necrosis
- Lymphocele
- Acute rejection – occurs in approximately 20% of patients
- Primary non-function (the kidney never functions)
- Delayed graft function.

Late

- Chronic allograft nephropathy
- Vascular – renal artery stenosis
- Urological – ureteric stenosis (obstruction)
- Recurrent disease
- Infections (see below)
- Malignancy (see below).

Results

- 85–90% 1-year graft survival
- 75% 5-year graft survival.

LIVER TRANSPLANT

Recipient

Those with primary biliary cirrhosis, sclerosing cholangitis, chronic hepatitis, alcoholic cirrhosis, metabolic disease, biliary atresia in children. Hepatic resection where possible is preferred for malignant disease owing to the high recurrence rate post-transplant. Fulminant hepatic failure following hepatitis or drug overdose may be treated by liver transplantation.

Donor

Blood group match. No HLA or cytotoxic crossmatch currently undertaken. Size compatibility required. Preservation can be undertaken for up to 20 h using University of Wisconsin solution. Liver reduction techniques have been developed based on segmental anatomy of the liver such that parts of adult livers may be used in paediatric patients. Living related liver transplantation may also be undertaken, usually using the left lateral segment.

Operation. This is an orthotopic operation. The recipient's liver is removed. The donor vena cava is anastomosed to the recipient vena cava above and below the liver. The portal veins are anastomosed end-to-end. The donor hepatic artery on a patch of aorta is anastomosed to the common hepatic artery. End-to-end biliary tract anastomosis across a T tube is carried out.

Diagnosis of rejection. Reduced bile output of poor quality down the T tube. Deteriorating LFTs. Biopsy.

Complications
Early
- Vascular – bleeding, hepatic artery thrombosis, hepatic artery stenosis and portal vein thrombosis
- Biliary – biliary leaks and strictures
- Acute rejection – occurs in as many as 70% of patients
- Primary graft non-function – rare.

Late
- Chronic rejection – 'vanishing bile duct syndrome'
- Recurrent disease
- Infections (see below)
- Malignancy (see below).

Results
- 1-year graft survival depends upon the underlying liver disease. For chronic liver disease the 1-year graft survival is in excess of 80% but for fulminant hepatic failure is around 50%.
- 5-year graft survival. This is around 70% for chronic liver disease but only around 45–50% for fulminant hepatic failure.

Some individuals have lived for more than 25 years after liver transplantation. Late graft loss is less common than for other forms of solid organ transplantation. About 20% of liver transplants at 5 years post-transplant appear to accept their liver grafts without the need for continuing immunosuppression. However, there are no criteria for defining this group prospectively.

HEART AND HEART/LUNG TRANSPLANT

Recipient
End-stage heart disease with survival of 1 year unlikely, e.g. viral myocarditis, cardiomyopathies, severe IHD. Heart/lung transplants are usually carried out for cardiac problems associated with pulmonary vascular hypertension. The four possible lung transplant operations are heart/lung, double lung, sequential single lung, or single lung transplantation. The procedure used depends upon the lung condition. The commonest causes for lung transplantation in general are cystic fibrosis, bronchiectasis, primary pulmonary hypertension, emphysema, and idiopathic pulmonary fibrosis.

Donor
Blood group match. No HLA or cytotoxic crossmatch. Size compatibility important. A safe time limit for cold ischaemia for the heart is 4–6 h. The lungs are less tolerant of ischaemia than the heart. The lungs are usually ventilated with 80% oxygen and kept semi-inflated during storage.

Operation
Heart. This is an orthotopic operation, the recipient's heart being removed. The recipient pulmonary veins are anastomosed to the left atrium and the recipient right atrium to the donor right atrium. The aorta and pulmonary arteries are

anastomosed end-to-end to the corresponding recipient vessels. The operation is carried out on cardiopulmonary bypass.

Lung. The technique depends upon whether it is a double lung transplant, sequential single lung transplant, or single lung transplant. A single lung transplant offers the advantage of maximum use of donor organs and relative technical simplicity. Cardiopulmonary bypass is not required. The main disadvantage of the single lung transplant is that there is only a limited amount of lung tissue and complications may result from the remaining diseased lung. The operation is therefore unsuitable for infective lung conditions such as bronchiectasis or cystic fibrosis.

Diagnosis of rejection

Heart. Cardiac arrhythmias. Regular endomyocardial biopsies via forceps inserted via the external jugular vein and guided to the endocardium under radiographic control.

Lung. Acute rejection is characterized by fever, lethargy, hypoxia and infiltrates on CXR. The diagnosis is confirmed by biopsy (bronchoscopic and transbronchial).

Complications

Heart. Cardiac arrhythmias and death. Sepsis. Chronic rejection with small vessel disease and recurrent angina.

Lung. Late complications include infection, obliterative bronchiolitis and malignancy.

Results

Heart, heart/lung
- 85% 1-year graft survival
- 73% 5-year graft survival.

Lung
- 70% 1-year graft survival
- 50% 5-year graft survival.

PANCREATIC TRANSPLANTATION

Recipient

These are juvenile-onset diabetics who have concomitant renal failure and require kidney transplantation in addition. The aim is to prevent the development of other microangiopathic complications. The kidney and pancreas from the same donor are usually transplanted simultaneously, one organ into the RIF, the other into the LIF. The use of pancreatic transplantation alone to attempt to prevent the complications of diabetes is increasing.

Donor

Blood group match. No history of diabetes. No family history of diabetes. Normal blood sugar.

Operation. This is usually a heterotopic transplant, the pancreas being placed in either the right or the left iliac fossa. The majority of pancreatic transplants are whole pancreatic transplants with bladder or enteric exocrine drainage. The pancreas is removed with a duodenal segment, the latter being anastomosed to the bladder or the terminal ileum. The vascular anastomoses are based on the splenic artery, superior mesenteric artery and portal vein. These are anastomosed to the iliac vessels.

Diagnosis of rejection. Isotope scans. Reduction in urinary amylase where the pancreas is drained into the bladder. Biopsy.

Complications. Bleeding, graft thrombosis, graft pancreatitis, pancreatic fistulae, peri-graft collections, fibrosis.

Results. According to the expertise of the centre where the transplant is carried out, there is a 50–80% 1-year graft survival. In centres with considerable experience of pancreatic transplantation, where the pancreas and kidneys are transplanted simultaneously the 1-year graft survival is 80%, with a 5-year graft survival of 65%. Where pancreas transplantation alone is carried out, the 1-year graft survival is only around 50%.

The poor results and complications have encouraged an attempt to transplant isolated islets of Langerhans. These are injected via the portal vein into the liver. Encouraging results are being reported.

SMALL BOWEL TRANSPLANTATION

Approximately 300 small bowel transplants have been performed worldwide. The main indication is intestinal failure (usually from short bowel syndrome) where complications secondary to total parenteral nutrition (TPN) have developed, i.e. no vascular access. The surgical technique may be via an isolated intestinal graft (superior mesenteric artery and vein anastomosed to the recipient aorta and IVC, respectively, the intestine being anastomosed to the native bowel and the distal end brought out as a stoma). Alternatively, a liver–intestine graft may be carried out. A few cases of living donation have been reported. The main complications are graft thrombosis, rejection, sepsis and GVH disease. Graft survival is around 60% at 1 year.

GENERAL COMPLICATIONS

These include infection and malignancy.

INFECTION

Infection post-transplant may be dangerous and life-threatening and is related to use of immunosuppression. Infections may be bacterial, viral, fungal or protozoal. These include:

- ***Bacterial***, e.g. coliform urinary tract infections, septicaemia, chest infections, e.g. ***Staph. pneumoniae***, tuberculosis
- ***Viral***, e.g. herpes simplex (cold sores on lips), herpes zoster, CMV, the latter giving rise to pneumonia, encephalitis and deterioration of graft function and BK polyoma virus leading to interstitial nephritis and ureteric strictures
- ***Fungal***, e.g. oral, oesophageal and vaginal candidiasis, aspergillosis, ***Pneumocystis carinii***
- ***Protozoal***, e.g. toxoplasmosis.

Management of infection

When a transplant patient develops a fever and rejection has been excluded, aggressive investigation should be undertaken to elucidate the cause. Investigations include swabs of wound discharge, urine cultures, sputum cultures, blood cultures, viral studies, CXR, USS, CT scan, bronchoscopy, bronchial washings, lung biopsy. Treatment may have to be started on a 'best guess' basis. Appropriate therapy should be started as soon as laboratory confirmation of the diagnosis has been obtained. In severely ill patients with overwhelming infection, immunosuppressive drugs should be reduced or stopped until the infection is under control.

MALIGNANCY

The incidence of malignancy is increased in all immunosuppressed transplant patients and therefore long-term follow-up is mandatory. Primary cancers develop in 5% of all recipients. There is a 100-fold increase compared with age-match controls. Altered immunity with depressed tumour surveillance is an aetiological factor.

Skin cancers are the most common, followed by non-Hodgkin's lymphomas. In ciclosporin-treated patients, non-Hodgkin's lymphoma occurs earlier in the post-transplant patient than with steroid and azathioprine therapy. Other cancers occur more commonly in transplant patients than in the general population.

Malignancy in transplant patients should be treated by standard methods. A decision to withdraw immunosuppression as part of the treatment of cancer is difficult. In general, patients with localized disease should be continued on immunosuppressive therapy, while the development of metastases is an indication for withdrawal of immunosuppression. However, decisions must depend on a careful consideration of the individual case.

Long-term follow-up of transplant patients

Any patient who has had a transplant should be followed up long-term by the Transplant Unit. Patients remain on immunosuppression for life and long-term complications may develop. Surveillance for development of malignancies is important. Other important factors involve prompt and appropriate treatment of infection; advice on vaccination procedures (live vaccine should never be given to immunosuppressed patients); contact with infectious disease; travel abroad; pregnancy.

Gynaecology

Between 10% and 20% of patients admitted with acute abdominal pain have a gynaecological cause. It is therefore important for the surgeon to be able to distinguish between surgical causes and gynaecological causes of acute abdominal pain. Gynaecological conditions which may be admitted as surgical emergencies include ectopic pregnancy, ovarian cyst (torsion or rupture), salpingitis, dysmenorrhoea, endometriosis, Mittelschmerz and complications of fibroids. Ruptured ectopic pregnancy is a life-threatening condition and requires urgent gynaecological referral.

ECTOPIC PREGNANCY

This occurs when the conceptus implants outside the uterus, e.g. fallopian tube, ovary or abdominal cavity. Over 95% occur in the fallopian tube. Risk factors for ectopic pregnancy include use of IUD, after pelvic inflammatory disease, after pelvic surgery and increasing maternal age.

Symptoms and signs. In the early stages, there may be no symptoms. Vaginal bleeding and iliac fossa pain are the commonest symptoms. Later, a mass may be palpable arising out of the pelvis associated with abdominal pain. Ruptured ectopic pregnancy presents with sudden severe pain gradually spreading across the abdomen. Signs of shock may be present with sweating, tachycardia and hypotension. Shoulder tip pain may be present due to irritation of the diaphragm by intraperitoneal blood.

Investigations
- Hb: may be low or may be normal after sudden bleed
- βhCG elevated
- USS: foetus in fallopian tube, intraperitoneal free fluid
- Laparoscopy.

Treatment. Salpingectomy or salpingostomy by laparoscopy or laparotomy.

OVARY

OVARIAN CYST

An ovarian cyst is any collection of fluid within an ovary. The classification of ovarian cyst is beyond the scope of this chapter and the reader is referred to a textbook of gynaecology. Most ovarian cysts are benign.

Symptoms and signs. May be found incidentally during routine abdominal or pelvic examination. Dull ache in the lower back or thighs. Pressure, fullness or pain in the abdomen. Dyspareunia. Painful periods and abnormal bleeding. Severe pain may arise from rupture, torsion or haemorrhage into a cyst. Intraperitoneal bleeding may occasionally mimic ruptured ectopic pregnancy. An abdominal mass is palpable when the cyst becomes large. Pressure effects on the bladder may cause frequency of micturition and, on the colon, constipation. Rarely, there may be hormonal symptoms due to secretion by the tumour of androgens or oestrogens. Rarely, ovarian cysts may become massive and fill the whole abdomen. Examination may reveal a mass arising out of the pelvis which it is impossible to get below. Maybe shifting dullness of ascites (malignancy or Meigs syndrome). Bimanual examination: mobility, consistency, nodules in the pouch of Douglas (with malignancy). Hard, irregular fixed mass likely to be malignant.

Investigations
- Hb: ↓ bleeding, malignancy
- WCC ↑ infarction due to torsion
- CA125: ↑ ovarian carcinoma
- USS: abdominal or transvaginal
- CT/PET: assess extent of condition especially if malignancy suspected.

Treatment. Depends on severity of symptoms, age of patient, risk of malignancy, desire for further children. In the case of acute presentation, treatment involves ultrasound guided cyst aspiration, laparoscopy or laparotomy.

OVARIAN CANCER

Ovarian cancer often presents late. It frequently causes non-specific symptoms which contribute to diagnostic delay resulting in it presenting at a late stage and therefore having a poor prognosis.

Symptoms and signs. Often asymptomatic in early stages. Abdominal pain, discomfort. Bloating, back pain, urinary frequency, constipation, abnormal vaginal bleeding, weight loss. Examination may reveal an abdominal mass or ascites. Pelvic examination may reveal an ovarian mass or secondaries in the pouch of Douglas.

Investigations
- Hb
- CA125
- USS: abdominal and transvaginal
- CT/PET scan: staging
- Laparoscopy.

Treatment. Depends on stage of disease. Oophorectomy. Bilateral salpingo-oophorectomy. In advanced disease, tumour debulking. Chemotherapy.

PELVIC INFLAMMATORY DISEASE

Pelvic inflammatory disease (PID) is a generic term for inflammation of the uterus, fallopian tubes and ovaries. The infection usually spreads from the vagina and cervix. PID is most commonly caused by a sexually transmitted infection, usually *chlamydia* or gonorrhoea. Childbirth, termination of pregnancy, insertion of an intrauterine contraceptive device and sexual intercourse during menstruation may all increase the risk of bacterial infection spreading from the vagina and causing PID.

Symptoms and signs. Lower abdominal or pelvic pain ranging from mild to severe. Abnormal vaginal discharge. Abnormal vaginal bleeding. Dyspareunia. Low back pain. Fever. Lower abdominal tenderness. Rarely a palpable mass if tubal abscess. Bimanual examination – cervical motion tenderness (cervical excitation) with or without and adnexal tenderness.

Investigations
● Hb
● FBC: WCC ↑
● High vaginal swab: *trichomonas vaginalis* (bacterial vaginosis)
● Endocervical swabs: chlamydia, *neisseria gonorrhoeae*
● Laparoscopy.

Treatment
Ambulant patients with mild symptoms. Treat to cover *Chlamydia*, gonorrhoea and anaerobes. Treatment is with doxycycline 100 mg b.d. 14 days plus 5 days metronidazole 400 mg b.d. If gonorrhoea is suspected add ciprofloxacin 500 mg as a single dose.

Patient systemically unwell. Admit. Intravenous antibiotics. Laparoscopy. Drainage of tubal abscess.

DYSMENORRHOEA

Dysmenorrhoea is painful menstruation. It may be primary or secondary. It is an extremely common complaint experienced by up to 95% of women of reproductive age. It typically consists of cramping suprapubic pain which starts at the onset of the menstrual flow and lasts for up to 72 h. It may be so severe that it mimics a lower abdominal emergency. Primary dysmenorrhoea has no associated organic pathology. Secondary dysmenorrhoea is associated with identifiable pathology, e.g. endometriosis, pelvic inflammatory disease, adenomyosis.

ENDOMETRIOSIS

Endometriosis is the presence of endometrium outside the lining of the uterine cavity. Of the women presenting with gynaecological symptoms, 10–15% have this condition. The condition may also be seen in asymptomatic women at laparoscopy or laparotomy.

Symptoms and signs. Symptoms are extremely variable. They include dysmenorrhoea, lower abdominal and pelvic pain. Dyspareunia. Low back pain. Infertility. Abdominal tenderness. PV – tenderness, thickening and nodularity in the Pouch of Douglas, ovarian mass, fixed retroverted uterus. Endometriosis may affect the urinary tract giving rise to haematuria, dysuria or ureteric obstruction. It may also affect the gastrointestinal tract causing cyclical rectal bleeding or obstruction. Rarely, it can affect the lungs causing haemoptysis. It may also occur in surgical scars and umbilicus causing cyclical pain and bleeding.

Investigations
- Laparoscopy: Gold Standard
- Transvaginal ultrasound: useful in diagnosis of ovarian endometrioma
- MRI: subperitoneal deposits
- CA125: limited value as screening test or diagnostic test.

Treatment. Analgesics. Combined oral contraceptive agents. Progestogens. Gonadotrophin-releasing hormone agonists. Surgery – conservative surgery to eradicate lesions with diathermy or laser. Radical surgery – hysterectomy, bilateral salpingo-oophorectomy.

Complications. Adhesion formation. Sub-fertility.

UTERINE FIBROIDS

A fibroid is a benign tumour of uterine smooth muscle termed a leiomyoma. They are the most common benign neoplasm in females. There are four types named according to where they are found.

1. Intramural fibroids are found in the wall of the uterus and are the most common type.
2. Subserosal fibroids are found growing outside the wall of the uterus and can become very large. The latter may become pedunculated and therefore subject to torsion.
3. Submucosal fibroids are found in the muscle beneath the epithelium of the womb.
4. Cervical fibroids are found in the wall of the cervix.

Symptoms and signs. Often asymptomatic. Menorrhagia leading to anaemia. Abdominal discomfort. Pressure on bladder, causing frequency. Pressure on rectum, causing constipation. Severe pain, torsion or degeneration. Palpable abdominal mass. Palpable mass on bimanual examination. Severe abdominal pain due to torsion of a pedunculated fibroid or degeneration of a fibroid following disruption of blood supply.

Investigations
- Hb: anaemia
- USS: abdominal and transvaginal
- MRI.

Treatment

Surgery. Myomectomy (hysteroscopic), laparoscopic, laparotomy. Hysterectomy (vaginal or transabdominal).

Uterine artery embolization.

MITTELSCHMERZ

This is a term for ovulation pain or mid-cycle pain. It is experienced by about 20% of women either in every cycle or intermittently.

Symptoms and signs. Lower abdominal and pelvic pain occurring midway through the menstrual cycle. It usually appears suddenly and subsides within hours, although sometimes it may last up to 72 h. The patient may be able to localize it to a particular ovary.

Investigations. USS: to exclude other causes of abdominal pain.

Treatment. Pain relief. Contraceptive pill to prevent ovulation.

INDEX

Note: Page numbers followed by *f* indicate figures and *t* indicate tables.